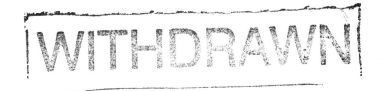

Treatment of Sex Offenders

D. Richard Laws • William O'Donohue

Editors

Treatment of Sex Offenders

Strengths and Weaknesses
in Assessment and Intervention

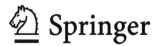 Springer

Editors
D. Richard Laws
Pacific Behavioural Assessment
Victoria, BC, Canada

William O'Donohue
Department of Psychology
University of Nevada
Reno, NV, USA

ISBN 978-3-319-25866-9   ISBN 978-3-319-25868-3   (eBook)
DOI 10.1007/978-3-319-25868-3

Library of Congress Control Number: 2016932375

Springer Cham Heidelberg New York Dordrecht London

Printed on acid-free paper

Springer International Publishing AG Switzerland is part of Springer Science+Business Media (www.springer.com)

Preface

It can be wise for a field to take stock from time to time. What do we, as a field, know? What do we not know? What are our challenges? What is controversial and what is not controversial in the field? To what extent are we meeting our stakeholders' expectations (and indeed what exactly are these)? How effective are our treatments? How well do we understand the etiology of the problems we treat? How accurate are our clinical predictions? How valid are our assessment devices? Are our diagnostic criteria clear and accurate? Do we have the right balance between prevention, treatment, and a public health perspective? Are the laws and policies involved in our field reasonable or do these need improvement? These sorts of questions can guide critically important decisions regarding funding priorities, research priorities, the reactions of others to our field, as well as public policy. Of course any field has problems but a key issue are these problems clearly recognized and is progress being made on these? All these questions deserve honest, direct, and detailed responses.

The field of the assessment and treatment of sexual offenders is certainly an important one. A number of diverse stakeholders are deeply concerned that this work is done well. Our failures can have devastating personal consequences. There can be a lot of emotions around these phenomena—one can see this around civil commitment, relapse rates in treatment, and even in the definition and diagnosis of a paraphilia. Practitioners and researchers work in a difficult context. There are a number of value issues that can generate considerable heat. And it is fair to say that what we want to accomplish, i.e., to prevent sexual offending, to measure a number of important dimensions regarding sexuality, to treat it with 100 % effectiveness, etc. has proven to be difficult tasks.

Clearly the field has made progress. For example, Laws (2016) provided a brief description of current best practice interventions:

> While there are some minor variations in the specifics of treatment programs across the world, any credible program will typically have the following structure, orientation, and elements. Following a comprehensive assessment period where static and dynamic risk factors are assessed and overall level of risk determined, offenders are allocated into a treatment stream. The default ecological assumption appears to be that sexual offending is a

product of faulty social learning and individuals commit sexual offenses because they have a number of skill deficits that make it difficult for them to seek reinforcement in socially acceptable ways. Thus the primary mechanisms underpinning sexual offending are thought to be social and psychological.... Furthermore, treatment is typically based around an analysis of individuals' offending patterns and takes a cognitive-behavioral/relapse prevention perspective. The major goal is to teach sex offenders the skills to change the way they think, feel, and act and to use this knowledge to avoid or escape from future high-risk situations. There are usually discrete treatment modules devoted to the following problem areas: cognitive distortions, deviant sexual interests, social skill deficits, impaired problem solving, empathy deficits, intimacy deficits, emotional regulation difficulties, lifestyle imbalance, and post-offense adjustment or relapse prevention.... (T)he length of treatment programs vary but for a medium-risk or higher offender will likely be at least 9 months in duration and frequently quite a bit longer. A treatment program that follows the model described is likely to produce results with moderately motivated offenders who actively participate in the program modules. Numerous meta-analyses attest to treatment success producing modest rates of recidivism (cited in Laws, 2016, in press).

This edited book was designed to explicate and discuss the state of the field. It will examine what we see as the key challenges. It is designed to have experts in important specialties give honest evaluations of the strengths and challenges of key dimensions of the field of sexual offending. In addition, these experts were encouraged to give their recommendations for the agenda for the future including research priorities, policy priorities, and funding priorities. It is relevant to understanding current views on best practices and thus ought to be informative to the practitioner. We can all agree that the field of sexual offending is both challenging and vitally important to accomplish its tasks in the most effective way possible.

Victoria, BC, Canada   D. Richard Laws
Reno, NV, USA   William O'Donohue

Reference

Laws, D. R. (2016). *Social control of sex offenders: A cultural history*. London: Palgrave Macmillan.

Contents

Contributors

Adam J. Carter, Ph.D. National Offender Management Service, London, UK

Leam A. Craig Forensic Psychology Practice Ltd., Sutton, Coldfield, UK

Centre for Forensic and Criminological Psychology, University of Birmingham, Edgbaston Birmingham, UK

School of Social Sciences, Birmingham City University, Birmingham, UK

Kresta N. Daly Barth Daly LLP., Sacramento, CA, USA

Yolanda Fernandez, C.Psych. Correctional Service CanadalService Correctionnel Canada, Regional Headquarters (Ont)lBureau Régional (Ont), Kingston, ON, Canada

Don Grubin, M.D., F.R.C.Psych. Institute of Neuroscience, Newcastle University, Gosforth, Newcastle upon Tyne, UK

Northumberland, Tyne and Wear NHS Trust, St Nicholas Hospital, Gosforth, Newcastle upon Tyne, UK

Leslie-Maaike Helmus Forensic Assessment Group, Nepean, ON, Canada

Drew A. Kingston, Ph.D., C.Psych. Brockville, ON, Canada

Robert J.B. Lehmann Institute of Forensic Psychiatry, Charité University Medicine Berlin, Berlin, Germany

Jill S. Levenson, Ph.D., L.C.S.W. Barry University, Miami Shores, FL, USA

Caroline Logan Greater Manchester West Mental Health NHS Foundation Trust, Prestwich Hospital, Prestwich, Manchester, UK

University of Manchester, Manchester, UK

Patrick Lussier, Ph.D. School of Social Work (Criminology program), Université Laval, Pavillon Charles-De Koninck, Quebec City, QC, Canada

Ruth E. Mann, Ph.D. National Offender Management Service, London, UK

Kieran McCartan, Ph.D. Health and Applied Social Science, University of the West of England, Bristol, UK

Michael H. Miner, Ph.D. Program in Human Sexuality, Department of Family Medicine and Community Health, University of Minnesota, Minneapolis, MN, USA

William O'Donohue, Ph.D. University of Nevada, Reno, NV, USA

Ryan Panaro LCSW, Boston, MA, USA

Martin Rettenberger Centre for Criminology, Wiesbaden, Germany

Department of Psychology, Johannes Gutenberg-University Mainz (JGU), Mainz, Germany

Daniel Rothman, Ph.D. Forensic Psychological Services — Ellerby, Kolton, Rothman & Associates, Winnipeg, MB, Canada

Joan Tabachnick DSM Consultants, Northampton, MA, USA

Tony Ward, M.A.(Hons.), Ph.D., Dip.Clin.Psyc. (Canty.), M.N.Z.C.C.P. School of Psychology, Victoria University of Wellington, Wellington, New Zealand

Gwenda M. Willis, Ph.D., P.G.Dip.Clin.Psyc. School of Psychology, University of Auckland, Tamaki Innovation Campus, Auckland, New Zealand

Robin J. Wilson, Ph.D., A.B.P.P. Wilson Psychological Services LLC, Sarasota, FL, USA

Department of Psychiatry and Behavioural Neurosciences, McMaster University, Hamilton, ON, Canada

Pamela M. Yates, Ph.D. Cabot Consulting and Research Services, Eastern Passage, NS, Canada

Chapter 1
Problems in the Classification and Diagnosis of the Paraphilias: What Is the Evidence That the DSM Warrants Use?

William O'Donohue

A classification system in science or an applied science is designed to achieve several intellectual as well as practical goals. When it is successful at achieving these goals it is an invaluable and even essential contribution to both basic and applied pursuits. When it fails to accomplish these it can be an impediment to progress as well as competent, safe practice. When the classification system is attempting to demarcate behavioral health problems such as the DSM-V (American Psychiatric Association, 2015) the extent to which these ends are achieved has a direct impact on the beneficial or iatrogenic effects of professional behavior. Therefore, it is important to critically evaluate the quality of any proffered classification system.

This chapter reviews the quality of the DSM5 diagnostic categories of the paraphilias. Some of these problems are shared by other diagnostic categories and some are unique to the paraphilias. The major unsolved problems include:

1. It is unclear whether the paraphilias are natural kinds or social constructions.
2. It is unclear whether the paraphilias are better construed as categorical or dimensional entities.
3. It is unclear if each paraphilia is properly subtyped—especially as there is some unexplained variance in the way the DSM5 provides subtypes for each paraphilia.
4. The definitional strategy for each paraphilia is unclear, particularly whether each ought to be defined by necessary and sufficient criteria, by attributes as open concepts, by prototypes, or by an explication of their human history as social constructs. No argument is provided for the definitional strategy utilized.

W. O'Donohue, Ph.D. (✉)
University of Nevada, Reno, NV 89503, USA
e-mail: wto@unr.edu

© Springer International Publishing Switzerland 2016
D.R. Laws, W. O'Donohue (eds.), *Treatment of Sex Offenders*,
DOI 10.1007/978-3-319-25868-3_1

5. It is unclear who ought to properly define these and what interests these may represent and serve. It is possible that the conventional analysis of special interests do not apply to these constructs.

6. There are controversies whether the revisions were made with an open, transparent, fair, and reasonable process that was evidence-based. Explicit referencing of claims is not provided in the DSM5.

7. The justification supplied in the DSM5 for the revisions—i.e., that there was such significant progress in genetics, brain imaging, cognitive neuroscience and epidemiology that a revision became necessary does not seem to apply to the paraphilias.

8. The definition of mental disorders given in the DSM5 might possibly exclude some paraphilias as this definition specifically excludes sexual behavior that is socially deviant unless the deviance is due to dysfunction in the individual— and the exact nature of this internal dysfunction is not specified or known.

9. The general definition of mental disorder provided in the DSM5 necessitates that all mental disorders arise from a dysfunction ("in the psychological, biological or developmental processes underlying mental functioning") in the individual but the diagnostic criteria of the paraphilias fails to specify this dysfunction.

10. Strangely, instead of relying on the general definition of mental disorders the DSM5 surprisingly provides two problematic candidates for demarcating the paraphilias—their commonness (relative to other paraphilias) and their noxiousness/illegality. There at least is some tension with the earlier exclusionary criteria of "social deviance."

11. The DSM5 diagnostic criteria for paraphilia seem to be developmentally naïve. It is unclear how these diagnoses relate to the developmental spectrum although the DSM5 at times indicates that special consideration ought to be given to "old people."

12. The DSM5 states that for actual diagnoses to be made the clinician must consider predisposing, precipitating, and protective factors yet this is impossible for the paraphilias as these are unknown.

13. There seems to be no clearly explicated relationships between the individual paraphilia diagnostic categories. These seem to be more of a heap than systematic network of interrelated constructs.

14. Importantly, the interrater reliability of these diagnostic categories is unknown and has been for at least a third of a century.

15. These diagnostic categories have unknown construct validity and predictive validity.

16. Each of the paraphilias now requires a problematic distinction between a paraphilic orientation and a paraphilic disorder. It is unclear that a paraphilic orientation is actually benign and the interrater reliability of this distinction is unknown.

17. It is unclear if all the paraphilias are included in the DSM5; for example an attraction to rape—a nonconsenting partner is not included.

18. There is a possible overconcern with false positives in diagnostic categories due to the miscategorization of homosexuality as a paraphilia in past editions of the DSM.

19. There is an overreliance in the diagnostic criteria that rely on notoriously prob-
    lematic self-report. In some paraphilic diagnoses—but not others—a simply
    denial seems sufficient for ruling out a diagnosis.
20. Other constructs commonly used in the diagnostic criteria of the paraphilias are
    also problematic—why is the duration 6 months?—why must the behavior be
    recurrent?—what does "acting upon" these exactly mean?—don't we all act on
    our sexual interests?
21. Why must a person be distressed by these to have this reach diagnostic signifi-
    cance? For example, isn't not being distressed by a sexual attraction to a child
    more of a problem instead of less of one—especially as the DSM5 acknowl-
    edges that Antisocial Personality Disorder is a common comorbid condition?
22. In places the DSM5 seems to claim that if the paraphilic interests are less
    intense than what it vaguely calls "normophilic interests" then this obviates a
    diagnosis—although why this is the case is unclear, not clearly specified in the
    individual diagnostic criteria, and it now requires the clinician to measure the
    intensity—whatever this means exactly—of all the client's sexual interests and
    behaviors. There is no evidence that intensity can be validly measured.
23. The DSM5 makes strange, unclear, vague, and undocumented epidemiological
    claims.
24. The DSM5 in its epidemiological claims seems to hide an important point made
    by the feminists—that sexual problems are a gendered problem—these are pos-
    sessed by males and their victims are females.
25. Finally, the DSM seems at time to be clinically naïve—for example requiring
    masochists to be distressed by their preference for pain.

Classification, Taxonomies and the DSM5

What are the overarching goals of a sound classification system? These are commonly taken to include: (1) an attempt to "carve nature at its joints" and both create
classificatory categories that function as a placeholder for all entities that ought to
be categorized *as well as facilitating the proper placement of all entities in the taxonomy*. These categories generally should be exhaustive (the classification system
should leave out no entity that ought to be classified), mutually exclusive (generally
an entity ought to belong to one and only one category), clear (an entity ought to be
able to be reliably placed within the structure of the classification system) and,
finally, ideally based on sound principles of classification (important distinctions
are made while trivial ones are avoided). For example, a biological taxonomy would
enumerate all key distinctions such as kingdoms, phyla, species, etc. and place these
categories in their proper position relative to one another, as well as be conducive to
the reliable and valid classification of phenomena within this structure, e.g., whether
the entity to be classified is in plant kingdom or animal kingdom, vertebrates or
nonvertebrates, mammals or nonmammals, etc. Thus, a classification system provides a comprehensive organization that reveals interrelationships. (2) In addition, a

sound classification system provides a *common language* and thus a system for cataloging and communicating knowledge. For example, in the periodic table of elements one knows clearly what is meant by when the term "oxygen" is used; and one even knows the scientific principles by which oxygen is placed between nitrogen and fluorine in the classification system. The organization of the periodic table of elements is founded on a deeper scientific knowledge of the phenomena to be classified—i.e., the atomic structure of these elements. In this sense, there is an important reflexive relationship between classification and basic science—carving nature at its joints allows scientific regularities to be found—but discovered scientific regularities also allows nature to be carved at its joints. (3) Finally, a classification system can function as a *useful inference generator* to lawful relations when it is based on these sound underlying scientific regularities. For example, the biological classification system allows the inference that species cannot interbreed and produce reproductively viable offspring. Elements with certain positions in the periodic table allows one to make inferences about which elements can combine with other elements and what kind of chemical bonds will be utilized.

However, it is also important to note that there are also some general controversies about taxonomies and classification in science:

1. *Natural kinds vs. social constructions*. There has been a significant debate in the last few decades in the philosophy of science whether the categories found in classification systems in science are "natural kinds," i.e., roughly that these categories describe what actually exists in reality in an objective way or, on the other hand, whether scientific entities are merely convenient verbal social creations or "social constructions"—i.e., conventions that are to some degree useful but have no real objective existence beyond these linguistic agreements (see for example, Foucault, 1990). For example, classifying balls and strikes in baseball are clearly social conventions—these can be alternatively defined and were created at a point in time and thus have a contingent human history. On the other hand, those that argue that science reveals natural kinds—objective "real" categories found in nature as opposed conventions created by humans, suggest that entities like sulfuric acid have a real, independent existence apart from human conventions—no matter how we divide the world in a linguistic system the kind of thing called sulfuric acid in high concentrations will damage or destroy human tissue. No words or changes in language can change this reality. The issue for our purposes is: Are mental disorders as defined in the DSM natural kinds or social constructions? Or more specifically for our interests in this chapter, are paraphilias natural kinds or social constructions? Given how few scientific regularities have been found with these categories, currently it is hard to argue that there is clear evidence that these diagnostic categories are natural kinds. Moreover, in general, the field of sexology or psychology, due to a variety of considerations, has seemed to regard these categories more as natural kinds (but see Foucault, 1990). On the other hand, there does seem to be something distinct between say someone who exposes himself to unsuspecting women and someone who does

not, especially given reliable and robust gender and age differences in the frequency of this kind of behavior.

2. *Are the key distinctions to be made categorical or dimensional?* A second general controversy is whether these entities ought to be classified along dimensions or whether these form discrete categories. For example, we can consider night and day to be either two discrete categories defined by essential properties (e.g., the presence or absence of sunlight). This is a categorical distinction. On the other hand, when we consider phenomena like dusk or dawn—which seem to have properties of both day and night—we may consider it more useful to construe these as points on a dimension—i.e., that the amount of sunlight can be measured and then a range of values on this dimension can be reported rather than a simple bifurcation of day vs. night. Kinsey (1948), for example, suggested that sexual orientation ought to be dimensional rather than categorical (heterosexual vs. homosexual). Kinsey (1948) used a scale from 0 that signified exclusive heterosexuality to 6 which signified exclusive homosexuality. Kinsey (1948, p. 639; 656) arguing for a dimension approach stated:

> Males do not represent two discrete populations, heterosexual and homosexual. The world is not to be divided into sheep and goats. It is a fundamental of taxonomy that nature rarely deals with discrete categories... The living world is a continuum in each and every one of its aspects.
> While emphasizing the continuity of the gradations between exclusively heterosexual and exclusively homosexual histories, it has seemed desirable to develop some sort of classification which could be based on the relative amounts of heterosexual and homosexual experience or response in each history [...] An individual may be assigned a position on this scale, for each period in his life. [...] A seven-point scale comes nearer to showing the many gradations that actually exist. —Kinsey, et al. (1948). pp. (639, 656)

The practical issue then becomes, should mental disorders or a particular paraphilia be a categorical or a dimensional entity? The DSM5 apparently considers these to be categorical entities but does not provide a sound argument for this decision. Of course, if these are to be better construed as dimensional entities one needs to explicate what are the relevant dimensions and valid measurement operations to place entities on these dimensions. No clear candidates have been brought forward, although a Kinsey-like dimension could be used.

3. A third controversy is the problem of subtyping. This is essentially a problem of when to stop making distinctions and new categories—when a taxonomy has made all important distinctions. Assuming that there is a legitimate superordinate category—the questions then becomes, "Are there subtypes of this category—and then are there subtypes of these subtypes, and so on"? If so, how would one tell? If not, how does one tell? Let's take the example of pedophilia: Is incest versus nonbiological attraction an important subtype? Is age or age range (say, 3–5 versus 8–10) of the child who is of sexual interest an important additional principle of categorization? What about gender preference? Whether the person is interested in grooming the child or not? Whether violence is part of the attraction? Whether the person is in denial or not? Whether the person has exclusively this orientation or not? Whether the individual has acted on the interest or not?

And so on. Currently, for pedophilia the DSM5 recognizes only three subtyping distinctions (without presenting an argument for these): (1) exclusive versus nonexclusive; (2) attracted to males, females, or both; and (3) limited to incest. However it is interesting to note that for many other paraphilias, the DSM5 uses different categories used for subtyping. For example, most of the other paraphilic disorders listed in the DSM5 allow subtyping along the dimensions of in full remission or not; or whether the individual is in a controlled environment or not. Why the diagnostic category of pedophilia does not contain this subtyping but has a unique set of distinctions is none too clear.

4. *What ought a definition of a category or dimension look like?*—Ought each distinction list sufficient and necessary conditions like "bachelors are unmarried male adults" or "oxygen has 16 protons in its nucleus"? Or should the category have some sort of other definitional attributes? The cognitive psychologist Eleanor Rosch (1975) has suggested that humans categorize by the use of prototypes. For example, the prototype for must of us for the category of bird is a robin. We then judge whether or not other candidates fit into the category of bird by how closely the candidate seems to be to the robin prototype. Ought we to at least help categorization by including these core prototypes? On the other hand, Meehl (1990) has suggested that diagnostic categories cannot have such clear definitional properties but rather are "open concepts." Open concepts are characterized by (a) fuzzy boundaries, (b) a list of indicators (i.e., signs and symptoms)—none of which are essential and that are indefinitely extendable, and (c) have essentially an unclear nature. Finally, those who orient toward a social constructionist view would suggest explicating the history, contingency, social forces, and special interests that have come to construct the open concept is important and goes a long way to understanding and defining the category.

5. *A fifth, and final, controversy is who gets to decide on such categorization?* Sometimes this is relatively uncontroversial—no one is really questioning the authority of the periodic table of elements or claiming it is just a product of certain social or political interests. Why psychiatry largely controls the diagnostic system is unclear as is how the DSM committees are chosen and how they function. Post-modernist critics of science (see O'Donohue, 2013 for a summary) have suggested that scientists have interests—sometimes personal such as fame, power, or money but sometimes more social or political ones such as either maintaining or changing the status quo. So these philosophers suggest analyzing science from the point of view of "Cui bono?"—whose interests are being served? Revisions of the DSM have also been plagued by these kinds of criticisms. To what extent are these moves simply in the interests of organized psychiatry, Big Pharma, white males, or medicine more broadly? On the other hand, there is a mode of analysis that might be more unconventional but possibly more telling: to what extent have GLBT interest groups or other sexual "liberation" groups had direct or indirect influence on this taxonomy? To what extent is serving these interests legitimate?

Lilienfeld (2014) has argued more generally that the DSM has had "many masters" and represents a compromise between multiple competing demands and constituencies. The DSM-5 revision has been controversial not only for the content of proposed changes to diagnostic criteria but also for its process that occurred to produce these changes. Part of the problem is that the process was unclear and at times was not transparent. There have been accusations of secrecy, lack of adequate representation by various groups and interests (for example, social work seems to have been relatively ignored), lack of quality control, failure to generate and explicate comprehensive and critical literature reviews to justify the changes, and an unjustified "paradigm shift" toward incorporating a biological etiology for which the justifying scientific evidence does not exist. Interestingly, this criticism has not been coming from the usual anti-psychiatric interests but rather from some of the most eminent and respected DSM experts within psychiatry itself—such as the previous DSM editors. Both Allen Frances, the Editor of the DSM-IV (1994), and Robert Spitzer, the chief editor of DSM-III (1980) and DSM-III-R (1987) and the single person most responsible for creating the modern symptom-based descriptive DSM psychiatric approach to diagnosis, have been loud critics of the DSM5 revision.

Further Problems and Controversies

Why Was a Revision of the DSM Necessary?

The DSM5 makes rather expansive claims that do not clearly apply to the paraphilia diagnoses such as "However, the last two decades since DSM-IV was released have seen real and durable progress in such areas as cognitive neuroscience, brain imaging, epidemiology and genetics" (p. 5). This sort of claim is the rationale for why a new edition of the DSM is needed. However, the section on paraphilias in the DSM5 is certainly devoid of any specifics regarding the alleged scientific progress on the cognitive neuroscience, brain imaging, epidemiology or genetics of the paraphilias. It is unfortunate that this general claim about scientific progress is not qualified to be more in line with at least some of the state of science in these disorders, especially because dysfunctions in these are the key properties proffered by the DSM to define mental disorders.

What Is a Mental Disorder According to the DSM5 and Do Paraphilias Fall Under This Definition?

The DSM5 defines a mental disorder as:

> A mental disorder is a syndrome characterized by clinically significant disturbance in an individual's cognition, emotional regulation, or behavior that reflects a dysfunction in the psychological, biological or developmental processes underlying mental functioning.

Mental disorders are usually associated with significant distress or disability in social, occupational or other important activities. An expectable or culturally approved response to a common stressor or loss, such as the death of a loved one, is not a mental disorder, socially deviant behavior (e.g., political, religious, or sexual) and conflicts that are primarily between the individual and society are not mental disorders unless the deviance or conflict results from a dysfunction in the individual as described above (p. 20).

The question becomes, "What sorts of sexual behavior fit this general definition, and, more specifically, do the categories of paraphilia contained in the DSM5 actually fit this definition of a mental disorder"? Unfortunately the answers to these important questions are none too clear. The phrase in the definition above "... socially deviant behavior (e.g., political, religious or *sexual*, italics added) ... are not mental disorders unless the deviance or conflict results for a dysfunction in the individual as described above" adds considerable ambiguity and confusion. Why is the term "sexual" used here to exclude some socially deviant behavior from the realm of mental disorders? Unfortunately, no argument or further elucidation is given. How does one tell if the sexual issue is "primarily a conflict between the individual and society" or a "dysfunction in the individual"—and why are these regarded as mutually exclusive categories? What is the scope or extension of this exclusion—why does this not apply to all sexual deviation? If it does not apply to all sexual deviation, what principle demarcates those conditions that are internal dysfunctions versus those that are "societal conflicts" that are excluded? Finally, how exactly does one go about validly discerning if the sexual behavior "... results in a dysfunction in the individual as described above"? Presumably then this raises the question of, "Does this sexual behavior result from 'a syndrome characterized by clinically significant disturbance in an individual's cognition, emotional regulation, or behavior that reflects a dysfunction in the psychological, biological or developmental processes underlying mental functioning'"? Given our very poor understanding of the etiology of the paraphilias, this again is none too clear. In fact, Moser and Kleinpelz (2005) have suggested that since the paraphilias do not meet the general definition of mental disorder as contained in earlier editions of the DSM that the paraphilias be dropped from the DSM.

Paradoxically, later when the DSM5 turns to its section on the paraphilias it seems to ignore the definitional criteria it had earlier laid out for mental disorders. Thus, the DSM5 is not even internally consistent. Instead in this section the DSM states,

"These disorders (i.e., paraphilias) have traditionally been selected for specific listing and assignment of explicit diagnostic criteria in the DSM for two main reasons: they are relatively common, in relation to other paraphilic disorders, and some of them entail actions for their satisfaction that because of their noxiousness or potential harm to others are classed as criminal offenses" (p. 685).

This shift is very strange indeed. Suddenly there is no talk about progress in cognitive neuroscience, brain imaging, genetics, predisposing or protective factors and disturbances in these resulting in disorders but rather the relatively pedestrian notions that the paraphilias are "relatively common" (whatever that precisely means and why something being common is considered to be disordered is somewhat paradoxical) and that they are noxious (noxious to whom? and why is this dimension picked out to define a problem—many find metallic rock and roll noxious but certainly this—offensive taste—ought not be the criterion for a category of mental disorders). And that which is criminal ought not to determine that which is a health problem. Stealing is relatively common but not regarded as a mental disorder.

Further, the DSM5 (p. 685) states "The term paraphilia denotes any intense and persistent sexual interest other than sexual interest in genital stimulation or preparatory fondling with phenotypically normal, physically mature, consenting human partners." This seems to be a reasonable candidate for distinguishing abnormal from abnormal behavior. However, some additional issues could include: (1) explicating how this criterion obviates concerns expressed earlier in the DSM5 about conflicts between an individual and society; (2) how this generally meets the DSM5 definition of mental disorder (i.e., it arises from a dysfunction within the individual), and (3) how this applies to adolescents and children (paraphilias are adult disorders but much attention is given to the treatment of juvenile offenders (see for example Bromberg & O'Donohue, 2012). Finally, the DSM5 asserts somewhat unclearly "With old people the term paraphilia may be defined as any sexual interest greater than or equal to normophilic sexual interests (p. 685)." It is not clear why "old people" are given this special consideration and this involves an additional difficult measurement task; measuring the magnitude of multiple different sexual interests.

In addition, the DSM5 states, "it requires clinical training to recognize when the combination of predisposing, precipitating, perpetuating, and protective factors has resulted in a psychopathological condition in which physical signs and symptoms exceed normal ranges" (p. 19). However, the truth of this statement is dependent upon whether the basic science has actually made sufficient progress to uncover the "predisposing, precipitating, perpetuating and protective factors" and whether enough is none about normal variability to make a sound actuarial judgment about exceeding "normal ranges." It is clear that these broad almost promissory statements made in the DSM5 do not apply to the paraphilias that again, because no such basic information exists. These sorts of statements in the DSM5 seem to have a broad rhetorical function rather than a more careful descriptive function about the actual state of scientific progress.

What Are the Relations Between Broad Categories of Mental Disorders in the DSM5 or Within Specific Disorders Within a Broad Category?

There seems to be no scientific principles that are relevant to the relations between broad diagnostic categories. Personality disorders, substance disorders, and the paraphilias are all broad diagnostic categories but their taxonomic relationship appears to be nonexistent. These are contained in the same manual but are in no hierarchical or other order. Moreover, there seems to be no organizing principle with allows the understanding of subcategories of these. Pedophilia, voyeurism, and fetishistic disorder are all subcategories of the superordinate category of paraphilia, but the relationship between these is totally unclear and unspecified. They are simply listed one after another in a seemingly arbitrary order.

Unknown Interrater Reliability of Each Paraphilic Disorder

There have been no field trials of the revisions contained in the DSM5 to show to what extent clinicians can make diagnoses of the paraphilias with acceptable inter-rater reliability. In fact although true, this statement is much too weak. For decades the paraphilias have been orphaned regarding studies of the diagnostic interrater reliability. Students of the history of the various versions of the DSM know that because of some evidence of the lack of diagnostic consistency in the first two versions of the DSM, the DSM-III was an attempt to correct this problem. It attempted to more clearly outline behavioral diagnostic criteria for reliable diagnosis. There was some evidence that this was at least partially successful for some of the major diagnoses such as depression and schizophrenia. However as Blanchard (2011) has astutely stated:

"One of the first questions one might ask about the field trials conducted for the DSM revisions is how many patients with diagnoses of paraphilia were studied." The field trials for DSM-III, which were sponsored by the National Institute of Mental Health, included three patients with paraphilias (Appendix F, Tables 1 and 2, pp. 470–471). That's it. Paraphilia diagnoses were not included in the field trials for DSM-III-R (American Psychiatric Association, 1987, Appendix F, pp. 493–495) or for DSM-IV (see O'Donohue, Regev, & Hagstrom, 2000, p. 98). Thus, the sum total of patients who have been studied in conjunction with revising the DSM diagnostic criteria for the paraphilias is 3. That is fewer than half the number of paraphilia diagnoses listed in the DSM. That means that most of the paraphilias diagnostic criteria were never looked at with a single patient as part of the DSM production process ever.

Unfortunately, this number—3—has not changed with the DSM5. In fact, there are reasons to think this concern over diagnostic interrater reliability has actually intensified. The DSM5 know requires the clinician to make a further distinction between a *paraphilic orientation* and a *paraphilic disorder*. And these concerns are multiplied because this applies to each diagnostic category, i.e., to a fetishitic orientation versus a fetishitic disorder or to an exhibitionistic orientation versus an exhibitionistic disorder, and so on. There are of course obvious reliability questions concerning this clinical judgment. Thus, to date, it is clear that for nearly a third of a century there has been no evidence that the paraphilias can be reliably diagnosed. Despite this important lacuna it has been the major diagnostic system used, with no real competitors. It is astonishing that there has been so little progress on this basic psychometric issue that has obvious implications for practice. If someone were to ask the question: "Is there scientific evidence that if a person were to receive a paraphilic diagnosis from one clinician that they would receive the same diagnosis from another clinician?" the answer is "No." Surprisingly, in contrast to worries about this fundamental issue, the revisions contained in the DSM5 may make the psychometric issue more complex by calling for further distinctions and attendant judgments that can add to further unreliability.

Unknown Validity

Although the interrater reliabilities of the DSM5 paraphilic diagnoses are unknown it must be remembered that because validity is not a prerequisite for reliability, extremely high reliability can exist without validity. That is, another gap in our knowledge of the quality of the DSM5 paraphilic categories is that we have little evidence about their construct or predictive validity. It is difficult to make valid inferences from diagnostic categories when little is know about the etiology, treatment course, protective factors, or other regularities involving the entities.

Robins and Guze (1970) described several essential criteria for determining the extent to which a diagnosis is valid. Validity refers to the extent to which a diagnosis actually captures what it purports to measure. A valid diagnosis is "honest" in that it correlates in expected directions with external criteria. Robins and Guze specified four requirements for the validity of psychiatric diagnoses:

1. Clinical description, including symptomatology, demographics, precipitants, and differences from seemingly related disorders. The last-named task of distinguishing a diagnosis from similar diagnoses is called differential diagnosis.
2. Laboratory research, including data from psychological, biological, and laboratory tests.
3. Natural history, including course and outcome.
4. Family studies, especially studies examining the prevalence of a disorder in the first-degree relatives of probands—that is, individuals identified as having the diagnosis in question.

Some authors also have suggested that a valid diagnosis should ideally be able to predict the individual's response to treatment (Waldman, Lilienfeld, & Lahey, 1995). Unfortunately, nearly all of this information is missing in the paraphilic diagnoses contained in the DSM5. No genetic studies are described. Very little information is given about course and outcome. No laboratory research—either physiological or psychological—is described. Some descriptive psychopathology is given although at times (more below) only very vague statements are made which are either heavily qualified or have such a range that the information has very limited use. Thus, there is little information in the diagnostic categories that support the validity of these.

Are All Paraphilic Diagnostic Categories Included?

Two categories that have not been included are a "rapist" diagnostic category—roughly either those that are attracted to sex with a nonconsenting individual or can maintain arousal through active nonconsent. In addition, Blanchard et al. (2009) has advocated a hebephilic diagnostic category—or expanding the pedophilic category to something along the lines of "hebopedophilia" to combine both a sexual attraction to pre-pubescent and early pubescent children by someone who is at least 5 years older. Because no clear candidate for a demarcation of "abnormal sexuality" has been explicated in the DSM—it is more difficult to understand the rationale for why these categories have been excluded.

What Is the Justification for the Diagnostic Categories That Are Included?

It is reasonable to hypothesize that the field is very sensitive to the mistake that in the past homosexuality was regarded as a mental disorder. There is very little dissent that this was a horrible mistake and one that should be avoided in the future at all costs. This may be called the problem of the false positive—i.e., that some entity is considered a mental disorder and perhaps especially a paraphilia when it actually is not. Humans can have the tendency to overcorrect mistakes and it may be the case that this is happening now in the field. There seems to be more concern about falsely categorizing something as deviant sexual behavior than the converse: not calling something deviant sexuality when it actually is. It appears that each paraphilia has its corresponding "sexual liberation" movement which argues that the same mistake of falsely categorizing this behavior as a mental disorder is being made. Part of this seems to be reflected in the new distinction between a so called "paraphilic orientation" and a "paraphilic disorder." This is a new distinction in this edition—which again there is no evidence can be reliably made by clinicians. However, what about its validity—why is such a distinction valid? These are important issues made all the more difficult by the DSM's conflicting and unclear or sometimes absent statements about why a particular paraphilia is in fact to be properly considered a mental disorder. However, it appears that the field is a bit weak kneed about this: and perhaps this is due to being overly impacted about the past mistake of miscategorizing homosexuality. It seems like an important intellectual task to more clearly demarcate why each paraphilia is indeed a mental disorder (using better criteria than they are "common" or "noxious" or are based on a "dysfunction" in the individual).

Difficulties Applying the DSM5 Diagnostic Criteria of Paraphilia

O'Donohue, Regev, and Hagstrom (1990) have previously suggested that there are ambiguities that lead to assessment problems for the clinician that can lead to inter-rater reliability problems contained in the DSM-IV. It appears that most of these concerns still apply to the DSM5. First, part of the difficulty involves that some sexual behavior is covert—it is experienced in heads and thus is not readily observable by others. Sexual fantasies, sexual dreams, sexual intentions, cognitive arousal, etc. are all not observable by others. Yet these are all relevant to understanding and evaluating the extent to which a person's sexual behavior or orientation is disordered or not. If a client fully and accurately reported this covert behavior there would be little problem. However, because we know that many individuals with paraphilias are in denial or directly lie about their behavior, the field faces an important measurement problem related to defining diagnostic categories that rely on covert behavior and hence accurate self-report. A fundamental strategic and conceptual question is as follows: To what extent should covert behavior which often is not reported accurately—and to which that field really has no validity check—ought to be part of the DSM5 diagnostic criteria? There seems to be an essential tension between recognizing that such covert behavior is an important part of one's sexuality but at the same time including it in diagnostic criteria when there is motivation to distort and being unable to check the validity of any self-report.

Most strangely of all at times the DSM5 seems to take self-report as face valid and appears to be uninterested in its accuracy. For example, for Sexual Masochism Disorder it states, "The diagnostic criteria for Sexual Masochism Disorder are intended to apply to individuals who freely admit to having such paraphilic interests" (p. 694). Thus, a simple denial (even a false one) is sufficient to exclude this diagnosis! This is quite strange.

However more specifically, the diagnostician faces further ambiguities:

1. Most diagnoses require that the other diagnostic criteria persist over a period of 6 months. Why "over a period of 6 months"? The basic idea in all likelihood is to show some temporal stability. However is this really necessary—are there actually cases where someone was attracted to children for a 2 month period and then it spontaneously remitted? It seems that these problems are chronic not acute. In addition, why 6 months as opposed to some other time period? No justification is given in the DSM5.

2. The DSM5 requires that the behavior be "recurrent"? Does that simply mean more than once? For example for Exhibitionistic Disorder the DSM5 states "'Recurrent' genital exposure to unsuspecting others (i.e., multiple victims, each on a separate occasion) may, as a general rule, be interpreted as three or more victims on separate occasions." Why three victims? Why isn't doing this one time sufficiently noxious, criminal, or indicating a dysfunction in the individual? What if a person exposed themselves hundreds of times to only one victim? They still wouldn't deserve a diagnosis? Why isn't two victims sufficient—especially as we know that it is usually the case that known victims are usually much less than all victims?

3. The DSM5 requires the behavior to be "intense"? How is intensity to be assessed? Intense relative to what? There is no objective valid way to measure this. Again, this wording forces the field to rely on self-report. In addition, there is a principle of assessment that we ought to not ask what clients are unable to tell us. Here we need to ask if the person's fantasies, urges or behaviors were "intense." What if they were to ask, "What exactly do you mean by intense, and how would I tell if my fantasy yesterday met this criterion or criteria?" It would seem that we could

not answer this. Moreover, do we really want to say that repeated "nonintense" sexual fantasies regarding children do not meet the diagnostic threshold?

4. What is "sexual behavior"? Or more specifically, what exactly is the extension of this term? It seems clear that intercourse would be included, but what about other possible candidates for "behavior"? Is "flirting" with a child sexual behavior? Is looking at an attractive person sexual behavior? Is smiling at an attractive person sexual behavior? Is placing a towel at a beach so an attractive person can be more easily viewed a sexual behavior? Is buying a present for a person you are attracted to a sexual behavior? Is choosing to be a school bus driver a sexual behavior? Again, the scope of this term is none too clear. It can even be argued that all our behaviors are sexual behaviors in that our sexual orientation is a deep and pervasive part of our personality.

5. What does "acting on" mean? How is this causal relation to be assessed? Don't we all act on our sexual interests in many ways? Isn't it impossible not to? Aren't all these "micro-sexual behaviors" listed above examples of acting on? However, there are other difficult questions: what about unintentional behaviors such as sexual dreams, would these be acting on? Or does acting on mean only an illegal act or an act involving genitals?

The DSM5 requires that the condition cause "marked distress" or "interpersonal difficulties"? Why? Why can't these conditions be pathological in and of themselves? O'Donohue et al. (2000) suggested that this part of the definitional criteria would rule out a "contented pedophile" and raise the question of why someone who is not distressed by this ought to be regarded as more pathological not less. The DSM5 states "… a paraphilia by itself does not nearly justify or require clinical intervention" (p. 686). Thus, the DSM5 paradoxically would indicate that someone who is sexually attracted to children does not need therapy. It views this proclivity to harm children as not sufficient for intervention. It seems to assume that individuals can over prolonged periods of time, not act on their sexual interests, although the evidence for this is not given. Or the individual needs to be personally distressed by this—the distress of parents or children is irrelevant. For example, the DSM5 states that Antisocial Personality Disorder is a relatively common comorbid condition with pedophilia but apparently not recognizing that when this condition is comorbid it is also less likely that the this person would be distressed by his pedophilic interests. In addition, there is also the issue of what kinds of distress and what levels. Finally, it is difficult to parse "interpersonal difficulties" as sometimes these seem legitimate but in other situations these are not. Being African-American in the South has caused individuals "interpersonal difficulties" as does homosexuality but these as seen not the individual's problem but really the problem of others. Beyond parsing whose fault the interpersonal difficulties are to be attributed, the question becomes also, what kinds of interpersonal difficulties, what levels of these, and how they are to be measured. The DSM5 states further: "a paraphilic disorder is a paraphilia that is currently causing distress or impairment to the individual or a paraphilia whose satisfaction has entailed personal harm, or risk of harm to others" (p. 685–686). Are "interpersonal difficulties" to be confined to personal harm or risk of harm to others? Finally, the DSM5 states for exhibitionistic disorders: "since these individuals deny having urges or fantasies involving genital exposure, it follows that they would also deny feeling subjectively distressed or socially impaired by such impulses. Such individuals may be diagnosed with exhibitionistic disorder despite their negative self report" (p. 690)—this seems perfectly reasonable why this statement is only included for exhibitionistic disorder and not for other paraphilic disorders. The same phenomena of denial would be observed. This inconsistency is none too clear.

Can Stronger "Normophilic" Sexual Interests Obviate a Paraphilic Sexual Interest?

The DSM5 also states problematically:

> "the most widely applicable framework for assessing the strength of a paraphilia itself is one in which examinees paraphilic sexual fantasies, urges or behaviors are evaluated in relation to their normophilic sexual interests and behaviors. In a clinical interview or on self administered questionnaires, examinees can be asked whether their paraphilic sexual fantasies urges or behaviors are weaker than, approximately equal to, or stronger than their normophilic sexual interests and behaviors. The same type of comparison can be and usually is employed in psychophysiological measures of sexual interest such as penile plethysmography in males or viewing time in males and females (p. 686)."

It seems that the DSM5 is saying that if a person has a paraphilic sexual interest that is weaker than a normophilic sexual interest that this has some diagnostic relevance-perhaps even obviating a paraphilic diagnosis. This is troublesome for two major reasons. First, it presents a difficult assessment task to the clinician: he or she must accurately measure the strength of two sexual interests. The DSM5 hints that this might be done through self-report—but this seems naïve psychometrically especially in forensic cases. However, secondly, it seems confused. Is a person not to be diagnosed with a paraphilic interest if this interest is less than his interest in normal sexual behavior? If a person says he would prefer having sex 10 times a week with adults but only 6 times a week with children, does this person then not deserve a pedophilic diagnosis? It would seem that this issue of the relative strength of the paraphilic sexual interest is a red herring—if it is present it is sufficient for a diagnosis—a stronger "normophilic" interest is not an overriding mediator.

Strange or at Least Surprising Epidemiological Claims

It is unfortunate that the DSM5 does not use normal referencing procedures so that the warrant for its assertions could be understood and evaluated. It makes strange claims about the incidence and prevalence of the paraphilias. For example the DSM5 states that "frotteuristic acts" … "may occur in up to 30% of adult males in the general population" (p. 692). Of course the word "may" is a bit of a weasel word in this context but this seems quite high. In addition sometimes the range of prevalence is extremely large: for example for Sadism the DSM5 states unhelpfully that the range is between 2 and 30 %. Finally, at times it is not as clear as it could be that paraphilias are very uncommon in females. Feminists have pointed out that many sexual problems are gendered: it is males who are the perpetrators and females who are the victims. The DSM5 seems to obscure this fundamental point. For example, with voyeurism the DSM5 states "… in nonclinical samples, the highest possible lifetime prevalence for voyeuristic disorder is approximately 12% in males and 4% in females" (p. 688). This implies that males suffer from this at three times the frequency of females. This ratio is surprising and seems way too low. Based on arrest rates and clinical presentation it would seem that males are aroused by viewing unsuspecting individuals at ratios much greater than 3 to 1. Exhibitionistic acts according to the DSM5 occur in a 2:1 male to female ratio—again what appears to be a sex ratio that is way too low. Similar questions could be raised about making more explicit gender statements in other areas such as pedophilia.

A Lack of Clinical Astuteness and Understanding Reflexivity

The DSM5 states for the diagnostic criteria for Sexual Masochism Disorder: "the diagnostic criteria for sexual masochism disorder are intended to apply to individuals who freely admit to having such paraphilic interests …. In contrast, if they declare no distress, exemplified by anxiety, obsessions, guilt or shame, about these paraphilic impulses and are not hampered by them in pursuing other personal goals, they could be ascertained as having masochistic sexual interest but should *not* be diagnosed with sexual masochism disorder." (p. 694).

Does this not miss perhaps how masochistic tendencies may play a role in the larger personality? Would a person who enjoys pain—even if it largely confined to sexual pain—perhaps also have less of a tendency to report being bothered by the sequelae of such interests and behaviors? Could again, this be an additional part of the problem and not an obviating condition? Ought at least this sort of issue be considered in the diagnostic criteria—a lack or normal reporting of distress due to perhaps more generalized masochistic tendencies?

Conclusions

The DSM5 diagnostic categories of the paraphilias face a myriad of problems. Taken individually these 25 problems are all significant but taken collectively they represent a serious indictment of the DSM5. Unfortunately, there seems to be little progress from the DSM4 to the DSM5 meaning that there has been little improvement in a third of a century. Some of may be due to a failure to recognize these problems, but some of this seems to be that the field ignores these problems. The DSM5 paraphilia diagnoses seem to mainly be used because of their inclusion in a document that has strengths associated with other diagnostic categories (although many other problems in other diagnostic categories) and because of its lack of competitors. However, it is perplexing that although this emperor has no clothes, few have pointed this out and attempted to remedy these problems. Rather it seems that the social forces associated with the influence of this document rather than the scientific adequacy of these categories have functioned to persuade.

Classification is an important scientific pursuit — it provides the fundamental entities for a field. When early chemistry thought there were four fundamental elements — earth, fire, air, and water — little progress occurred because of this fundamental error related to carving nature at its joints. These problems in the DSM5 classification system surely have direct implications for other problems in the field. One needs valid classification in order to do meaningful treatment outcome studies. One needs valid classification in order to devise accurate and meaningful assessment devices. And most importantly one needs valid classification in order to both help individuals and to protect the interests of other members of society. Clearly overcoming the problems in the classification of the paraphilias ought to be more of a priority.

References

American Psychiatric Association. (1987). *The diagnostic and statistic manual-IVTR*. Washington, DC: American Psychiatric Association Press.

American Psychiatric Association. (2015). *The diagnostic and statistic manual-5*. Washington, DC: American Psychiatric Association Press.

Blanchard, R., Lykins, A. D., Wherrett, D., Kuban, M. E., Cantor, J. M., Blak, T., et al. (2009). Pedophilia, Hebephilia, and the DSM-V. *Archives of Sexual Behavior, 38*(3), 335–350.

Blanchard, R. (2011). Letter to the editor. A brief history of field trials of the DSM diagnostic criteria for paraphilias. *Archives of Sexual Behavior, 40*, 861–862.

Bromberg, D., & O'Donohue, W. (2012). *Juvenile sexual offending*. New York, NY: Springer.

Foucault, M. (1990). *The history of sexuality*. New York, NY: Vintage.

Kinsey, A. C. (1948). *Sexual behavior in the human male*. Bloomington, IN: Indiana University Press.

Lilienfeld, S. O. (2014). DSM5: Centripetal scientific and centrifugal antiscientific forces. *Clinical Psychology, 21*(3), 269–279.

Moser, C., & Kleinplatz, P. J. (2005). Does heterosexuality belong in the DSM? *The Lesbian and Gay Psychology Review, 6*(3), 261–267.

O'Donohue, W., Regev, L., & Hagstrom, A. (2000). Problems with the DSM-IV diagnosis of pedophilia. *Sex Abuse, 12*(2), 95–105.

O'Donohue, W. (2013). *Clinical psychology and the philosophy of science*. New York, NY: Springer.

Robins, E., & Guze, S. B. (1970). Establishment of diagnostic validity in psychiatric illness: Its application to schizophrenia. *Am J Psychiatry, 126*(7), 983–987.

Waldman, I. D., Lilienfeld, S. O., & Lahey, B. B. (1995). Toward construct validity in the childhood disruptive behavior disorders: Classification and diagnosis in DSM-IV and beyond. In T. H. Ollendick & R. J. Prinz (Eds.), *Advances in clinical child psychology* (Vol. 17, pp. 323–364). New York, NY: Plenum Press.

Chapter 2
A Brief History of Sexual Offender Risk Assessment

Leam A. Craig and Martin Rettenberger

Introduction

Assessing the risk of further offending behavior by adult sexual perpetrators is highly relevant and important to professionals involved in public protection, and accurate risk assessment is one of the most important developments for the field since the early 1900s (Barbaree, Langton, Gopnik-Lewinski, & Beach, 2013; Craig, Browne, & Beech, 2008). The goal of any risk assessment is to establish the likelihood of future occurrences of sexual offending behavior and to identify strategies that will reduce this potential (Hanson & Morton-Bourgon, 2005; Hart, Laws, & Kropp, 2003; Quinsey, Harris, Rice, & Cormier, 2006). There are three general accepted principles in this evaluation. First, the risk assessment must consider individual characteristics of the offender, called *risk factors*, which have an empirically demonstrated relationship with recidivism. Second, there is no single risk factor sufficiently related to recidivism that it should be considered on its own; a combination of factors is required to conduct a valid risk assessment. Third, structured approaches for the combination of risk factors such as actuarial risk assessment instruments (ARAIs) or professional judgment tools are more accurate than unstructured clinical opinions alone (Hanson & Morton-Bourgon, 2009).

L.A. Craig (✉)
Forensic Psychology Practice Ltd., Sutton Coldfield, UK

Centre for Forensic and Criminological Psychology, University of Birmingham, Edgbaston, Birmingham, UK

School of Social Sciences, Birmingham City University, Birmingham, UK
e-mail: leamcraig@forensicpsychology.co.uk

M. Rettenberger
Centre for Criminology, Wiesbaden, Germany

Department of Psychology, Johannes Gutenberg-University Mainz (JGU), Mainz, Germany
e-mail: martin.rettenberger@uni-mainz.de

© Springer International Publishing Switzerland 2016
D.R. Laws, W. O'Donohue (eds.), *Treatment of Sex Offenders*,
DOI 10.1007/978-3-319-25868-3_2

Over the last three decades, great advances have been made in what we know about sexual offending behavior and how to assess sexual recidivism risk, and the development and promulgation of ARAIs is certainly one of the most important advances. Criminal justice professionals have increasingly endorsed actuarial measures of risk as the most reliable predictive instruments for decision making (Ericson & Haggerty, 1997; Hannah-Moffat & Shaw, 2001).

The fervor toward using ARAIs has permeated the entire criminal justice system with specific reference being made to relevant legislative acts in the USA, Canada, the UK, and other European countries. For example, the USA has enacted legislation allowing for the postprison civil commitment of sex offenders as *sexually violent predators* (SVPs; Covington, 1997; Doren, 2002; Miller, Amenta, & Conroy, 2005). Consequently, the judicial system relies heavily on the opinions of psychologists and other expert witnesses who testify at commitment hearings often citing the use of actuarial tests for the prediction of sexual recidivism. In Canada, the National Parole Board (NPB) notes, "…There are numerous actuarial risk assessment instruments that exist and which the Board must consider in its decision-making process" (National Parole, 2004, p. 20). In order to help the NPB members get a better understanding of these various actuarial risk assessment tools, the NPB invited several forensic psychologists to research and develop a guide on these risk assessment tools. In England and Wales, directions to the Parole Board under Section 32(6) of the Criminal Justice Act 1991 (issued August 2004) regarding the release and recall of life sentence prisoners states the Parole Board must take into account "…any indication of predicted risk as determined by a validated actuarial risk predictor model or any other structured assessment of risk and treatment needs."

In this chapter, we briefly summarize the history and early development of risk assessment from clinical intuition and observation to the development of different "generations" of risk assessment instruments.

Risk Estimation Through Clinical Observation

Before 1950, there was little structured research focusing on outcome and follow-up recidivism data with any follow-up studies focusing on violence (dangerousness) in mentally disordered offenders. Although not sophisticated by today's standards, the early identification of sexual recidivism risk was usually based on clinical observations in patients and changes in environmental factors. For example, Ernits (1922) found that after the legalization of alcohol sales in 1920 in Estonia, [sexual] assaults on women increased by more than double for the first half of the year. An enlarged prostate gland was alleged to be a common cause of sexual crime in elderly men, and the proposal put forward, and practiced in Germany, is that castration should be adopted as a preventative measure against sexual crimes. It was also noted that in homosexuality, the attractive appearance and physique of the accomplice may be an important causal factor but not in heterosexuality.

In his anthropological study of the American criminal, Hooton (1939) found a great excess of unmarried men among criminals in general, and Bonger (1936) believed that important factors include inadequate housing accommodation, which brings children into close contact with sex life, and low mental standing of parents as predictors of sexual risk.

East and Hubert (1939) suggested that sexual offending risk may be linked to the early experience of perverse activity arising before the ordinary sexual pattern of activity has been established or from a more recent happening which actively repels the normal heterosexual expression. East (1949) commented that psychopathic personalities—a constitutional psychic inferior group—often commit sexual offenses. It was argued that psychoneurotic persons sometimes show their sexual inferiority and strive for superiority by committing a sexual murder or other sexual crimes and that an anxiety state may be a causal factor of a sexual offense. Alcoholic psychoses and schizophrenia were reported to be frequently associated with sexual crime and sexual murder, and morbid impulsive sexual conduct was argued to be an early manifestation of later sexual offending behavior.

Some early references to the examination of risk factors associated with general criminal recidivism were by Glueck and Glueck *500 Criminal Careers* (1930), a pioneering work in the field. Although not specific to sexual recidivism, their research focused on juvenile delinquency from which they developed the "Social Prediction Tables" model for predicting the likelihood of delinquent behavior in youth based on a number of static risk factors, many of which are still relevant today (Table 2.1). For the juvenile delinquents, they made attempts to predict criminality using statistics, followed by the likelihood of their rehabilitation upon release. Glueck and Glueck (1930) were the first criminologists to perform studies of chronic juvenile offenders and among the first to examine the effects of psychopathy among the more serious delinquents and claimed that potential deviants could be identified by as young as 6 years of age.

However, these risk observations were primarily based on unstructured clinical opinion, which has since been shown to be unreliable (Meehl, 1954; Hanson & Morton-Bourgon, 2009; Quinsey et al., 2006). Arguments for and against mechanical prediction had been published since the 1920s with one of the first attempts to introduce an actuarial prediction method into parole which was the "experience table" (Hart, 1924). In a study looking into the factors determining parole, Warner (1923) concluded that life history and background factors were of little value in predicting parole outcome. Reanalyzing Warner's data, Hart (1924) found that the accuracy of the prognostic score could be significantly improved if individual predictors were pooled. The method of using such experience tables has remained largely the same.

In the first large-scale study, Burgess (1928) examined the relationship between offenders' background factors and parole outcome. This study resulted in the development of a prototype expectancy table which was derived from computations of the degree to which violation rates of subpopulations with specific background characteristics deviated from the average violation rate of a given parolee population. Where the subpopulation violation rate was lower than that of the total parolee

Table 2.1 Glueck and Glueck's (1930) risk factors

	1930—500 Criminal Careers	1934—1000 Juvenile Delinquents	1950—Unraveling Juvenile Delinquency
Family	– Official record of arrest among family members – Economic hardship – Poor parental education – Abnormal or unhealthy home situation – Long/complete absence of parents – Intemperate (excessive use of alcohol, violent behavior) – Immoral mother – Foreign or mixed parentage – Child moved about during childhood or adolescence – Child left parental home prior to sentence	– Very large family – Poor parental education – Parents separated/divorced – Parents unduly quarrelsome – Insufficient parental supervision/discipline – Parents' excessive use of alcohol/violence – Parents' immoral, foreign, or mixed marriage	– Insufficient parental discipline – Poor supervision – Very large family – Low family cohesiveness
School	– Educational retardation	– Educational retardation – Leaving school early in life – Truancy	
Lifestyle	– Elicits heterosexual relations – Gambling – Alcoholism – Keeping bad company – Infrequent church attendance – Open conflict with social authorities—school/law	– Hanging around streets during leisure time	– Restless – Impulsive – Extroverted – Aggressive – Destructive
Personality/ intelligence	– Dull or borderline intelligence – Psychotic or psychopathic – Neuropathic traits – Extreme suggestibility – Emotional instability – Impulsiveness	– Subnormal intelligence – Marked emotional and personality handicaps	– Hostile – Defiant – Resentful – Suspicious – Stubborn – Assertive – Adventurous – Not submissive to authority, tendency to think in concrete not abstract terms
Employment	– Unskilled/semiskilled work prior to incarceration	– Unskilled/semiskilled work prior to incarceration	

population, the corresponding background factor was considered a favorable one. All positive factors were incorporated into an experience table, and a candidate for parole was assigned one point for each favorable factor in his background. A table giving the violation rate for offenders with different numbers of favorable factors was derived for the population under study. Burgess (1928) found that an experience table was more accurate than a probation officer's predictions of parole success. Similarly, Sarbin (1942) and Wittman and Steinberg (1944) also found that statistical methods are more accurate in outcome predictions. Sarbin (1944) argued a priori for the superiority of mechanical prediction, as not doing justice to the potential flexibility of clinical judgments and that the clinician engages in a weighting-and-adding process used in statistical prediction formulas, but clinicians calculate less reliably and so are less accurate (Grove & Lloyd, 2006).

Although proponents of the clinical judgment continued to emphasize the value of professional intuition, the emphasis in risk prediction slowly changed following Meehl's (1954) publication. Meehl's (1954) seminal book made four major contributions to the clinical-statistical debate which was to advance the field beyond recognition:

1. Distinguished data gathering from data combination, focusing on the accuracy of clinical versus mechanical methods for combining data.
2. A convincing refutation that the clinical-statistical antithesis is artificial, although in his later work he argued against using both together (Grove & Meehl, 1996).
3. A recognition of a clinician's potential for creative insight.
4. Comparisons of clinical and statistical prediction strongly favored statistical prediction.

We will now consider the impact of Paul E. Meehl's contribution to the field of risk prediction in the development of ARAIs for sexual offenders.

Risk Estimation Through Mechanical Prediction

Meehl (1954) encouraged applying actuarial prediction to clinical assessment in the 1950s. He was one of the first to introduce the idea of mechanical risk assessment tools based on known recidivism factors. Here, Meehl (1954) suggested that mechanical risk assessment tools have explicit item rules as well as clear definitions for combining the item scores into a total score. Using experience tables, these total scores are then translated into probabilistic estimates of risk, a core feature of his definition of an actuarial risk assessment procedure and a method still employed in several modern ARAIs (Hanson & Thornton, 2000; Thornton et al., 2003).

Meehl and Rosen (1955) were among the first to consider the effect of base rates on prediction and adequate sampling methodology in order to enhance predictive accuracy. All actuarial risk instruments are ultimately derived from base rates, which are usually recorded as reoffense or recidivism. So a base rate of 10 % usually means that 10 % of a group of sexual offenders can be expected to reoffend within a given time period. However, base rates are inherently ambiguous, unreliable, and unstable (Koehler, 1996). It is well documented that base rates differ between ages and subgroups of offenders, increase with longer follow-up periods (Grubin, 1998; Hanson, 1997a; Hood, Shute, Feilzer, & Wilcox, 2002; Prentky, Lee, Knight, & Cerce, 1997), and vary between sexual recidivism studies from 0.10 to 0.40 (Barbaree, 1997). For example, the base rate for rapists (17.1 %) is higher than that of intrafamilial offenders (8.4 %) but less than that of extrafamilial offenders (19.5 %) (Hanson, 2001). Although the recidivist rate for intrafamilial offenders was generally low, those aged between 18 and 24 years are at greater risk of recidivism (30.7 %) (Hanson, 2001).

Szmukler (2001) illustrates how low base rates increase the probability of making a false-positive error prediction. With a base rate of 6 %, an ARAI with good predictive accuracy (e.g., $r = 0.70$; see Janus & Meehl, 1997) would be wrong nine times out of 10. Using Szmukler's positive predictive value model, given the base rate for sexual offense recidivism in the UK fluctuates around 3 % (Falshaw, 2002), the same ARAI would be wrong 94 times out of 100 (Craig, Browne, Stringer, & Beech, 2004).

Conversely, raising the base rate increases the probability of making a false-negative error prediction, thus predicting a large number of people will not fail when in fact they will. In reality, the difficulty of predicting events increases as the base rate differs from 0.50 (Meehl & Rosen, 1955). Therefore, the accuracy of our predictions is greatest when the base rate is roughly 50 %. As the base rate drops below 50 % or rises above 50 %, we begin to make more errors, and importantly, we begin to shift the region of error (Prentky & Burgess, 2000). Low-frequency events are difficult to predict, but high-frequency events are easy to predict, and decision-making methods are hardest and need to be highly accurate when predicting the opposite to the predominant pattern. With very infrequent events, the probability of making false-positive errors will be high. Therefore, in attempting to predict failure (i.e., sexual recidivism) when the base rate is small, we end up predicting that a large number of individuals will reoffend when in fact they will not. The probability that a positive result is true varies with the base rate of the group to which to the test is being applied. With rare conditions, even the most accurate test will produce lots of "false positives," and the large number outside the condition serves to magnify even small errors in the test (Janus & Meehl, 1997).

Based on Meehl's (1954) work about the comparison between actuarial and clinical prediction methods, two core variables of ARAIs are that they use explicit methods of combining the risk factors and that the total score which resulted usually from adding up the individual item scores to a total sum score is linked to an empirically derived probability figure (Dawes, Faust, & Meehl, 1989; Hanson & Morton-Bourgon, 2009). Referring to Sawyer (1966), Hanson and Morton-Bourgon (2007) differentiated risk assessment into one of the four following categories depending whether the risk factors are empirically or conceptually derived and whether the final judgment is determined by a structured professional judgment (SPJ)-related procedure or by an explicit algorithm: empirical actuarial, conceptual actuarial, SPJ, and unstructured. The empirical actuarial approach proposed by Hanson and

Morton-Bourgon (2007) is most comparable with the abovementioned historical definition of actuarial assessment by Meehl (1954). In this approach, the items are selected based on the observed relationship with outcome (i.e., recidivism risk), and explicit rules are provided for combining the items into an overall risk judgment (e.g., the Sex Offender Risk Appraisal Guide [SORAG]; Quinsey et al., 2006; or the Static-99; Hanson & Thornton, 2000). In the conceptual actuarial approach, the final judgment is determined by explicit rules, but the items are selected based on theory or on a combination of theory and empiricism. Popular examples of conceptual actuarial risk assessment instruments for sexual offenders are the Structure Risk Assessment (SRA; Thornton, 2002) or the Violence Risk Scale—Sexual Offender Version (VRS-SO; Wong, Olver, Nicholaichuk, & Gordon, 2003).

In their updated meta-analysis, Hanson and Morton-Bourgon (2009) propose two further categories of standardized risk assessment instruments which could be more or less actuarial in terms of Meehl (1954): mechanical and adjusted actuarial. Mechanical risk assessment tools have explicit item rules as well as clear definitions for combining the item scores into a total score. However, they did not provide a table which linked the total scores to empirically derived recidivism probabilities which was a core feature of Meehl's (1954) definition of an actuarial risk assessment procedure. Furthermore, mechanical instruments selected their items based primarily on theory or literature reviews instead of empirical investigations about the relationships between predictors and outcome (Hanson & Morton-Bourgon, 2009). SPJ instruments like the Sexual Violence Risk-20 (SVR-20: Boer, Hart, Kropp, & Webster, 1997) could become mechanical risk assessment tools in this sense if—which is not uncommon in clinical practice—the user omits the SPJ-related final risk judgment and instead of this simply adds up the single item scores to a total score (Hanson & Morton-Bourgon, 2007; Rettenberger, Boer, & Eher, 2010).

The adjusted actuarial risk assessment method is based on the total scores of actuarial or mechanical tools but provides the additional judgment option of a so-called clinical override. In this case, the evaluator is allowed to overrule the actuarially derived final judgment by external factors which are usually not specified in advance. Furthermore, the method of combining the external factors with the results of the actuarial tool is also not predetermined (Hanson & Morton-Bourgon, 2009). The clinical override is one core feature of most SPJ instruments (Boer & Hart, 2009) and is also included in the VRS-SO (Wong et al., 2003).

However, care must be taken when using clinical override in SPJ, and in particular with ARAIs, as any deviation from the empirically approved methodology runs the risk of invalidating the scale (Craig & Beech, 2010). Furthermore, Hanson and Morton-Bourgon (2009) identified at that time only three direct empirical investigations of the clinical override beyond actuarial or mechanical judgment (Gore, 2007; Hanson, 2007; Vrana, Sroga, & Guzzo, 2008) but concluded nevertheless that the result pattern is quite clear: Clinically, adjustments of actuarial and mechanical instruments lead usually to a decrease of predictive accuracy. Therefore, Hanson and Morton-Bourgon (2009) stated that "the simplest interpretation is that the overrides simply added noise" (p. 9). In a recently published study, Wormith, Hogg, and Guzzo (2012) investigated the clinical override option for a relatively new instrument, the

Level of Service/Case Management Inventory (LS/CMI; Andrews, Bonta, & Wormith, 2004), and noted that this clinical feature reduced the predictive validity of the instrument.

Meehl (1954) already claimed that the best prediction scheme is the one that produces the smallest error for each client. This might involve using clinical prediction in one case and statistical prediction in another case. However, to choose the data combining method on a case-by-case method, the assessor would have to know, in advance, which combination method would produce the best result for the individual case (Grove, 2005).

Generations of Risk Assessment

Based on Andrews and Bonta's (2006) *The Psychology of Criminal Conduct* (PCC), the focus on the conceptualization of different "generations" of risk assessment is that risk assessment should not only provide as much as possible predictive accuracy but also information about the opportunities of risk management, i.e., about the potential risk-reducing influence of (therapeutic) interventions and sanctions (Boer & Hart, 2009; Hanson & Morton-Bourgon, 2009; Wong et al., 2003). Andrews and Bonta (2006) proposed three generations of risk assessment: first, intuitive clinical judgment; second, actuarial risk assessment methods based on predominantly or exclusively static risk factors; and third, risk assessment methods based on dynamic factors (Harris & Hanson, 2010). A fourth generation of risk assessment tools pretends to integrate more systematically data about the intervention and monitoring process with a comprehensive permanently up-to-date assessment (i.e., in terms of a "case management" procedure; Andrews, Bonta, & Wormith, 2006). The most prominent example of a fourth-generation risk assessment instrument is the above-mentioned LS/CMI (Andrews et al., 2004).

The proliferation of the second-generation risk assessment instruments as well as the development of third- and fourth-generation risk assessment instruments was strongly influenced and supported by the Risk-Need-Responsivity (RNR) model of offender rehabilitation (Andrews & Bonta, 2006; Harris & Hanson, 2010a, 2010b). Andrews and Bonta (2006) suggested that an effective intervention has to focus on risk (i.e., the risk potential of the single offender for committing new offenses), need (i.e., consideration of empirically proven criminogenic needs in terms of particular treatment goals), and responsivity (i.e., the use of intervention techniques and treatment programs to which the individual offender's abilities, learning style, motivation, and strengths respond).

Today, the RNR model is regarded as probably the most influential model for the assessment and treatment of offenders (Bonta & Andrews, 2007; Ward, Mesler, & Yates, 2007) and was also successfully proven for sexual offenders (Hanson, Bourgon, Helmus, & Hodgson, 2009). Hanson et al. (2009) reported that treatment programs which adhered to the RNR principles showed the best results in reducing recidivism in sexual offenders. Because of the consistency of these findings with the general offender rehabilitation literature (Andrews & Bonta, 2006; Bonta & Andrews, 2007; Craig, Dixon, & Gannon, 2013), the authors suggested that the RNR model should be the most relevant aspect in the design and implementation of interventions for sexual offenders (Hanson et al., 2009). Obviously, the use of ARAIs could, therefore, be able to improve the risk-reducing results of treatment programs by measuring accurately the individual level of risk with second-generation risk assessment instruments and by defining treatment targets in terms of criminogenic needs with third (or fourth)-generation risk assessment instruments. Indeed, this is a model adopted by the UK National Offender Management Service (NOMS) as part of the Structured Assessment of Risk and Need: Treatment Needs Analysis (SARN-TNA) as well as by other European countries (e.g., Eher, Matthes, Schilling, Haubner-MacLean, & Rettenberger, 2012).

Taken together, the current state of research indicated that actuarially based instruments are today the best available instruments for the prediction of recidivism risk in sexual offenders (Grove & Meehl, 1996; Hanson & Morton-Bourgon, 2009). Furthermore, the use of these instruments has to be regarded as a necessary precondition for the implementation and application of the treatment programs for sexual offenders (Andrews & Bonta, 2006; Bonta & Andrews, 2007; Hanson et al., 2009).

We will now briefly summarize some of the internationally most commonly used second- and third-generation actuarial risk assessment instruments for sexual offenders. Because of the currently already overwhelming and permanently increasing state of empirical knowledge about ARAIs, it is certainly not possible to give a complete review about all existing validation studies of every instrument. However, the aim of the following overview is to give insight into the most important instruments and their scientific and empirical foundation.

Second-Generation Risk Assessment

The literature has witnessed a proliferation of ARAIs for estimating sexual recidivism risk; probably the most well known include Risk Matrix 2000/Sexual (RM2000-S; Thornton et al., 2003), extensively used in the UK; the Rapid Risk Assessment for Sexual Offense Recidivism (RRASOR; Hanson, 1997b), the Static-99 (Hanson & Thornton, 2000), the Static-2002/R (Phenix, Doren, Helmus, Hanson, & Thornton, 2008), and the Sex Offender Risk Appraisal Guide (SORAG; Quinsey et al., 2006) are also well-known and used scales. Table 2.2 contains a description of scales and the items that make up each of these scales.

Validation studies for second-generation ARAIs have consistently demonstrated predictive accuracy across samples and countries including Australia (Allan, Dawson, & Allan, 2006), Austria (Rettenberger, Matthes, Boer, & Eher, 2010), Belgium (Ducro & Pham, 2006), Brazil (Baltieri & de Andrade Baltieri & de Andrade, 2008), Canada (Kingston, Yates, Firestone, Babchishin, & Bradford, 2008), Denmark (Bengtson, 2008), Germany (Stadtland et al., 2005), New Zealand (Skelton, Riley, Wales, & Vess, 2006), and the UK (Craig et al., 2006a, 2006b).

Table 2.2 List of items in ARAIs for sexual offenders

Risk instrument	Scale description
Rapid Risk Assessment for Sexual Offense Recidivism Hanson (1997)	This scale was developed in Canada using predominantly North American samples but has since been validated in England and Wales using a prison sample. RRASOR contains four items, past sexual offenses, age at commencement of risk, extrafamilial victims, and male victims. Offenders are allocated points according to the presence of these and given a risk categorization on this basis. Based on a system of assigning points to the presence of such variables, the scale ranges from 0 (first-time incest offenders, over the age of 15) to 6 (extrafamilial boy victim pedophiles with four or more previous convictions and released prior to the age of 25) The scoring manual for RRASOR is available online from Public Safety Canada
Static-99 Hanson and Thornton (2000)	Static-99 consists of ten items: prior sex offenses, prior sentencing occasions, convictions for noncontact sex offenses, index nonsexual violence, prior nonsexual violence, unrelated victims, stranger victims, male victims, lack of a long-term intimate relationship, and offender aged under 25 on release (or now, if the offender is in the community) The revised 2003 coding rules for Static-99 are available from www.static99.org
Static-2002 Hanson and Thornton (2003)	Static-2002 is an actuarial risk tool for evaluating the risk of sexual and violent recidivism among adult male sexual offenders and should be considered a separate instrument to Static-99. Static-2002 predicts sexual, violent, and any recidivism as well as other actuarial risk tools commonly used with sexual offenders and is slightly better than Static-99. Static-2002 is intended to assess some theoretically meaningful characteristics presumed to be the cause of recidivism risk (persistence of sexual offending, deviant sexual interests, general criminality). Static-2002 has 14 items, with some items modified from Static-99. For example, the item "young" on Static-2002 has four age categories rather than two. New items not included in Static-99 are "any juvenile arrest for sexual offense," "rate of sexual offending," "young, unrelated victims," "any community supervision violation," and "years free prior to index." Static-2002 items are grouped into five domains: age, persistence of sex offending, deviant sexual interests, relationship to victims, and general criminality. Total scores can range from 0 to 14. Several studies have provided support for the predictive validity of Static-2002 (Haag, 2005; Langton, Barbaree, Hansen, Harkins, & Peacock, 2006; Langton, Barbaree, Seto, et al., 2007) with AUC values ranging from 0.71 to 0.76 The scoring manual for the Static-2002 is available online from www.static99.org
Risk Matrix 2000 Thornton et al. (2003)	This scale has separate indicators for risk of sexual recidivism (RM2000-S), and overall violence (RM2000-V), and can be combined to give a composite risk of reconviction for sexual or nonsexual assaults—Risk Matrix 2000/Combined (RM2000-C). This scale is used in prison, probation, and other mental health settings in the UK, as it is a widely cross-validated, static risk assessment for sex offenders (Harkins & Beech, 2007). An individual's level of sexual violence risk (low, medium, high, very high) is ascertained by a two-stage process. The first stage involves scoring individuals on three easily obtainable items: (1) age at commencement of risk, (2) sexual appearances, (3) and total criminal appearances. From the total score from these three items, an individual is initially rated as low, medium, high, or very high risk. The second stage of RM2000 contains four aggravating factors, said to contribute to elevated risk: (1) male victim, (2) stranger victim, (3) noncontact sexual offenses, (4) and lack of a long-term intimate relationship. If two of these aggravating factors are identified, in an individual's psychosocial history, their risk category is raised one level from Stage 1 of the process and two levels if all four items are present. In a cross-validation study, the RM2000-S obtained moderate (AUC 0.68) accuracy in predicting sexual reconviction, whereas the RM2000-V obtained good accuracy in predicting violent and sexual/violent (combined) (AUC 0.87 and 0.76) reconviction (Craig, Beech, & Browne, 2006a, 2006b)
	The RM2000 scoring guide is available from www.cfcp.bham.ac.uk

(continued)

Table 2.2 (continued)

Risk instrument	Scale description
Sex Offender Risk Appraisal Guide (SORAG) Quinsey et al. (1998)	SORAG was designed to predict at least one reconviction for a sexual offense. Developed from a version used for violent offenders (Violent Risk Appraisal Guide, VRAG; see Quinsey, et al. 1998), SORAG contained 14 static risk factors including lived with biological parents, elementary school maladjustment, alcohol problems, marital status, criminal history for violent and nonviolent offenses, history of sexual offenses [against girls under 14 years], age at index offense, criteria for any personality disorder, schizophrenia, phallometric test results, and psychopathy (PCL-R, Hare, 1991) scores

The predictive accuracy of the various ARAIs, using the AUC[1] indices, typically fall between 0.65 and 0.80 with some studies reporting AUC indices of 0.90 for the SORAG (Harris & Rice, 2003) and 0.92 for the Static-99 (Thornton, 2001; for a review see, for example, Craig et al., 2008).

While ARAIs are undoubtedly superior to that of clinical judgment, the use of ARAIs is not without its limitations (Craig et al., 2004; Hart, Laws, & Kropp, 2003). Nevertheless, ARAIs provide a baseline of risk, differentiating between high-, medium-, and low-risk estimations from which more detailed assessments can be conducted, in keeping with the RNR principles.

Third-Generation Risk Assessment

Dynamic risk factors or the so-called criminogenic needs are the core construct of third-generation instruments (Harris & Hanson, 2010a, 2010b). The central difference between static risk factors captured in the second-generation ARAIs and third-generation dynamic risk factors is that they are amenable to changes based on interventions which can lead to risk-related changes in the individual offender. The most prominent examples for third-generation instruments are the Stable-2007 and the Acute-2007 (Eher et al., 2012; Hanson, Harris, Scott, & Helmus, 2007; Harris & Hanson, 2010a, 2010b). Another dynamic treatment and risk-need assessment framework which will be discussed in more detail on the following pages is the SARN-TNA framework, which is widely used within the National Offender Management Service (NOMS) in England and Wales. Table 2.3 lists the risk items shared by the SARN and Stable-/Acute-2007 dynamic frameworks.

---

[1] The area under the curve (AUC) of the receiver operating characteristic (ROC) analysis is a comparison of the sensitivity (true positive divided by the sum of the true positive and false negatives) with specificity (true negative divided by the sum of the false positive and false negative), i.e., hit rate against the false alarm rate.

Referring to Cohen (1992), Rice and Harris (2005) formulated the following interpretation criteria for AUC values: Results of 0.71 or above are classified as "good" and numbers between 0.64 and 0.71 are classified as "moderate." Significant AUC values that are below the value of 0.64 are classified as "small."

Table 2.3 Risk items from third-generation dynamic frameworks

	Third-generation dynamic frameworks		
Stable dynamic factors	SRA/SARN (Thornton, 2002; Webster et al. 2006)	Stable-2007 (Hanson et al., 2007)	Acute-2007 (Hanson et al., 2007)
Sexual interests (obsession/preoccupation)	Sexual preoccupation (obsession) Sexual preference for children Sexualized violence Other offense-related sexual interests (fetish)	Sexual preoccupation/sex drive Sex as a coping strategy Deviant sexual interests	Victim access Hostility sexual preoccupation
Attitudes supportive of sexual offense	Adversarial sexual attitudes Sexual entitlement Child abuse-supportive beliefs The belief women are deceitful	Sexual entitlement Pro-rape attitudes Child molester attitudes	
Relationships/socio-affective functioning (intimacy deficits)	Personal inadequacy Emotional congruence with children Grievance stance Emotional loneliness (lack of intimate relationships)	Lack of lovers/intimate partners Emotional identification with children Hostility toward women General social rejection/loneliness Lack of concern for others	Collapse of social supports
Self-regulation/self-management	Impulsive, unstable lifestyle Not knowing how to solve life's problems Out of control emotions or urges (emotional dysregulation)	Impulsive acts Poor cognitive problem-solving skills Negative emotionality/hostility	Rejection of supervision Emotional collapse Substance abuse

Stable-2007 and Acute-2007

One of the most influential research projects about dynamic risk factors in sexual offenders was the Dynamic Predictors Project (DPP; Hanson & Harris, 2000; Hanson et al., 2007; Harris & Hanson, 2010a, 2010b). The starting point for this research was a study published by Hanson and Harris (2000) where they investigated the differences between two approximately equally large samples of sexual offenders known to have reoffended sexually while on community supervision ($n = 208$) and of sexual offenders who have not reoffended ($n = 201$). With a focus specifically on the risk factors which could have changed in the time periods proceeding the reoffense, Hanson and Harris (2000) identified two separate types of dynamic risk factors: on the one hand relatively stable enduring traits (e.g., attitudes, cognitive distortions, or self-regulation deficits) and, on the other hand, temporally rapidly changeable acute risk factors located rather in the environment and situational context. This led to the development of the Sex Offender Risk Assessment Rating (SONAR; Hanson & Harris, 2001) which consisted of five stable dynamic risk factors (intimacy deficits, social influences, attitudes, and general as well as sexual self-regulation) and four acute dynamic risk factors (substance abuse, negative mood, anger/hostility, and opportunities for victim access).

Due to conceptual and clinical concerns, the SONAR was later separated into two measures, the Acute-2000 and Stable-2000. In 1999, Hanson et al. (2007) initiated the Dynamic Supervision Project (DSP), a prospective longitudinal field trial examining the reliability, validity, and clinical utility of the Acute-2000 and Stable-2000. A total of 156 parole and probation officers from every Canadian province as well as from the US states of Alaska and Iowa who were trained in the application of the Static-99, the Stable-2000, and the Acute-2000 completed risk assessments on $N = 997$ sexual offenders. After an average follow-up of 3 years, the accuracy of the Static-99 for the prediction of sexual recidivism was expectably high ($AUC = 0.74$). The same was true for the Acute-2000 ($AUC = 0.74$) although the Stable-2000 ($AUC = 0.64$) performed less well. For the Stable-2000, not all risk factors showed the hypothesized linear relationship with recidivism or any incremental predictive accuracy beyond the Static-99. In a subsequent revision, the three attitude items were dropped due to a lack of prognostic relevance, and the revised Stable-2007 demonstrated higher predictive accuracy ($AUC = 0.67$) and incremental predictive power beyond the Static-99 alone (Hanson et al., 2007).

The Acute-2000 was only a subset of the included risk factors which was significantly related to all outcome measures (sexual, violent, and general criminal recidivism). This result led to a revision (e.g., Acute-2007) which separated two different factors: factors relevant for the prediction of violent and sexual recidivism (victim access, hostility, sexual preoccupation, and rejection of supervision) and general criminality factor which contains all seven abovementioned specified risk factors. The option of an eighth unspecified unique risk factor was dropped in the revised Acute-2007 version. Another interesting, and especially for policy makers in applied risk assessment settings, relevant finding was that the Static-99/Stable-2007 risk prediction system showed higher predictive accuracy (up to $AUC = 0.84$) when used by "conscientious" officers who were defined by the fact that they have submitted complete datasets without missing data (Hanson et al., 2007).

The Stable-2007 has been cross-validated in only a few independent studies, while the Acute-2007 has yet to be cross-validated. Nunes and Babchishin (2012) conducted a construct validity study about the Stable-2000 and the Stable-2007 by examining correlations between selected items of the risk tools and validated independent measures of relevant constructs. The authors concluded that the results generally supported the construct validity of the stable risk measures, but the degree of convergence was lower than expected (Nunes & Babchishin, 2012). Eher et al. (2012) investigated the predictive and incremental validity of the Stable-2000 and the Stable-2007 in a prison-released sample of sexual offenders from Austria ($N=263$) by using a prospective longitudinal research design. After an average follow-up period of 6.4 years, the Stable-2007 was significantly related to all outcomes (AUC=0.67–0.71), whereas the Stable-2000 showed only weak predictive accuracy for the prediction of sexual recidivism (AUC=0.62). Furthermore, the study provided additional evidence for the incremental validity of the Stable-2007 beyond the second-generation static risk factors (Eher et al., 2012). In a further cross-validation study from Austria, Eher et al. (2013) investigated the predictive accuracy of the Static-99 and the Stable-2007 in a sample ($N=96$) of released male forensic patients hospitalized under mandatory treatment who committed sexually motivated offenses. The Static-99 (AUC=0.86) and the Stable-2007 (AUC=0.71) were significantly related to sexual reoffending after an average follow-up period of approximately 7 years. Again, the Stable-2007 provided evidence for the incremental predictive accuracy beyond the Static-99 (Eher et al., 2013). In a currently published German study, Briken and Müller (2014) examined the utility of risk assessment instruments like the Stable-2007 for assessing the criminal responsibility and the necessity for placement in a forensic psychiatric hospital according to the German penal code. The authors concluded that specific items of the Stable-2007 (e.g., deviant sexual interests, sexual preoccupations, or relationship deficits) and the Acute-2007 (e.g., sexual preoccupation, emotional collapse, or collapse of social support) could be used as empirically well-established proxy variables beyond and additionally to formal diagnosis according to the International Classification of Diseases (ICD) and the *Diagnostic and Statistical Manual of Mental Disorders* (DSM) criteria, in order to assess the severity of paraphilic disorders (Briken & Müller, 2014).

Structured Assessment of Risk and Need: Treatment Needs Analysis (SARN-TNA)

The SARN-TNA framework is widely used within the National Offender Management Service (NOMS) in England and Wales. The SARN-TNA is an "empirically guided" process for identifying factors related to risk. That is, it directs the assessor to consider only factors that are known to affect the likelihood of further offending. The framework consists of the actuarial RM2000 (Thornton et al., 2003) assessment and the SARN-TNA, which is used routinely alongside sex offender treatment in order to identify treatment needs. Typically, TNA grid is "opened" before the treatment program and is based on a structured interview and collateral information in order to identify deficits in the offender's *generality* (which refers to the existence of the factor in contexts other than offending) and *offense chain* (which refers to the sequence of situations, thoughts, feelings, and behaviors leading to offenses, including lifestyle features that made the chain more likely to start).

The SARN-TNA comprises 15 dynamic risk factors organized into four domains:

Sexual Interests Domain: This domain refers to both the direction and strength of sexual interests and considers offense-related sexual preferences and sexual pre-occupation both factors identified as predictive of sexual recidivism (Hanson & Bussière, 1998; Hanson & Morton-Bourgon, 2005; Pithers, Kashima, Cumming, & Beal, 1988; Proulx, Pellerin, McKibben, Aubut, & Ouimet, 1999).

Offense-Supportive Attitudes Domain: This domain refers to sets of beliefs about offenses, sexuality, or victims that can be used to justify sexual offending behavior. Denial or minimization of a particular offense is not considered relevant unless it can be linked to more general attitudes. Distorted beliefs in sexual offenders are well supported within the literature (Beech, Fisher, & Beckett, 1999; Hanson & Harris, 2000; Hanson & Scott; 1995; Pithers et al., 1988; Ward, Louden, Hudson, & Marshall, 1995) as offense precursors consistent in both child molesters (Beech et al., 1999; Hanson & Scott, 1995) and rapists (Malamuth & Brown, 1994; Hanson & Scott, 1995). Consistent with this, Hanson and Morton-Bourgon (2005) found denial and minimization unrelated to sexual recidivism, while more general attitudes tolerant of sexual crime were associated with sexual recidivism.

Relationships Domain: This refers to the ways of relating to other people and to motivating emotions felt in the context of these interactions. Negative emotional states such as anxiety, depression, and low self-esteem (Pithers et al., 1988; Proulx et al., 1999), and especially anger (Hanson & Harris, 2000), have been found to be offense precursors. Factors such as low self-esteem, loneliness, and external locus of control seem to distinguish child molesters from comparison groups (Beech et al., 1999). Thornton (2002) argues that at least four aspects of socio-affective functioning are relevant to sexual offending: inadequacy (external locus of control, low self-esteem, and loneliness), emotional congruence (being more emotionally open to children than adults), lack of emotional intimate relationships with adults (shallow relationships or the absence of relationships and emotional loneliness), and aggressive thinking (rumination of anger, suspiciousness, sense of grievance, a tendency to rehearse negative emotion, reluctance to see others' point of view). Meta-analytical results support the recidivism relevance of emotional congruence with children and to a lesser extent hostility (Hanson & Morton-Bourgon, 2005).

Self-Management Domain: This refers to an individual's ability to plan, problem solve, and regulate dysfunctional impulses that might otherwise lead to relapse (Pithers et al., 1988; Ward, Hudson, & Keenan, 1998). Antisocial behavior and lifestyle impulsivity have been identified as precursors of sexual reoffending

(Prentky & Knight, 1991). Thornton (2002) likens this construct to that of Factor 2 in the Hare Psychopathy Checklist-Revised (PCL-R; Hare, 1991) which has been found to predict sexual recidivism (Firestone et al., 1999; Rice & Harris, 1997).

An Initial Deviancy Assessment (IDA) is calculated from the SARN-TNA and organized into three levels of deviance: *low* deviance, when no dynamic marked risk factors are apparent (i.e., no risk factor within any SARN-TNA domain scores a 2 in both generality and offense chain); *moderate* deviance, where only one domain contains a risk factor/risk factors scoring a 2 in both generality and offense chain; and *high* deviance, where there are two or more domains containing a risk factor with a score of 2 for both generality and offense chain. This is translated to *low*, *medium*, or *high* dynamic risk/treatment need. Assessors are trained in applying the framework and have to pass a competency test and checked for inter-rater reliability. A triangulation method of assessment is used including psychometric evidence, official records (court documents, prison or probation files, treatment logs and reports, prison wing records), and offender interviews (Tully, Browne, & Craig, in press).

Despite its wide use within NOMS, research into the SRA and adapted SARN framework as a risk assessment tool is limited. In one of the two studies described in the original paper, Thornton (2002) compared offenders with previous convictions for child molestation (repeat) against offenders who had been convicted for child sexual offenses for the first time (current only). Using psychometric measures to approximate three of the four domains, Thornton found that the repeat offenders demonstrated more distorted attitudes, more socio-affective dysfunction, and poorer self-management.

In a follow-up study using a similar methodology, Thornton and Beech (2002) found that the number of dysfunctional domains made a statistically significant contribution to prediction over and above the Static-99 risk category. Craig, Thornton, Beech, and Browne (2007) conducted similar research into psychometrically assessed deviant domains in a sample of 119 sexual offenders and found that the SRA deviancy index predicted sexual reconviction independent of the Static-99 (SRA AUC=0.69). Craig et al. (2007) calculated a Psychological Deviance Index (PDI) by standardizing each of these scale scores for a domain. Of the four dynamic risk domains, the *Sexual Interests* domain obtained a large effect in predicting sexual reconviction over 2-year (AUC=0.86) and 5-year follow-up periods (AUC=0.72). The *Self-Management* factor obtained moderate results (AUC=0.71) in predicting sexual reconviction at 2 years. In comparison, Static-99 obtained moderate accuracy in predicting sexual reconviction, at 2 years (AUC=0.66) and 5 years (AUC=0.60). When the rates of sexual recidivism were compared with the PDI, it was found that the increase in rates of sexual recidivism mirrored the increase in the degree of PDI. As the PDI increased from zero, one, two, three, and four, the rates of reconviction were 3 %, 10 %, 8 %, 14 %, and 26 %, respectively. However, when the PDI was grouped into low (0), moderate (1–2), and high (3+) categories, it was found the degree of PDI and rates of reconviction were linear at 3 %, 18 %, and 40 %, respectively.

Wakeling, Beech, and Freemantle (2013) recently examined the relationship between psychometric changes in treatment and recidivism in a sample of 3773 sex offenders based on the SARN-TNA deviancy domain framework. They reported a 2-year sexual reconviction rate of 1.7 % with a sexual and violent reconviction rate combined of 4.4 %. Clinically significant changes were calculated for the psychometrics. They found that those whose scores were in the "normal range" before and after treatment were reconvicted at a significantly lower rate than those whose scores were not in the "normal range" after treatment on selected psychometric scales. Additionally, participants who were deemed "changed" overall on three of the four risk domains were reconvicted at a lower rate than those who were deemed not to have changed on these domains. Consistent with Craig et al. (2007), psychometric measures of sexual obsession and paraphilia obtained the highest AUC values of 0.71 and 0.62 on average, respectively, in predicting sexual and violent reconviction.

As part of a review and revision of the SARN framework, protective factors are incorporated into the dynamic framework, making more explicit issues of responsivity as well as factors of desistance (see Laws & Ward, 2010), in keeping with the RNR principles (Andrews & Bonta, 2006). This has led to a new needs analysis tool to help guide treatment planning, Risk and Success Factors Analysis (RSFA), and a new risk assessment report format to bring all the evidence together, Structured Assessment of Risk, Need, and Responsivity (SARNR). The framework continues to be centered on the four core domains as well as an additional item, *purpose*, aimed at being a responsible member of society, sticking to the rules, and getting on with the people (good citizenship). The assessment methodology adopts a triangulation of evidence to identify an individual's risk factors based on interview data, observation, file review, treatment program products, and psychometric measures.

This revision explicitly incorporates ideas in the Good Lives Model (GML: Ward, 2002; Ward & Maruna, 2007) emphasizing the importance of life experiences. Incorporating a measure of *purpose* in the SARNR promotes appropriate relationships, contact with the community, and pro-social influences which are often considered important areas for assessment and treatment intervention.

Sexual Violence Risk-20 (SVR-20)

The SVR-20 (Boer et al., 1997) developed more as a set of guidelines and assesses the risk of sexual violence by selecting 20 factors, from an extensive list, that could be comprehensively divided into three main sections to formulate sexual violence risk. Factors include: (a) *Psychological Adjustment*—sexual deviation, victim of child abuse, cognitive impairment, suicidal/homicidal ideation, relationship/employment problems, previous offense history (nonsexual violent, nonviolent), psychopathy, substance use problems, and past supervision failure; (b) *Sexual Offending*—such as high-density offenses, multiple offenses, physical harm to victims, use of weapon, escalation, and cognitive distortions; and (c) *Future Plans*—whether the offender lacks realistic plans and has negative attitudes toward instruction. The AUC indices for the SVR-20 in predicting sexual reconviction are mixed. Craig et al. (2006a, 2006b) as well as Sjöstedt and Långström (2002) found that the SVR-20 was a better predictor of violent reconviction than of sexual reconviction. Barbaree et al. (2008) reported an AUC of 0.63 in a sample of 468 Canadian sexual offenders, while Rettenberger et al. (2010) reported an AUC of 0.71 in a sample of 394 Austrian sexual offenders. In a Dutch study using a sample of 122 sexual offenders admitted to a forensic psychiatric unit, de Vogel, de Ruiter, van Beek, and Mead (2004) found that the SVR-20 final risk judgment is a better predictor for sexual recidivism than Static-99. In this study, the SVR-20 obtained higher AUC scores for total score (AUC=0.80) and final risk judgment (AUC=0.83) than comparable results for Static-99 (AUC=0.71).

Rettenberger et al. (2011) examined the predictive accuracy and psychometric properties of the SVR-20 in a sample of 493 male sexual offenders assessed between 2001 and 2007 at the Federal Evaluation Centre for Violent and Sexual Offenders (FECVSO) in the Austrian prison system. Sexual reconviction data was examined over a 3- and 5-year period. In measuring predictive accuracy of the scale, Rettenberger et al. (2011) reported encouraging results for the total sample (AUC=0.72) as well as for the rapist subgroup ($n=221$, AUC=0.71) and the child molester subsample ($n=249$, AUC=0.77). Of the three subscales, the Psychosocial Adjustment scale produced the most promising results significantly predicting general sexual recidivism (AUC=0.67) for the entire sample.

Adaptations to the SVR-20 have been made in order to make the scale more relevant to sexual offenders with intellectual disabilities (Boer, Frize, Pappas, Morrissey, & Lindsay, 2010), although these have yet to be empirically validated. Furthermore, the SVR-20 is currently under revision (Boer, Hart, Kropp, & Webster, 2015). The revised SVR-20 (second edition) follows a clear multidimensional focus, all items having both dynamic and static features and all items having variable components (i.e., a continuum exists within items and issues where items interact to produce the complexities we see in the individual case—with some examples within and between items). A convergent approach is recommended—using an appropriate actuarial baseline to provide an anchor for structured clinical evaluation (Boer, 2006; Singer, Boer, & Rettenberger, 2013). Many of the original 20 items remain the same than in the first version although some items have changed or been replaced, allowing for the inclusion of new items. As Boer (2010) noted, given the existing research base for the original SVR-20, to change the scale beyond recognition would invalidate much of the research base. In the Psychosocial Adjustment section, new items "sexual health problems" and "past nonsexual offending" have been included, the latter replacing "past nonsexual violent" and "past nonviolent offenses." The item "past supervision failure" has been moved to the Future Plans section and renamed. In describing the changes to the Psychosocial Adjustment section, Boer (2010) argued it is common for "sexual health problems" to decrease risk and it is also common that sexual desire and ability decrease with age. Thus, this item measures *normal* decreases in risk with aging for all individuals. There are also some individuals who have sexual health disorders that increase their risk if a sexual assault occurs, e.g., HIV. HIV+ persons are not at any greater risk to offend than anyone else, but if an HIV+ person does sexually offend, the victim may be lethally affected. Boer (2010) argued there are some unique cases in which older individuals offend in nonsexual ways due to impotence and there are some individuals who actually do not start offending until they are much older. Within the Sexual Offenses section, a new item "diversity of sexual offending" replaces "multiple offense types," "actual or threatened physical harm to victim" replaces "physical harm to victim(s)," and "psychological coercion in sexual offenses" replaces "use of weapons of threats of death." It is argued that persons who have committed multiple types (as determined by differing victim characteristics and varying in nature) of sexual offenses are at increased risk for sexual recidivism. This is a risk factor that likely reflects the presence of sexual deviation and attitudes that support or condone sexual violence. Psychological coercion refers to coercive tactics ranging from grooming of victims through the use of gifts or additional privileges for a victim to threats of family separation or abandonment—all of which serve to provide the offender with victim access while protecting the offender's behavior from discovery. Boer (2010) noted this item is supported more by the clinical treatment literature than from the meta-analyses per se. This is a risk factor that likely reflects the presence of sexual deviation (e.g., sadism) and attitudes that support or condone sexual violence. The Future Plans section includes three items (instead of two in the 1997 version). As well as continuing to have "realistic future plans" and "negative attitudes toward intervention," a new item, "negative attitudes toward supervision," has been added. It is argued that noncompliance with supervision is related to recidivism of a general, violent, and sexually violent nature, and persons who reject or do not comply with supervision are at increased risk for criminality and violence. Such attitudes may be related to future sexual violence by resulting in inadequate professional support, leading to increasing sexual deviance, increased distress, or increased risk for exposure to destabilizing influences such as drugs, alcohol, or potential victims. The scoring system has also altered to reflect changes (reductions, no change or increases) in a risk-relevant item over a specified period of time.

Risk for Sexual Violence Protocol (RSVP)

The RSVP (Hart et al., 2003) can be seen as a variation and evolution of earlier SPJ guidelines. Like the SVR-20, the RSVP does not employ actuarial or statistical methods to support decision making about risk. Rather, it offers a set of guidelines for collecting relevant information and making structured risk formulations. The RSVP is an evolved form of the SVR-20 and is based on a rejection of actuarial approaches to the assessment of risk of sexual violence. Similar to the SVR-20, the RSVP identifies the potential risk factors (presence) and makes a determination of their importance to future offending (relevance). However, in addition to the SVR-20, the RSVP provides explicit guidelines for risk formulation, such as risk scenarios and management strategies.

The RSVP assumes that risk must be defined in the context in which it occurs and regards the primary risk decision as preventative and considers steps which are required to minimize any risks posed by the individual. The RSVP is a 22-item protocol divided into five domains including sexual violence history, psychological adjustment, mental disorder, social adjustment, and manageability. The RSVP should not be used to determine whether someone committed (an) act(s) of sexual violence in the past, and it does not provide an estimate of specific likelihood or probability that someone will commit acts of sexual violence in the future. The authors suggest that the RSVP is designed to highlight information relating to clinical problems rather than producing an overall risk score. Information is structured in a number of steps: case information, presence of risk factors, relevance of risk factors, risk scenarios (possible futures), risk management strategies, and summary judgments. Until now, there has been little cross-validated research reporting on the predictive accuracy or psychometric properties of the RSVP.

Conclusions

Since the early days of unstructured clinical intuition, the field of risk assessment and the subsequent development of ARAIs for estimating sexual recidivism risk have changed beyond recognition. Following the work of Meehl (1954) and others, the development of mechanical tools to predict outcome events has consistently demonstrated superiority over unstructured clinical intuition. Advances in meta-analytical technologies have led to highly structured and defined ARAIs consisting of factors positively associated with sexual recidivism risk and based on experience tables, from which probabilistic estimates of risk can be derived (Hanson & Morton-Bourgon, 2009). While these measures continue to outperform clinical judgment, they are criticized for failing to adequately explain the risk presented by an individual. Addressing these limitations, clinicians and researchers are looking to third-generation risk assessments. Many third-generation risk assessment frameworks begin with an actuarial estimation of risk followed by a more detailed assessment of criminogenic factors or psychological vulnerabilities (Hanson et al., 2007; Mann, Hanson, & Thornton, 2010; Ward & Beech, 2004), which better target resources and interventions to those who need it, in keeping with the RNR principles of offender rehabilitation. These frameworks (SARNR and Stable-/Acute-2007) are, at present, the best efforts in structuring dynamic risk-related information in a way that both targets treatment need as well as identifies risk scenarios. It is insufficient to simply estimate a level of risk using ARAIs without considering changing dynamic factors, conditions, and events (acute risk) in which the individual's risk is elevated. For practitioners in the field, this is community case management.

A promising area of research will be the development and validation of fourth-generation measures, such as the Level of Service/Case Management Inventory (LS/CMI; Andrews et al., 2004). However, until such time as fourth-generation measures demonstrate predictive validity over and above second-generation measures, ARAIs are, at the present time, the most accurate in estimating sexual recidivism risk in sexual offenders. Combining the use of ARAIs, accompanied with third-generation assessment framworks, as part of a convergent approach (using a variety of tests that "converge" on the issue at hand; see Boer, 2006; Singer et al., 2013) will likely aid in identifying and targeting treatment need, risk assessment and case management.

References

Allan, A., Dawson, D., & Allan, M. M. (2006). Prediction of the risk of male sexual reoffending in Australia. *Australian Psychologist, 41*, 60–68. doi:10.1080/00050060500391886.

Andrews, D. A., & Bonta, J. (2006). *The psychology of criminal conduct* (4th ed.). Cincinnati, OH: Anderson.

Andrews, D. A., Bonta, J., & Wormith, S. J. (2004). *The level of service/case management inventory (LS/CMI)*. Toronto, ON: Multi-Health Systems.

Andrews, D. A., Bonta, J., & Wormith, S. J. (2006). The recent past and near future of risk and/or need assessment. *Crime and Delinquency, 52*, 7–27. doi:10.1177/0011128705281756.

Baltieri, D. A., & de Andrade, A. G. (2008). Comparing serial and nonserial sexual offenders: Alcohol and street drug consumption, impulsiveness and history of sexual abuse. *Revista Brasileira de Psiquiatria, 30*, 25–31. doi:10.1590/S1516-44462006005000067.

Barbaree, H. E. (1997). Evaluating treatment efficacy with sexual offenders: The insensitivity of recidivism studies to treatment effects. *Sexual Abuse, 9*, 111–128.

Barbaree, H. E., Langton, C. M., Blanchard, R., & Boer, D. P. (2008). Predicting recidivism in sex offenders using the SVR-20: The contribution of age-at-release. *International Journal of Forensic Mental Health, 7*, 47–64.

Barbaree, H., Langton, C. M., Andres Gopnik-Lewinski, A., & Beach, C. A. (2013). Risk assessment of sex offenders. In H. Bloom & R. D. Schneider (Eds.), *Law and mental disorder: A comprehensive and practical approach*. Toronto, ON: Irwin Law Inc.

Beech, A. R., Fisher, D., & Beckett, R. (1999). Step 3: *An Evaluation of the prison sex offenders treatment program*. London: HMSO. UK. Home Office Occasional Report. Home Office Publications Unit, 50, Queen Anne's Gate, London, SW1 9AT, England. Retrieved April 10, 2005, from www.homeoffice.gov.uk/rds/pdfs/occ-step3.pdf.

Bengtson, S. (2008). Is new better? A cross-validation of the Static-2002 and the Risk Matrix 2000 in a Danish sample of sexual offenders. *Psychology, Crime & Law, 14*, 85–106.

Boer, D. P., Frize, M., Pappas, R., Morrissey, C., & Lindsay, W. R. (2010). Suggested adaptations to the SVR-20 for offenders with intellectual disabilities. In L. A. Craig, W. R. Lindsay, & K. D. Browne (Eds.), *Assessment and treatment of sexual offenders with intellectual disabilities: A handbook* (pp. 177–192). Chichester: Wiley-Blackwell.

Boer, D. P., & Hart, S. D. (2009). Sex offender risk assessment: Research, evaluation, "best-practice" recommendations and future directions. In J. L. Ireland, C. A. Ireland, & P. Birch (Eds.), *Violent and sexual offenders. Assessment, treatment and management* (pp. 27–42). Cullompton, UK: Willan Publishing.

Boer, D. P., Hart, S. D., Kropp, P. R., & Webster, C. D. (1997). *Manual for the sexual violence risk-20: Professional guidelines for assessing risk of sexual violence*. Vancouver, Canada: The Mental Health, Law and Policy Institute.

Boer, D. P., Hart, S. D., Kropp, P. R., & Webster, C. D. (2015). *Sexual violence risk-20, Version 2*. Burnaby, Canada: Mental Health, Law, & Policy Institute, Simon Fraser University.

Bonger, W. A. (1936). *Introduction to Criminology, tr.* London: E. Van Loo.

Bonta, J., & Andrews, D. A. (2007). *Risk-need-responsivity model for offender assessment and rehabilitation (User Report 2007–06)*. Ottawa, ON: Public Safety Canada.

Briken, P., & Müller, J. L. (2014). Beurteilung der Schuldfähigkeit bei paraphiler Störung. Kann der Schweregrad der Störung mithilfe von Kriterien aus Prognoseinstrumenten erfasst werden? [Assessment of criminal responsibility in paraphilic disorder. Can the severity of the disorder be assessed with items of standardized prognostic instruments?]. *Nervenarzt, 85*, 304–311. doi:10.1007/s00115-013-3901-x.

Burgess, E. W. (1928). Factors determining success or failure on parole. In A. A. Bruce (Ed.), *The workings of the indeterminate sentence law and the parole system in Illinois*. Springfield, MA: Illinois State Board of Parole.

Covington, J. R. (1997). Preventive detention for sex offenders. *Illinois Bar Journal, 85*, 493–498.

Craig, L. A., & Beech, A. R. (2010). Towards a best practice in conducting actuarial risk assessments with adult sexual offenders. *Aggression and Violet Behavior, 15*, 278–293.

Craig, L. A., Beech, A. R., & Browne, K. D. (2006a). Cross validation of the risk matrix 2000 sexual and violent scales. *Journal of Interpersonal Violence, 21*(5), 1–22.

Craig, L. A., Beech, A. R., & Browne, K. D. (2006b). Evaluating the predictive accuracy of sex offender risk assessment measures on UK a samples: A cross-validation of the risk matrix 2000 scales. *Sex offender treatment, 1,* 1–16. Retrieved from http://www.sexual-offender-treatment. org/14.0.html

Craig, L. A., Browne, K. D., Stringer, I., & Beech, A. (2004). Limitations in actuarial risk assessment of sexual offenders: A methodological note. *The British Journal of Forensic Practice, 6,* 16–32.

Craig, L. A., Browne, K. D., & Beech, A. R. (2008). *Assessing risk in sex offenders: A practitioner's guide.* Hoboken, NJ: John Wiley & Son.

Craig, L. A., Dixon, L., & Gannon, T. A. (2013). *What works in offender rehabilitation: An evidenced based approach to assessment and treatment.* Wiley-Blackwell: Chichester.

Craig, L. A., Thornton, D., Beech, A., & Browne, K. D. (2007). The relationship of statistical and psychological risk markers to sexual reconviction in child molesters. *Criminal Justice & Behavior, 34*(3), 314–329.

Dawes, R. M., Faust, D., & Meehl, P. E. (1989). Clinical versus actuarial judgment. *Science, 243*(4899), 1668–1674.

de Vogel, V., de Ruiter, C., van Beek, D., & Mead, G. (2004). Predictive validity of the SVR-20 and Static-99 in a Dutch sample of treated sex offenders. *Law and Human Behavior, 28,* 235–251.

Doren, D. M. (2002). *Evaluating sex offenders: A manual for civil commitments and beyond.* Thousand Oaks, CA: Sage Publications Inc.

Ducro, C., & Pham, T. (2006). Evaluation of the SORAG and the Static-99 on Belgian sex offenders committed to a forensic facility. *Sexual Abuse: A Journal of Research and Treatment, 18,* 15–26. doi:10.1177/107906320601800102.

East, N. (1949). *Society and the criminal.* London: H.M.S.O.

East, W. N., & Hubert, W. H. (1939). *Psychological treatment of crime.* HMSO, London.

Eher, R., Matthes, A., Schilling, F., Haubner-MacLean, T., & Rettenberger, M. (2012). Dynamic risk assessment in sexual offenders using STABLE-2000 and the STABLE-2007: An investigation of predictive and incremental validity. *Sexual Abuse: A Journal of Research and Treatment, 24,* 5–28. doi:10.1177/1079063211403164.

Eher, R., Rettenberger, M., Gaunersdorfer, K., Haubner-MacLean, T., Matthes, A., Schilling, F., & Mokros, A. (2013). Über die Treffsicherheit der standardisierten Risikoeinschätzungsverahren Static-99 und Stable-2007 bei aus einer Sicherungsmaßnahme entlassenen Sexualstraftätern [On the accuracy of the standardized risk assessment procedures Static-99 and Stable-2007 for sexual offenders released from detention]. *Forensische Psychiatrie, Psychologie, Kriminologie, 7,* 264–272. doi: 10.1007/s11757-013-0212-9

Ericson, R. V., & Haggerty, K. D. (1997). *Policing the risk society.* Toronto, ON: University of Toronto Press.

Ernits, V. (1922). *Rev internat contre l'alcoolisme, 4,* 178.

Falshaw, L. (2002). *Assessing reconviction, re-offending and recidivism in a sample of UK sexual offenders.* Paper presented at the eleventh annual conference of the division of forensic psychology, Manchester, April 2002.

Firestone, P., Bradford, J. M., McCoy, M., Greenberg, D. M., Larose, M. R., & Curry, S. (1999). Prediction of recidivism in incest offenders. *Journal of Interpersonal Violence, 14,* 511–531.

Glueck, S., & Glueck, E. (1930). *500 criminal careers.* Philadelphia, PA: Alfred A Knopf Press.

Grove, W. M. (2005). Clinical versus statistical prediction: The contribution of Paul E. Meehl. *Journal of Clinical Psychology, 61*(10), 1233–1243.

Gore, K. S. (2007). Adjusted actuarial assessment of sex offenders: The impact of clinical overrides on predictive accuracy. *Dissertation Abstracts International, 68*(07), 4824B. UMI No. 3274898.

Grove, W. M., & Meehl, P. E. (1996). Comparative efficiency of informal (subjective, impressionistic) and formal (mechanical, algorithmic) prediction procedures: The clinical-statistical controversy. *Psychology, Public Policy, and Law, 2,* 293–323. doi:10.1037/1076-8971.2.2.293.

Grove, W. M., & Lloyd, M. (2006). Meehl's contribution to clinical versus statistical prediction. *Journal of Abnormal Psychology, 115*, 192–194.

Grubin, D. (1998). Sex offending against children: Understanding the risk. *Home Office Research Development and Statistics Directorate Research Findings, Police Research Series,* Paper 99.

Haag, A. M. (2005). Do psychological interventions impact on actuarial measures: An analysis of the predictive validity of the Static-99 and Static-2002 on a re-conviction measure of sexual recidivism. *Dissertation Abstracts International, 66*(08), 4531B. UMI No. NR05662.

Hannah-Moffat, K., & Shaw, M. (2001). *Taking risks: Incorporating gender and culture into the classification and assessment of federally sentenced women in Canada.* Ottawa, ON: Status of Women Canada.

Hanson, R. K. (1997a). *The development of a brief actuarial risk scale for sexual offense recidivism (User Report No. 1997-04).* Ottawa, ON: Department of the Solicitor General of Canada.

Hanson, R. K. (1997b). *The development of a brief actuarial risk scale for sexual offense recidivism (User Report No. 1997-04).* Ottawa, ON: Department of the Solicitor General of Canada.

Hanson, R. K. (2001) *Age and sexual recidivism: A comparison of rapists and child molesters.* (Cat No.: JS42-96/2001). Department of the Solicitor General of Canada. http://www.sgc.gc.ca/EPub/Corr/eAge200101/eAge200101.htm

Hanson, R. K. (2007, March). *How should risk assessments for sexual offenders be conducted?* Paper presented at the Fourth Annual Forensic Psychiatry Conference, Victoria, British Columbia, Canada.

Hanson, R. K., & Harris, A. J. R. (2001). A structured approach to evaluating change among sexual offenders. *Sexual Abuse, 13*, 105–122.

Hanson, R. K., Bourgon, G., Helmus, L., & Hodgson, S. (2009). The principles of effective correctional treatment also apply to sexual offenders: A meta-analysis. *Criminal Justice and Behavior, 36*, 865–891. doi:10.1177/0093854809338545.

Hanson, R. K., & Bussière, M. T. (1998). Predicting relapse: A meta-analysis of sexual offender recidivism studies. *Journal of Consulting and Clinical Psychology, 66*, 348–362.

Hanson, R. K., & Harris, A. J. R. (2000). Where should we intervene? Dynamic predictors of sexual offence recidivism. *Criminal Justice and Behavior, 27*, 6–35. doi:10.1177/0093854800027001002.

Hanson, R. K., Harris, A. J. R., Scott, T. L., & Helmus, L. (2007). *Assessing the risk of sexual offenders on community supervision: The Dynamic Supervision Project (Corrections research user report 2007-05).* Ottawa, ON: Public Safety Canada. Retrieved from http://www.public-safety.gc.ca/res/cor/rep/_fl/crp2007-05-en.pdf.

Hanson, R. K., & Morton-Bourgon, K. (2005). *Predictors of sexual recidivism: An updated meta-analysis* (Corrections Research, Public Safety and Emergency Preparedness Canada, Ottawa, Canada). Retrieved April 6, 2005, from http://www .psepc-sppcc.gc.ca/publications/corrections/pdf/200402_e.pdf

Hanson, R. K., & Morton-Bourgon, K. (2007). *The accuracy of recidivism risk assessment for sexual offenders: A meta-analysis (Corrections Research User Report No. 2007-01).* Ottawa, ON: Public Safety Canada.

Hanson, R. K., & Morton-Bourgon, K. (2009). The accuracy of recidivism risk assessments for sexual offenders: A meta-analysis of 118 prediction studies. *Psychological Assessment, 21*, 1–21. doi:10.1037/a0014421.

Hanson, R. K., & Scott, H. (1995). Assessing perspective-taking among sexual offenders, non-sexual criminal and non-offenders. *Sexual Abuse: A Journal of Research and Treatment, 7*, 259–277.

Hanson, R. K., & Thornton, D. (2000). Improving risk assessment for sex offenders: A comparison of three actuarial scales. *Law and Human Behavior, 24*, 119–136. doi:10.1023/A:1005482921333.

Hare, R. (1991). *Manual for the psychopathy checklist-revised (PCL-R).* Toronto, ON: MultiHealth Systems, Inc.

Hart, H. (1924). Predicting parole success. *Journal of Criminal Law and Criminology, 1*, 405–414.

Harris, A. J. R., & Hanson, R. K. (2010). Clinical, actuarial, and dynamic risk assessment of sexual offenders: Why do things keep changing? *Journal of Sexual Aggression, 16*, 296–310. doi:10.1080/13552600.2010.494772..

Harris, G. T., & Rice, M. E. (2003). Actuarial assessment of risk among sex offenders. In R. A. Prentky, E. S. Janus, & M. C. Seto (Eds.), *Sexually coercive behavior: Understanding and management* (Vol. 989, pp. 198–210). New York, NY: New York Academy of Sciences.

Hart, S. D., Kropp, P. R., Laws, D. R., Klaver, J., Logan, C., & Watt, K. A. (2003). *The risk for sexual violence protocol (RSVP): Structured professional guidelines for assessing risk of sexual violence*. Burnaby: Mental Health, Law, and Policy Institute, Simon Fraser University.

Hart, S., Laws, D. R., & Kropp, P. R. (2003). The promise and the peril of sex offender risk assessment. In T. Ward, D. R. Laws, & S. M. Hudson (Eds.), *Sexual deviance: Issues and controversies* (pp. 207–225). Thousand Oaks, CA: Sage Publications.

Hood, R., Shute, S., Feilzer, M., & Wilcox, A. (2002). Sex offenders emerging from long-term imprisonment—A study of their long-term reconviction rates and of parole board members' judgements of their risk. *British Journal of Criminology, 42*(2), 371–394.

Hooton, E. A. (1939). *The American criminal. An anthropological study. vol. 1. The native criminal of native parentage*. Cambridge, MA: Harvard University Press.

Janus, E. A., & Meehl, P. E. (1997). Assessing the legal standard for predictions of dangerousness in sex offender commitment proceedings. *Psychology, Public Policy and Law, 3*, 33–64.

Kingston, D. A., Yates, P. M., Firestone, P., Babchishin, K., & Bradford, J. (2008). Long term predictive validity of the Risk Matrix 2000: A comparison with the Static-99 and the Sex Offender Risk Appraisal Guide. *Sexual Abuse: A Journal of Research and Treatment, 20*, 466–484. doi:10.1177/1079063208325206.

Koehler, J. J. (1996). The base rate fallacy reconsidered. Descriptive, normative, and methodological challenges. *Behavioral and Brain Sciences, 19*, 1–17.

Langton, C. M., Barbaree, H. E., Harkins, L., & Peacock, E. J. (2006). Sexual offenders' response to treatment and its association with recidivism as a function of psychopathy. *Sexual Abuse, 18*, 99–120.

Langton, C. M., Barbaree, H. E., Seto, M. C., Peacock, E. J., Harkins, L., & Hansen, K. T. (2007). Actuarial assessment of risk for reoffense among adult sex offenders: Evaluating the predictive accuracy of the Static-2002 and five other instruments. *Criminal Justice and Behavior, 34*, 37–59.

Laws, D. R., & Ward, T. (2010). *Desistance from Sex offending: Alternatives to throwing away the keys*. New York City: Guilford Press. Desistance from sexual offending.

Malamuth, N. M., & Brown, L. M. (1994). Sexually aggressive men's perception of women's communication: Testing three explanations. *Journal of Personality and Social Psychology, 67*, 699–712.

Mann, R. E., Hanson, R. K., & Thornton, D. (2010). Assessing risk for sexual recidivism: Some proposals on the nature of psychologically meaningful risk factors. *Sexual Abuse: A Journal of Research and Treatment, 22*, 191–217. doi:10.1177/1079063210366039.

Meehl, P. E. (1954). *Clinical versus statistical prediction: A theoretical analysis and a review of the evidence*. Minneapolis, MN: University of Minnesota Press.

Meehl, P. E., & Rosen, A. (1955). Antecedent probability and the efficiency of psychometric signs, patterns or cutting scores. *Psychological Bulletin., 52*, 194–216.

Miller, H. A., Amenta, A., & Conroy, M. (2005). Sexually violent predator evaluations: Empirical evidence, strategies for professionals, and research directions. *Law and Human Behavior, 29*, 29–54.

National Parole Board, (2004). *Evaluation report for the national parole board's effective corrections and citizen engagement initiatives 2000–2003*. Retrieved electronically on 30th October 2008. Retrieved from: http://www.npbcnlc.gc.ca/rprts/pdf/ecce_2000_2003/ecce_2000_2003_e.pdf

Nunes, K. L., & Babchishin, K. M. (2012). Construct validity of stable-2000 and stable-2007. *Sexual Abuse: A Journal of Research and Treatment, 24*, 29–45. doi:10.1177/1079063211404921.

Phenix, A., Doren, D., Helmus, L., Hanson, R. K., & Thornton, D. (2008). *Coding rules for Static-2002*. Retrieved June 2015, from http://www.static99.org/pdfdocs/static2002codingrules.pdf

Pithers, W. D., Kashima, K. M., Cumming, G. F., & Beal, L. S. (1988). Relapse prevention: A method of enhancing maintenance of change in sex offenders. In A. C. Salter (Ed.), *Treating child sex offenders and victims: A practical guide* (pp. 131–170). Newbury Park, CA: Sage.

Prentky, R. A., & Burgess, A. W. (2000). *Forensic management of sexual offenders: Perspectives in sexuality, behavior, research and therapy*. New York, NY: Kluwer Academic/Plenum Publishers.

Prentky, R. A., & Knight, R. A. (1991). Identifying critical dimensions for discriminating among rapists. *Journal of Consulting and Clinical Psychology, 59*, 643–661.

Prentky, R. A., Lee, A. F. S., Knight, R. A., & Cerce, O. (1997). Recidivism rates among child molesters and rapists: A methodological analysis. *Law and Human Behaviour, 21*(6), 635–659.

Proulx, J., Pellerin, B., McKibben, A., Aubut, J., & Ouimet, M. (1999). Recidivism in sexual aggressors: Static and dynamic predictors of recidivism in sexual aggressors. *Sexual Abuse: A Journal of Research and Treatment, 11*, 117–129.

Quinsey, V. L., Harris, G. T., Rice, M. E., & Cormier, C. A. (1998). *Violent offenders: Appraising and managing risk*. Washington, DC: American Psychology Association.

Quinsey, V. L., Harris, G. T., Rice, M. E., & Cormier, C. (2006). *Violent offenders: Appraising and managing risk* (2nd ed.). Washington, DC: American Psychological Association.

Rettenberger, M., Boer, D. P., & Eher, R. (2011). The predictive accuracy of risk factors in the Sexual Violence Risk-20 (SVR-20). *Criminal Justice and Behavior, 38*, 1009–1027. doi:10.1177/0093854811416908.

Rettenberger, M., Matthes, A., Boer, D. P., & Eher, R. (2010). Actuarial recidivism risk assessment and sexual delinquency: A comparison of five risk assessment tools in different sexual offender subtypes. *International Journal of Offender Therapy and Comparative Criminology, 54*, 169–186. doi:10.1177/0306624X08328755.

Rice, M. E., & Harris, G. T. (1997). Cross-validation and extension of the violence risk appraisal guide for child molesters and rapists. *Law and Human Behavior, 21*, 231–241.

Sarbin, T. R. (1942). A contribution to the study of actuarial and individual methods of prediction. *The American Journal of Sociology, 48*, 593–602.

Sarbin, T. R. (1944). The logic of prediction in psychology. *Psychological Review, 51*, 210–228.

Sawyer, J. (1966). Measurement and prediction: Clinical and statistical. *Psychological Bulletin, 66*, 178–200. doi:10.1037/h0023624.

Singer, J. C., Boer, D. P., & Rettenberger, M. (2013). A convergent approach to sex offender risk assessment. In K. Harrison & B. Rainey (Eds.), *The Wiley-Blackwell handbook of legal and ethical aspects of Sex offender treatment and management* (pp. 341–355). New York, NY: Wiley.

Sjöstedt, G., & Långström, N. (2002). Assessment of risk for criminal recidivism among rapists: A comparison of four different measures. *Psychology Crime and Law, 8*, 25–40.

Skelton, A., Riley, D., Wales, D., & Vess, J. (2006). Assessing risk for sexual offenders in New Zealand: Development and validation of a computer-scored risk measure. *Journal of Sexual Aggression, 12*, 277–286.

Stadtland, C., Hollweg, M., Kleindienst, N., Dietl, J., Reich, U., & Nedopil, N. (2005). Risk assessment and prediction of violent and sexual recidivism in sex offenders: Long-term predictive validity of four risk assessment instruments. *Journal of Forensic Psychiatry and Psychology, 16*, 92–108.

Szmukler, G. (2001). Violence risk prediction in practice. *British Journal of Psychiatry, 178*, 84–85.

Thornton, D. (2002). Constructing and testing a framework for dynamic risk assessment. *Sexual Abuse: A Journal of Research and Treatment, 14*, 139–153. doi:10.1177/107906320201400205.

Thornton, D., & Beech, A. R. (2002). Integrating statistical and psychological factors through the structured risk assessment model. *Paper presented at the 21st annual research and treatment conference, Association of the Treatment of Sexual Abusers*, 2–5 Oct, Montreal, Canada.

Thornton, D., Mann, R., Webster, S., Blud, L., Travers, R., Friendship, C., & Erikson, M. (2003). Distinguishing and combining risks for sexual and violent recidivism. In R. A. Prentky, E. S. Janus, & M. C. Seto (Eds.), *Sexually coercive behavior: Understanding and management* (Vol. 989, pp. 225–235). New York: New York Academy of Sciences.

Tully, R. J., Browne, K. D., & Craig, L. A. (2015). An examination of the predictive validity of the structured assessment of risk and need– treatment needs analysis (SARN-TNA) in England and Wales. *Criminal Justice and Behavior, 42*(5), 509–528.

Vrana, G. C., Sroga, M., & Guzzo, L. (2008). *Predictive validity of the LSI–OR among a sample of adult male sexual assaulters.* North Bay, ON: Nipissing University. Unpublished manuscript.

Wakeling, H., Beech, A. R., & Freemantle, N. (2013). Investigating treatment change and its relationship to recidivism in a sample of 3773 sex offenders in the UK. *Psychology Crime and Law, 19*(3), 233–252.

Ward, T. (2002). Good lives and the rehabilitation of offenders: Promises and problems. *Aggression and Violent Behavior, 7*, 513–528.

Ward, T., & Beech, A. R. (2004). The etiology of risk: A preliminary model. *Sexual Abuse: A Journal of Research and Treatment, 16*, 271–284.

Ward, T., & Maruna, S. (2007). *Rehabilitation: Beyond the risk assessment paradigm.* London, UK: Routledge Peterson & Co.

Ward, T., Hudson, S. M., & Keenan, T. (1998). A self-regulation model of the sexual offense process. *Sexual Abuse: A Journal of Research and Treatment, 10*, 141–157.

Ward, T., Louden, K., Hudson, S. M., & Marshall, W. L. (1995). A descriptive model of the offense chain for child molesters. *Journal of Interpersonal Violence, 10*, 452–472.

Ward, T., Mesler, J., & Yates, P. (2007). Reconstructing the risk-need-responsivity model: A theoretical elaboration and evaluation. *Aggression and Violent Behavior, 12*, 208–228. doi:10.1016/j.avb.2006.07.001.

Warner, S. B. (1923). Factors determining parole from the Massachusetts Reformatory. *Journal of Criminal Law and Criminology, 14*(2), 172–207.

Webster, S. D., Mann, R. E., Carter, A. J., Long, J., Milner, R. J., O'Brein, M. D., et al. (2006). Inter-rater reliability of dynamic risk assessment with sexual offenders. *Psychology Crime and Law, 12*, 439–452.

Wittman, M. P., & Steinberg, L. (1944). Follow-up of an objective evaluation of prognosis in dementia praecox and manic-repressive psychoses. *Elgin Papers, 5*, 216–227.

Wong, S. C. P., Olver, M. E., Nicholaichuk, T. P., & Gordon, A. (2003). *The violence risk scale: Sexual offender version (VRS-SO).* Saskatoon: Regional Psychiatric Centre and University of Saskatchewan, Saskatoon, Saskatchewan, Canada.

Wormith, S. J., Hogg, S., & Guzzo, L. (2012). The predictive validity of a general risk/needs assessment inventory on sexual offender recidivism and an exploration of the professional override. *Criminal Justice and Behavior, 39*, 1511–1538. doi:10.1177/0093854812455741.

Chapter 3
Strengths of Actuarial Risk Assessment

Robert J.B. Lehmann, Yolanda Fernandez, and Leslie-Maaike Helmus

Forensic assessment done well is a comprehensive process of obtaining information from diverse sources and creating an integrated conceptualization of the information in order to understand the client, inform decision makers, provide appropriate intervention, and manage future risk. This task is an important part of many legal decisions (e.g., civil commitment evaluations, end of sentence evaluations, and allocation of treatment) as the potential danger to society of individuals who are already known to have committed a violent offense constitutes a major concern for courts and forensic practitioners. A critical part of the process is risk assessment, which involves combining multiple risk factors together into an overall assessment of the likelihood of an outcome, such as recidivism (Hanson & Morton-Bourgon, 2009). Risk assessment and risk measures have evolved considerably over the last decades (e.g., Hanson, 2005; Harris & Hanson, 2010; Mann, Hanson, & Thornton, 2010) and distinct approaches to and generations of risk assessment can be differentiated (Andrews & Bonta, 2010; Bonta, 1996; Heilbrun, 1997).

Heilbrun (1997) argues that there are at least two models of risk assessment: the prediction and the management model. The prediction model focuses on maximizing the accuracy of the prediction of the outcome—in this model, it does not matter why something predicts the outcome, just that it does. The management model aims

R.J.B. Lehmann (✉)
Institute of Forensic Psychiatry, Charité University Medicine Berlin,
Oranienburger Straße 285, Berlin 13437, Germany
e-mail: R.Lehmann@charite.de

Y. Fernandez, C.Psych.
Correctional Service Canada|Service Correctionnel Canada, Regional Headquarters
(Ont)|Bureau Régional (Ont), Kingston, ON, Canada K7L 4Y8
e-mail: yolanda.fernandez@csc-scc.gc.ca

L.-M. Helmus
Forensic Assessment Group, 11 Aspen Grove, Nepean, Ottawa, ON, Canada
e-mail: Lmaaikehelmus@gmail.com

© Springer International Publishing Switzerland 2016
D.R. Laws, W. O'Donohue (eds.), *Treatment of Sex Offenders*,
DOI 10.1007/978-3-319-25868-3_3

at reducing the risk of the occurrence of a specified event's outcome (e.g., sexual recidivism). In contrast, Bonta (1996) has provided a similar but more nuanced characterization of the development of risk assessment in three generations. The first generation consists of unstructured clinical judgment (UCJ), where a clinician gathers information and forms a subjective risk assessment. The weaknesses of this method are its overreliance on personal discretion and its lack of accountability and replicability (Bonta, 1996).

The second generation of risk assessment relies on instruments that combine primarily static (i.e., historical and unchanging), empirically derived risk factors (Bonta, 1996). In these instruments (commonly referred to as actuarial), items are often scored with either a 0–1 dichotomy (absent-present) or with a specified weighting determined by the strength of the item's relationship to recidivism. The weakness in this generation is that the focus on static factors is assumed to preclude identification of areas to target in treatment to reduce risk and it cannot reflect positive changes (Bonta, 1996).

The third generation evolved from the second to incorporate criminogenic needs (Bonta, 1996), which are dynamic (i.e., changeable) risk factors that, if changed, should alter the likelihood of reoffending (Andrews et al., 1990). Examples of key criminogenic needs (Andrews & Bonta, 2010) include antisocial personality (e.g., aggression, impulsivity) and antisocial attitudes (e.g., negative attitudes toward the criminal justice system, identification with criminals). Third-generation scales are therefore sensitive to offender changes and they also tend to have a stronger basis in theories of offending, as well as empirical evidence (Bonta, 1996). Similar to the second generation, these tools are typically actuarial. Recently, Andrews, Bonta, and Wormith (2006) have suggested that a fourth generation of risk assessment has emerged, which provides a comprehensive guide for human service delivery that spans from intake through to case closure.

In terms of understanding dynamic risk factors (i.e., third- and fourth-generation approaches), Hanson and Harris (2000) have articulated a further distinction between stable and acute dynamic factors. Stable factors constitute relatively enduring problems (e.g., alcoholism, personality disorders) and acute risk factors are rapidly changing features indicating imminent risk of reoffending (e.g., intoxication, emotional collapse). Whereas the strength of stable risk factors is monitoring risk over the medium to long term (e.g., treatment change), acute risk factors are intended for monitoring current risk over a high-risk period (e.g., community supervision).

One area not addressed by Bonta's (1996) description is the status of structured professional judgment (SPJ). SPJ is a method of risk assessment where explicit risk factors (often both static and dynamic) are scored, but the combination of these items into an overall evaluation of risk is left to the judgment of the clinician (Boer, Wilson, Gauthier, & Hart, 1997). Proponents of SPJ argue that clinical judgment should be incorporated in risk assessment because the statistical approach of actuarial scales is not always appropriate in individual cases (Webster, Douglas, Eaves, & Hart, 1997). SPJ therefore has the greatest amount of flexibility to respond to unique case-specific factors. Other researchers, however, have been dismissive of SPJ (Andrews & Bonta, 2010; Bonta, 2002; Quinsey, Harris, Rice, & Cormier,

2006) and classify it as a variation of the first generation of risk assessment (Andrews et al., 2006).

Hanson and Morton-Bourgon (2009) have added to the classification of risk assessment methods by applying a more stringent definition of actuarial scales. Their definition is based on Meehl's (1954) criteria that actuarial scales involve explicit rules to combine pre-specified items into total scores and empirically derived estimates of recidivism probability linked to each total score (Hanson & Morton-Bourgon, 2009). Given that several tools satisfying the first criteria of actuarial scales do not include absolute recidivism estimates, Hanson and Morton-Bourgon (2009) made a distinction between actuarial scales (using Meehl's definition) and mechanical scales. Mechanical scales typically contain factors identified based on theory or previous literature reviews, which are combined into a total score based on explicit item weightings, but do not contain a table with recidivism estimates per score. If SPJ scales are used to sum items to produce a total score, without creating a summary professional judgment, this would be using the SPJ scale as a mechanical scale.

The purpose of this chapter is to discuss the strengths of actuarial risk assessment. First, we will provide greater discussion of ways to conceptualize risk factors that may be included in risk scales (actuarial or other approaches). Then, we will discuss what types of information can be provided by actuarial risk scales, how the greater objectivity inherent in actuarial risk scales contributes to understanding important psychometrics of the risk assessment approaches, and how the predictive accuracy of actuarial scales compares to other approaches. These sections will be applicable to any type of offender risk assessment (i.e., any scale designed to predict an outcome among offenders). In the next section, the reader will be introduced to a small sampling of sexual offender risk scales. Sex offender risk scales are focused on because we have greater familiarity with them and they will serve as examples of the types of scales that could be used with other offender types. Then, results of surveys will be highlighted to illustrate what scales are being used in practice and how the information is being used. Lastly, the practical clinical power of actuarial risk assessment instruments in everyday practice will be discussed.

Conceptualizing Risk Factors: Psychologically Meaningful Risk Factors

As discussed above regarding the generations of risk assessment (Bonta, 1996), risk factors have often been classified as either static or dynamic (with dynamic factors further classified as stable or acute). The assumption has been that only dynamic risk factors can identify treatment targets or be used in risk management models. As an alternative to the static/dynamic conceptualization of risk factors, however, another approach is to focus on psychologically meaningful risk factors (Mann et al., 2010), also sometimes called risk-relevant propensities. In this model, risk factors are indicators of underlying constructs/propensities. For example, self-regulation problems may be an underlying psychological propensity related to recidivism.

Certain past and present behaviors, such as substance abuse, job instability, getting into fights, and poor problem-solving, may all be indicators of this propensity. In this model, the distinction between static and dynamic risk factors is simply a heuristic to describe indicators, rather than a fundamental difference between the risk-relevant constructs. For example, a history of car accidents (a static variable) and current substance abuse (a dynamic variable) may both be indicators of the same underlying propensity (poor self-regulation). In other words, psychologically meaningful risk factors can be measured using either static or dynamic risk factors.

Nonetheless, even though static and dynamic risk factors may measure the same constructs, there are practical advantages to distinguishing between them in risk assessment. Conceptually, it is easy to divide risk factors into those that the offender cannot change or manage (static) versus those he/she can (dynamic), with the latter being easier to incorporate into treatment planning (though this does not mean that static risk assessment cannot also inform risk management). Also, the types of information used to assess these risk factors are different. Static risk factors are often easy and reliably coded based on fairly straightforward criminal history information, as well as offender and victim demographics. Interviews with the offender may not be required, which makes these items practical for correctional systems that need to assess and manage large populations with limited resources. In comparison, dynamic risk factors are often more time-intensive to assess. Credible assessments should minimally include detailed reviews of file information (criminal history and personal/social history) and ideally an interview with the offender (e.g., Fernandez, Harris, Hanson, & Sparks, 2014). Other sources of information (e.g., specialized testing, collateral interviews) can also enhance dynamic assessment.

Complicating this distinction further is recent research and theoretical work that suggests the existence of *protective* factors (e.g., Farrington & Ttofi, 2011; Lösel & Farrington, 2012), which may reduce the risk of recidivism or interact with a risk factor to decrease its association with recidivism. Although the attempt to focus on offender strengths in assessment is admirable and would likely increase the comprehensiveness of the assessment and improve the therapeutic climate, Harris and Rice (2015) have argued that current descriptions of supposedly protective risk factors are mostly just the opposite end of risk factors and do not reflect new constructs. Consequently, the idea of risk-relevant propensities (Mann et al., 2010) implies that static, dynamic, and/or protective factors can be used to assess the same risk-relevant contructs, thereby informing risk management practices. Certainly, however, assessing *changes* in risk would require some consideration of dynamic risk factors.

Crime Scene Behaviors as Indicators of Risk-Relevant Propensities

One neglected area of research has been to use crime scene behaviors as indicators of risk-relevant constructs. Enduring risk-related individual offender propensities (e.g., hostility) may manifest themselves in concrete offense behavior (e.g., excessive humiliation, genital injury). Consequently, research trying to understand offender characteristics from crime scene behavior may be relevant to risk assessment.

Canter and Heritage were among the first researchers to classify sexual offenders on the basis of observable or directly inferred crime scene behavior alone. In essence, this task consists of analyzing largely observable behaviors with inferences made about the latent (or unobservable) dimensions and themes within the data. Loosely, this process is referred to as Behavioral Thematic Analysis (BTA), a cornerstone of investigative psychology (IP) research (Canter, 2004). BTA has been used as a predictive tool exploring the relationship between behavioral themes and stranger offender characteristics with notable success (e.g., Goodwill, Alison, & Beech, 2009; Häkkänen, Puolakka, & Santtila, 2004; Mokros, 2007; Santtila, Häkkänen, Canter, & Elfgren, 2003).

Studies employing BTA of stranger rape offense details have found the presence of five (Canter & Heritage, 1990), four (Alison & Stein, 2001; Canter, Bennell, Alison, & Reddy, 2003) or three (Canter, 1994; Häkkänen, Lindlöf, & Santtila, 2004) themes of offense behavior. Although the BTA of these previous studies differed in interpretation, it is argued, in line with Wilson and Leith (2001), that each was consistent in finding themes of hostility, criminality, and pseudo-intimacy. The hostility theme is characterized by expressive, non-strategic aggression beyond that necessary to commit the offense. Here, the offender wants to hurt the victim and may perform brutal (sadistic) sexual acts. In the criminality theme, the sexual assault is considered one among many antisocial behaviors the offender commits. Whereas for stranger rapists the pseudo-intimacy theme may represent deviant sexual fantasies involving the victim receiving intense pleasure during the offense and falling in love with the offender, for the acquaintance rapist this theme may represent the misperception of the victim's sexual intent. However, during the offense both offender types show behaviors frequently present in consensual relationships.

Similarly, studies employing BTA of child molestation offenses have found the presence of three (Canter, Hughes, & Kirby, 1998) or four (Bennell, Alison, Stein, Alison, & Canter, 2001) offense themes. Here, it is argued that these themes can be summarized as fixated (i.e., love, intimate), regressed (i.e., autonomy), aggression (i.e., hostility), and criminality (i.e., control, criminal-opportunist). The themes of criminality and aggression show considerable overlap with the offense behaviors of rapists. The theme of fixation describes offenders actively creating opportunities to offend by grooming potential victims with attention, affection, and gifts and actively seeking suitable targets. The theme of regression describes offenders motivated by non-paraphilic sexual excitation and victim availability, who could choose children as an alternative to age-appropriate partners.

However, the relevance of these behavioral themes as indicators of enduring offender propensities in the context of risk assessment has been previously neglected. Therefore, based on theoretical considerations (e.g., Ward, Polaschek, & Beech, 2005) and the discussed empirical evidence (e.g., Canter et al., 2003), Lehmann and colleagues developed precise and detailed conceptualizations of target propensities and their theoretical contexts to define crime scene behavior-based indicators of these constructs. In a first step Lehmann and colleagues were able to demonstrate the construct validity of the behavioral themes through correlational analyses with known sexual offending measures, criminal histories, offenders' motivation, and offense characteristics. For stranger rapists (Lehmann, Goodwill, Gallasch-Nemitz, Biedermann, & Dahle, 2013), the analyses revealed three behavioral offender propensities: sexuality, criminality, and hostility. Statistical analyses indicated that the behavioral theme of criminality significantly predicted sexual recidivism (AUC=0.64) and added incrementally to Static-99. For acquaintance rapists (Lehmann, Goodwill, Hanson, & Dahle, 2015), results indicated that the behavioral themes of hostility (AUC=0.66) and pseudo-intimacy (AUC=0.69) predicted sexual recidivism, with the latter adding incrementally to Static-99. For child molesters (Lehmann, Goodwill, Hanson, & Dahle, 2014), the behavioral themes of fixation on child victims (AUC=0.65) and (sexualized) aggression (AUC=0.59) significantly predicted sexual recidivism and added incrementally to Static-99. Recently, the predictive validity of the behavioral theme of fixation was cross validated with an independent sample (Pedneault, 2014). In sum, the results indicate that crime scene information can be used to assess risk-relevant constructs. Also, crime scene information seems to be relevant external information to the results of actuarial scales.

What Types of Information Can Actuarial Risk Scales Provide?

Risk assessment can include static, dynamic, protective, or crime scene behavior factors as indicators of risk-relevant propensities. Regardless of what types of risk factors are used, how they are combined, or how accurate the scale is, appropriately reporting risk assessment results make little difference if the decision makers do not understand the information, which is a serious possibility (e.g., Varela, Boccaccini, Cuervo, Murrie, & Clark, 2014). Consequently, there have been essential developments in actuarial risk assessment research regarding optimal ways to report and interpret risk assessment information in clinical practice (for a review, see Hilton, Scurich, and Helmus, 2015). Hence, an important advantage of actuarial risk assessment instruments is that they allow their scores to be linked to different types of empirically derived quantitative indicators of risk. In contrast, other approaches to risk assessment (e.g., SPJ) solely provide nominal risk categories (e.g., low, moderate, and high risk)[1] with research indicating that nominal risk categories are interpreted inconsistently by professionals (Hilton, Carter, Harris, & Sharpe, 2008; Monahan & Silver, 2003). Three important metrics for risk communication are percentile ranks, risk ratios, and absolute recidivism rates.

---

[1] The only exception we are aware of is that the Spousal Assault Risk Assessment guide (SARA) includes percentile distributions for the total scores and number of risk factors present, although not for the overall summary judgment (Kropp & Gibas, 2010).

Percentiles

Percentiles communicate information about how common or unusual a person's score is in comparison to a reference population (Crawford & Garthwaite, 2009). Percentiles have the advantage of being fairly easily defined and communicated and are consistent with the communication of many types of psychology tests, such as intelligence tests (for more information, see Hanson, Lloyd, Helmus, & Thornton, 2012). They are particularly helpful in decisions for resource allocation. For example, if a correctional service has sufficient resources to offer treatment to 15 % of their offenders, then all the information required by an offender risk assessment may be a percentile (e.g., the highest risk 15 % should be prioritized for treatment).

Disadvantages of this metric are that the information provided is norm-referenced (i.e., relative to other offenders), when risk assessment is often intended to be criterion-referenced (i.e., focused on the likelihood of recidivism). Additionally, the relationship between percentiles and the ultimate outcome of interest (recidivism) is not necessarily linear. In other words, the difference between two risk scores in percentile units may have little to do with the difference between two risk scores in terms of the likelihood of recidivism. For example, in Static-99R, scores of −3 and −2 correspond to the 1st and 4th percentiles, respectively (with percentiles defined as a midpoint average; Hanson et al., 2012). In the higher risk range, scores of 7 and 8 correspond to the 97th and 99th percentile, respectively, which is a similar difference as scores of −3 compared to −2. In contrast, the expected recidivism rates in routine correctional samples for scores of −3 and −2 barely have a perceptible difference (0.9 % versus 1.3 %, respectively), whereas the difference in recidivism rates for scores of 7 and 8 is larger and more meaningful (27.2 % versus 35.1 %; Phenix, Helmus, & Hanson, 2015).

Risk Ratios

Risk ratios describe how an offender's risk of recidivism compares to some reference group (e.g., low risk offenders or offenders with the median risk score). For example, offenders with a Static-99R score of 4 are roughly twice as likely to sexually reoffend as offenders with a Static-99R score of 2 (Hanson, Babchishin, Helmus, & Thornton, 2013). Risk ratios are well-matched to the fundamental attribute being measured by risk scales (scorewise increases in relative risk for recidivism) and are robust to changes in recidivism rates across different samples as well as across different lengths of follow-up (Babchishin, Hanson, & Helmus, 2012a; Hanson et al., 2013). They also have the most potential for combining results from different risk scales because it is possible for them to have a common meaning across scales (Babchishin, Hanson, & Helmus, 2012b; Hanson et al., 2013; Lehmann et al., 2013).

Despite these advantages, risk ratios have rarely been developed or reported for forensic risk scales. They are, however, commonly used for medical risk communication. Possible barriers to their use include more complex calculations compared to other metrics for communicating risk (for an example of different types of risk ratios and other decisions required in their calculation, see Hanson et al., 2013), difficulty in communicating them to laypeople (e.g., Varela et al., 2014), and potential for misinterpretation. Specifically, risk is generally overestimated if risk ratios are not properly contextualized with information about base rates (Elmore & Gigerenzer, 2005). In the Static-99R example above, knowing that an offender with a score of 4 is twice as likely to reoffend as an offender with a score of 2 has a very different meaning if the recidivism rate for a score of 2 is 4 or 40 %.

Absolute Recidivism Estimates

Absolute recidivism estimates are by far the most frequent quantitative metric reported for actuarial risk scales. They are reported in approximately 90 % of assessment reports for preventative detention in Canada, compared to percentiles and risk ratios, which are reported in roughly 40 % and 0 % of cases, respectively (Blais & Forth, 2014). In a survey examining Static-99R reporting practices in sex offender civil commitment evaluations, absolute recidivism estimates were used by 83 % of respondents, compared to roughly one third who used either percentiles or risk ratios (Chevalier, Boccaccini, Murrie, & Varela, 2014).

Absolute recidivism estimates can be generated in a variety of ways, such as from observed recidivism rates for a group of scores (ideally requiring large sample sizes for each score) or using methods such as survival analysis or logistic regression (for discussion, see Hanson, Helmus, and Thornton, 2010). Absolute risk information is easy to understand but hard to obtain with high levels of confidence. Recidivism rates vary based on the follow-up length, so this must be specified. Additionally, there are several practical complications in obtaining good estimates of recidivism, including underreporting of offences, misclassification (e.g., sexual offences pled down to nonsexual violent offences), prosecutorial discretion, and legal/policy/cultural changes over time.

Likely due to the myriad factors that influence recidivism, research has found that absolute recidivism estimates were unstable across samples for the Static-99R and Static-2002R (Helmus, Hanson, Thornton, Babchishin, & Harris, 2012), as well as the MATS-1 (Helmus & Thornton, 2014) and the Risk Matrix 2000/Violence scale (but not the Risk Matrix 2000/Sex scale; Lehmann, Thornton, Helmus, & Hanson, 2015). Additional research has also raised concerns about the generalizability of the recidivism estimates for the VRAG (Mills, Jones, & Kroner, 2005; Snowden, Gray, Taylor, & MacCulloch, 2007). Moreover, analyses of two samples found that violent recidivism rates differed between samples after controlling for the VRS-SO pretreatment score (Olver, Beggs Christofferson, Grace, & Wong, 2014). Some solutions have been proposed for using absolute recidivism estimates in light of this variability (e.g., Hanson, Thornton, Helmus, & Babchishin, 2015), but the adequacy of these solutions is not yet known. Minimally, these findings of variability suggest that creating and reporting reliable and generalizable recidivism estimates for actuarial scales are more complicated than previously believed.

Psychometric Properties of Risk Scales

An important advantage of actuarial risk assessment is that (in contrast to UCJ) it is possible to test the psychometric properties of the risk scales. Compared to SPJ, the increased structure and availability of quantitative risk communication metrics in actuarial scales may provide more options and precision for evaluating psychometric properties, as well as stronger results. Professional standards dictate that forensic psychologists should have expertise on research related to the psychometric properties, appropriate uses, and strengths/weaknesses of risk assessment instruments they are using (American Psychological Association, 2013; Association for the Treatment of Sexual Abusers, 2014). The ability to comment on the psychometric properties of a risk scale is particularly important when risk decisions have to be defended in court; without this information, the method of risk assessment may be considered inadmissible evidence. This section discusses appropriate and inappropriate psychometric properties of actuarial risk scales and where applicable compares them to SPJ approaches.

Objectivity and Interrater Reliability

As actuarial risk assessment scales generally rely on explicitly defined predictor variables with specific scoring rules (e.g., how much weight to give the item), this facilitates more objective, transparent, standardized, and fair assessments. In contrast, UCJ has none of these features. SPJ scales may have explicitly defined predictor variables (contributing to greater objectivity than UCJ), but the subjectivity in how they influence the overall judgment should come at the expense of some objectivity, transparency, and standardization. This objectivity should increase interrater reliability, which refers to the consistency in scores across independent raters (i.e., if two different evaluators score the same individual, will they obtain the same results?). Not only does interrater reliability increase the general validity and defensibility of the assessment, but higher interrater reliability has also been associated with significantly higher predictive accuracy in some analyses (Hanson & Morton-Bourgon, 2009). Supporting the idea that the objectivity of actuarial assessment lends itself to higher interrater reliability is a finding from the Spousal Assault Risk Assessment guide (the SARA), where the interrater reliability of the SPJ summary risk rating was considerably lower than for the total score (summing the items; Kropp & Hart, 2000).

Internal Reliability

Another metric sometimes applied to risk scales is internal consistency, which refers to the degree of interrelatedness among the items (Cortina, 1993). Cronbach's α (Cronbach, 1951) is one of the most common indices of internal consistency. Unfortunately, despite its frequent use, internal consistency is not an informative metric for actuarial risk scales.

Developing a scale to predict an outcome (e.g., recidivism) is meaningfully different than classical scale construction in psychology. Specifically, most scales in psychology are norm-referenced, which means they are trying to capture how individuals display different amounts of some relevant construct (e.g., Aiken, 1985). Examples include tests of intelligence, ability, or personality. In contrast, risk assessment scales are inherently criterion-referenced, which means they are designed specifically to predict an outcome of interest. This means that some elements of test reliability and validity are not applicable (e.g., internal consistency; Aiken, 1985). In norm-referenced scales, internal reliability increases to the extent that multiple items are assessing the same construct (e.g., items are highly related to total scores); this may be achieved by including similar items but with different wordings or reverse-scored.

In contrast, the most important goal of criterion-referenced scales is to predict the outcome. For that reason, it does not make sense (and may be undesirable) to measure only one construct and to include multiple items assessing the same construct. Consequently, predictive accuracy and efficiency are maximized by including the smallest number of items measuring the most distinct constructs possible, instead of having multiple items assess a single construct. These goals would deliberately decrease internal consistency. Consequently, we do not recommend reporting internal consistency to evaluate the reliability of risk scales. Internal consistency is, however, useful for scales designed to assess a single construct (e.g., the Psychopathy Checklist-Revised; Hare, 2003).

Construct Validity

The results of risk scales should have greater meaning and clearer implications for case management decisions when the source of an offender's risk is identified and understood. This requires knowing what constructs are being measured by actuarial risk scales. Given that risk scales were designed as criterion-referenced (i.e., items were chosen based on their ability to predict the outcome), construct validity has been largely neglected in actuarial risk assessment scales. In recent years, however, greater attention has been paid to construct validity of actuarial risk scales (e.g., Babchishin et al., 2012b; Brouillette-Alarie, Babchishin, Hanson, & Helmus, 2015).

Specifically, items are assumed to predict the outcome because they are an indicator of some kind of latent underlying construct/propensity (Mann et al., 2010). Efforts to improve construct validity may focus on identifying the underlying constructs measured by the items, determining how well the items measure those constructs, and assessing how to best combine constructs into an overall assessment. Consequently, greater focus on construct validity should help improve predictive accuracy (by potentially identifying better indicators of constructs), resolve discrepancies in risk scales, identify optimal ways to combine risk scales, and better identify whether external information is likely to add to the results of an actuarial scale (e.g., Hanson, 2009).

Predictive Validity

Whereas reliability specifies the extent to which risk assessments give consistent results, predictive validity refers to the accuracy of measurement in predicting the outcome. For risk assessment, predictive validity (also called criterion-related validity) is most important. Discrimination and calibration are distinct indices of the predictive validity of a criterion-referenced scale (Altman, Vergouwe, Royston, & Moons, 2009).

Discrimination quantifies the model's ability to distinguish between recidivists and non-recidivists or in other words, to rank offenders according to their relative risk to reoffend. This indicates whether higher risk offenders are more likely to reoffend than lower risk offenders. The most commonly recommended and reported statistic for discrimination is the area under the curve from receiver operating characteristic curve analyses (AUC; Mossman, 1994; Swets, Dawes, & Monahan, 2000). For further discussion of the strengths and weaknesses of other discrimination statistics (such as correlations, Harrell's c index, and Cox and logistic regression), see Babchishin and Helmus (2015).

In contrast, there is little research on the calibration of risk scales, which refers to the ability of a risk scale to estimate absolute recidivism rates (Helmus, Hanson et al. 2012). Consequently, there are no well-established statistics for measuring calibration. For example, in 2009 there were at least 63 studies examining the discrimination of Static-99 (summarized in Hanson & Morton-Bourgon, 2009) but only two studies that examined its calibration (Doren, 2004; Harris et al., 2003). One promising statistic to assess calibration is the E/O index (Gail & Pfeiffer, 2005; Rockhill, Byrne, Rosner, Louie, & Colditz, 2003), which is the ratio of the predicted number of recidivists (E) divided by the observed (O) number of recidivists (Viallon, Ragusa, Clavel-Chapelon, & Bénichou, 2009; for more discussion of this statistic, see Helmus and Babchishin, 2014). Although calibration statistics have been historically neglected, they present one of the most promising advantages of actuarial risk scales. Discrimination can be examined with either SPJ or actuarial approaches, but calibration is a unique property of actuarial risk scales, as they are the only approach with empirically derived recidivism estimates associated with total scores.

Predictive Accuracy of Actuarial Scales Compared to Other Approaches

Research across a variety of disciplines (including offender risk assessment) supports the superiority of actuarial prediction schemes over professional judgment (Ægisdóttir et al., 2006; Bonta, Law, & Hanson, 1998; Dawes, Faust, & Meehl, 1989; Grove, Zald, Lebow, Snitz, & Nelson, 2000; Hanson & Morton-Bourgon, 2009; Mossman, 1994). Examining sex offender risk assessment, for example, recent meta-analytic research (Hanson & Morton-Bourgon, 2009), has found that actuarial measures had significantly higher accuracy in predicting sexual recidivism

($d=0.67$) than UCJ ($d=0.42$), whereas SPJ scales had accuracy closer to UCJ, but not significantly different than either of the two previous categories ($d=0.46$).

This cross-disciplinary literature contradicts the intuitive belief that the expertise of professionals should be better equipped to handle complex situations and case-specific factors (e.g., Boer et al., 1997). Paradoxically, it appears to be simultaneously correct that although level of expertise matters (e.g., experts generally outperform novices), actuarial decision algorithms outperform experts, but only under some conditions (Kahneman & Klein, 2009; Shanteau, 1992). An important question, then, is under what conditions?

In summarizing decision-making and cognitive science literature, Shanteau (1992) found evidence for good expert performance in weather forecasters, livestock judges, astronomers, test pilots, soil judges, chess masters, physicists, mathematicians, accountants, grain inspectors, photo interpreters, and insurance analysts. Poor professional judgments were noted for clinical psychologists, psychiatrists, astrologers, student admissions evaluators, court judges, behavioral researchers, counselors, personnel selectors, parole officers, polygraph judges, intelligence analysts, and stock brokers. Mixed performance was found for nurses, physicians, and auditors. Shanteau (1992) proposed a variety of task features that were associated with poorer performance from experts. He concluded that human behavior is inherently more unpredictable than physical phenomena and that decision-making is particularly difficult for unique tasks, when feedback is unavailable and when the environment is intolerant of error.

Kahneman (2011) provided a more updated summary of the performance of experts across a variety of tasks, with similar conclusions. According to Kahneman and Klein (2009), expert opinion can be expected to outperform actuarial decisions when the environment is regular (i.e., highly predictable), the expert has considerable practice, and there are opportunities to get timely feedback on decisions to learn from errors or false cues. These conditions are generally not present in offender risk assessment. The sheer number of diverse predictors of recidivism (e.g., see Andrews and Bonta, 2010, and Hanson and Morton-Bourgon, 2005) suggests that criminal behavior is not highly predictable (i.e., the number of contingencies are infinite; Hanson, 2009), and evaluators do not receive timely feedback on their decisions.

Professional Overrides

Another way to compare the predictive accuracy of actuarial approaches to SPJ is to examine "professional overrides." A professional override is when the results of an actuarial scale are adjusted based on professional judgment. The premise of SPJ scales is that the professional judgment is a helpful way to respond to case-specific factors or apply flexibility in terms of weighting items for a particular individual. Research, however, has consistently found that overrides to actuarial scales decrease their accuracy (Hanson, Helmus, & Harris, 2015; Hanson & Morton-Bourgon, 2009; Wormith, Hogg, & Guzzo, 2012). Research also demonstrates that professional judgment tends to be more conservative, less transparent, and less replicable than are actuarial measures (Bonta & Motiuk, 1990). Alexander and Austin (1992) have found that overrides also disproportionately are used to increase offenders' risk. If overrides are a necessary part of correctional policy (e.g., to introduce flexibility), Austin, Johnson, and Weitzer (2005) encourage adopting a general standard where only 5–15 % of final assessments should differ from initial actuarial results. Furthermore, the direction of inconsistencies should be balanced, where half are higher and half are lower than the original actuarial result. Overall, however, overrides may offer some advantages (e.g., flexibility), but the research seems clear that they have a negative impact on accuracy. One possible explanation for the disappointing results of professional judgment in this context is that the professionals may be able to accurately identify risk-relevant information that is not incorporated in the risk scale, but are unable to determine to what extent this new information is correlated with existing information in the scale or how much weight to give this new information.

Incremental Validity

Besides predictive accuracy, incremental validity which assesses the contribution of an additional measure to the prediction of an outcome (e.g., recidivism) is essential information in the context of risk assessment. Additional measures may add incrementally by either improving the measurement of constructs already included (e.g., attitudes, emotional regulation, intimacy deficits) or by the assessment of new risk-related constructs. The greater objectivity and structure of actuarial risk scales may facilitate easier interpretation of incremental results.

Incremental validity becomes increasingly important as the knowledge base for offender risk assessment expands. As risk scales become entrenched in practice, the threshold for newly developed scales should increase. In other words, if scales are already in use, the onus is on developers of new scales to demonstrate that their scale provides incremental accuracy to standard practice (Hunsley & Meyer, 2003). Unfortunately, statistical power is reduced for tests of incremental validity compared to bivariate predictive validity, and comparisons of scales may require sample sizes in the thousands (Babchishin et al., 2012b). This means that increasingly larger amounts of data are required for smaller gains in accuracy.

Combining Actuarial Risk Instruments

Generally, a comprehensive actuarial risk assessment of a range of psychological risk factors will yield better predictive accuracy than a less comprehensive assessment (Hanson & Morton-Bourgon, 2009; Mann et al., 2010). Accordingly, multiple risk measures are frequently used to assess offenders' risk for future offending (Jackson & Hess, 2007; Neal & Grisso, 2014). The use of multiple risk tools is justified on the grounds that they provide incremental information (Babchishin et al., 2012b; Welsh, Schmidt, McKinnon, Chattha, & Meyers, 2008). For some scales the developers propose starting with a commonly used risk scale and adjusting the overall rating based on the scores of an incrementally valid, additional risk instrument (e.g., Helmus, Hanson, Babchishin, & Thornton, 2014). Also, recent research indicates that averaging the risk ratios of different risk tools is a promising approach to obtaining a better overall evaluation of relative risk (Lehmann, Hanson et al. 2013), as opposed to other approaches, such as taking the highest or lowest risk estimate. Hence, a strength of actuarial risk assessment is the inclusion of a range of empirically validated risk factors or scales, which under certain circumstances (see Lehmann, Hanson et al. 2013) could be combined into an overall risk judgment of recidivism risk with better predictive accuracy than a single scale.

Selected Examples of Actuarial Risk Scales for Sex Offenders

Below, specific examples of risk scales for sex offenders will be discussed. Note that they are not meant as an exhaustive list of scales available—they are illustrative examples of scales we are most familiar with. This chapter was not intended to provide a detailed review of actuarial risk scales available.

The Static-99/R

The most commonly used static sex offender risk assessment tools in Canada and the United States are the Static-99 and Static-99R (Hanson & Thornton, 2000; Helmus, Thornton, Hanson, & Babchishin, 2012; Interstate Commission for Adult Offender Supervision, 2007; Jackson & Hess, 2007; McGrath, Cumming, Burchard, Zeoli, & Ellerby, 2010; Neal & Grisso, 2014). The Static-99/R is 10-item actuarial scales designed to assess sexual recidivism risk of adult male sex offenders. The items and scoring rules for Static-99 (Hanson & Thornton, 2000) and Static-99R (Helmus, Thornton et al., 2012) are identical with the exception of updated age weights for the Static-99R. The scale developers have recommended that Static-99R be used in place of the original scale (Helmus, Thornton et al., 2012). Static-99/R contains items covering the broad constructs of age and relationship status (i.e., whether the offender has ever lived with a lover for two or more years), sexual deviance (e.g., stranger victims, noncontact sexual offences, prior sex offenses), and general criminality (e.g., number of prior sentencing occasions, index nonsexual violence, prior nonsexual violence) identified in meta-analytic research (Hanson & Bussière, 1998; Hanson & Morton-Bourgon, 2005).

Accordingly, the strength of the risk tool is that it only uses risk factors empirically associated with sexual recidivism. Also, explicit rules for combining the factors into a total risk score are provided (A. Harris, Phenix, Hanson, & Thornton, 2003).

Other advantages are that with appropriate training, the scale can be scored quickly based on commonly available demographic and criminal history information, without a detailed file review or interview with the offender. The website for the scale (www.static99.org) contains an evaluator workbook that includes normative data for interpreting Static-99/R (nominal risk categories, absolute recidivism estimates, percentiles, and risk ratios) and sample reporting templates and is regularly updated with more recent research and normative data for the scale. Although Static-99R was designed to predict sexual recidivism, normative data for violent recidivism risk has previously been available for the scale as well. Most recently, Babchishin, Hanson, and Blais (2015) have found that the inclusion of so many items assessing sexual deviance overly dilutes the scale's predictive accuracy for violent recidivism. Consequently, the developers of Static-99R no longer recommend its use to comment on violent recidivism risk among sex offenders. Instead, they recommend using the BARR-2002R (Brief Assessment of Recidivism Risk-2002R), which was created form a subset of Static-2002R items (see Babchishin et al., 2015).

In terms of the psychometric properties of the risk scale, recent meta-analyses found moderate accuracy in predicting sexual recidivism for both Static-99 ($d=0.67$, $k=63$, $n=20{,}010$; Hanson & Morton-Bourgon, 2009) and Static-99R ($d=0.76$, $k=23$, $n=8106$; Helmus, Hanson et al. 2012). The interrater reliability for Static-99/R reported across different samples was found to be generally high (ICC>0.75; see Anderson & Hanson, 2010; Phenix & Epperson, 2015; Quesada, Calkins, & Jeglic, 2013). Risk ratios for Static-99R have been found to be highly stable across diverse samples and time period (Hanson et al., 2013), although the absolute recidivism rates per Static-99R score have significantly varied across samples (Helmus, Hanson et al. 2012), which complicates interpretation of the scale. Current recommendations for using Static-99R in light of this base rate variability are discussed by Hanson et al. (2015).

Risk Matrix 2000

The Risk Matrix 2000 (RM2000) has been adopted by the police, probation, and prison services of England, Wales, Scotland, and Northern Ireland (National Policing Improvement Agency, 2010; Social Work Inspection, HM Inspectorate of Constabulary for Scotland, & HM Inspectorate of Prisons, 2009). The RM2000 is an actuarial scale that assesses recidivism risk of adult male sexual offenders (Thornton et al., 2003). The scale is based on file information only and contains three separate sales: one for measuring risk of sexual recidivism (RM2000/S), one for measuring risk of nonsexual violent recidivism (RM2000/V), and one combination of the first two scales for measuring risk of any violent recidivism (RM2000/C).

The scoring of the RM2000/S includes two steps. In step 1 three risk items are scored (number of previous sexual appearances, number of criminal appearances, and age at next opportunity to offend) and offenders are assigned to four preliminary risk categories. In the second step four aggravating risk factors (any conviction for sexual offense against a male, any conviction for a sexual offense against a stranger, any conviction for a noncontact sex offense, and single – never been married) need to be considered. The presence of two or four aggravating factors raises the risk category by one or two levels, respectively. For the RM2000/V three items need to be scored (age on release, violent appearances, and any conviction for burglary) and offenders are also assigned to the four risk categories. The four nominal risk categories are low, medium, high, and very high risk. To get the score for the RM2000/C scale, the risk category points for the RM2000/S and RM2000/V need to be summed and converted into the four nominal risk categories.

In terms of the psychometric properties of the three risk scales, a recent a meta-analysis (Helmus, Babchishin, & Hanson, 2013) found moderate to high accuracy in predicting sexual recidivism for the RM2000/S (mean $d=0.74$ in both fixed-effect and random-effects models, $k=15$, $n=10,644$), in predicting nonsexual violent recidivism for the RM2000/V (after adjusting the largest study weight, mean fixed-effect $d=0.98$ and random-effects $d=0.96$, $k=10$, $n=9836$), and in predicting any violent recidivism for the RM2000/C (fixed-effect $d=0.81$ and random-effects $d=0.80$, $k=8$, $n=8277$).

Recently, Lehmann, Thornton et al. (2015) developed non-arbitrary metrics for risk communication for the RM2000 (i.e., percentiles, risk ratios, and absolute recidivism estimates) based on combining offenders from four samples of fairly routine (i.e., complete/unselected) settings: England and Wales, Scotland, Berlin (Germany), and Canada ($n=3144$). Although there were meaningful differences across these samples in the distribution of Risk Matrix scores, relative increases in predictive accuracy for each ascending risk category were remarkably consistent across samples. However, recidivism rates for the median risk category also showed some variability across samples for the Risk Matrix 2000 Violence and Combined scales, but not for the Sex scale (Lehmann, Thornton et al., 2015).

The Crime Scene Behavior Risk Measure

Whereas previous actuarial risk assessment instruments of static risk factors focused on the criminal history of sexual offenders, recent research indicates that sexual offender risk assessment can be improved by also utilizing crime scene behavior as indicators of risk for sexual recidivism. The seven items (explicit offense planning, sexualized language, actively seeking victim, no multiple juvenile offenders, approach-explicit, male victim at index offense, and hands-off: victim active) that comprise the Crime Scene Behavior Risk measure (CBR; Dahle, Biedermann, Lehmann, & Gallasch-Nemitz, 2014) showed high predictive accuracy for sexual recidivism with little variation between the development (c index[2]$=0.72$; $n=995$) and the replication sample (c index$=0.74$; $n=77$).

---

[2] Harrell's c index is an effect size analogous to the AUC, but it takes into account varying follow-up times. The c value can be interpreted in the same way as an AUC, with values of 0.56, 0.64, and 0.71 noting small, moderate, and large effect sizes.

The interrater reliability for the CBR total score ranged from moderate (ICC=0.60) in the development sample to excellent (ICC=0.89) in the cross-validation sample. For risk communication the authors provide estimated recidivism rates for each CBR score after 5 and 10 years. Further, the CBR was found to provide significant incremental validity and to improve the predictive accuracy of the Static-99R risk assessment tool (Dahle et al., 2014). Accordingly, the authors of the CBR recommend using the published nominal risk categories of the Static-99R (Helmus, Thornton et al., 2012) as an initial assessment of recidivism risk and adjusting the risk level according to the CBR score to obtain a better overall evaluation of recidivism risk. Hence, the assessment of sexual recidivism risk using different sources of information should yield a better understanding of the recidivism risk that emanates from a specific offender.

Stable-2007

The Stable-2007 (Hanson, Harris, Scott, & Helmus, 2007) is an interview- and file-review-based instrument designed to assess stable (i.e., medium- to long-term) dynamic risk factors for sexual recidivism, which are unlikely to change without deliberate effort (i.e., treatment targets; Hanson & Harris, 2013). Items are scored on a 3-point scale ranging from "0, no problem;" "1, maybe/some," to "2, yes, definite problem." The instrument contains 13 items divided into the 5 subsections of significant social influences, intimacy deficits (i.e., capacity for relationship stability, emotional identification with children, hostility toward women, general social rejection/loneliness, and lack of concern for others), sexual self-regulation (i.e., sex drive/preoccupation, sex as coping, and deviant sexual interests), general self-regulation (i.e., impulsive acts, poor cognitive problem-solving, and negative emotionality/hostility), and cooperation with supervision. The total score is obtained by summing all items and can range from 0 to 26 for offenders with a child victim and 0 to 24 for other offender types (the item *emotional identification with children* is scored only for offenders with a child victim). The Stable-2007 can inform decisions about treatment targets as well as about moderate- to long-term recidivism potential with higher scores indicating greater risk of sexual recidivism. In addition to detailed coding rules for each item, the Stable-2007 scoring manual also includes sample interview questions, practice cases, reporting suggestions, and advice for maintaining high quality risk assessments (Fernandez et al., 2014).

Excellent interrater reliability has been found for the Stable-2007 total score (ICC>0.75; Fernandez, 2008; Hanson et al., 2007). The predictive accuracy of the Stable-2007 for sexual recidivism was found to range from moderate (e.g., AUC=0.67; Hanson et al., 2015) to high (e.g., AUC=0.71; Eher, Matthes, Schilling, Haubner-MacLean, & Rettenberger, 2012).

For risk communication the authors provide nominal risk categories for the Stable-2007 as follows: 0–3=low need, 4–11=moderate need, and 12 or greater=high need, as well as percentiles (Fernandez et al., 2014). Hanson et al. (in press) found the Stable-2007 to add incrementally to the Static-99R and Static-2002R in most analyses. Of the scales, however, the Static-99R and Static-2002R had higher predictive accuracy than the Stable-2007. Consequently, the scale developers recommend using it in conjunction with a static scale (Hanson, Helmus, & Harris, 2015). The current evaluator workbook of Stable-2007 contains 1-year, 3-year, and 5-year recidivism estimates for risk categories based on combining Stable-2007 with either Static-99R, Static-2002R, or the Risk Matrix-2000 (Helmus et al., 2014; Helmus & Hanson, 2013).

Acute-2007

The Acute-2007 (Hanson et al., 2007) is an interview- and file-review-based instrument designed to assess acute dynamic (i.e., rapidly changing) risk factors for sexual recidivism which is essential to managing sexual offenders on community supervision. Items are scored on a 4-point scale ranging from "0, no problem;" "1, maybe/some;" "2, yes, definite problem;" to "3, intervene now." The Acute-2007 includes seven items (access to victims, sexual preoccupation, hostility, rejection of supervision, emotional collapse, collapse of social supports, and substance abuse), all of which are predictive of general recidivism. For predicting sexual or violent recidivism, however, a subscale of only four items is included (the first four listed above; Hanson et al., 2007). Some subsequent analyses have suggested that the four items of the sexual/violence subscale represent more of an approach trajectory toward offending, whereas the three additional items are more indicative of an emotional collapse/avoidant trajectory toward offending (Babchishin, 2013). Scores for the sex/violence subscale can range from 0 to 12, whereas the total of the general recidivism scale can range from 0 to 21, with higher scores indicating a higher likelihood of recidivism. The cut scores for the sex/violence subscale are $0 = $ low, $1 = $ moderate, and $2+ = $ high imminent recidivism risk. For the general recidivism scale, the recommended cut scores are reported as $0 = $ low, $1–2 = $ moderate, and $3+ = $ high.

In the development study the interrater agreement for the individual Acute items ranged from good to excellent with a median ICC of 0.90. Feedback from users suggested that the brevity of the item descriptions in the coding manual might be contributing to subjective variability in scoring some items. Consequently, a new manual with more comprehensive item descriptions along with examples for item scoring is in development. Both the general scale ($AUC = 0.72$) and the sex/violence subscale ($AUC = 0.74$) showed high ability to differentiate between the imminent sexual recidivists and the non-recidivists in the development sample (Hanson et al., 2007), though the three extra items of the general scale did not predict sexual recidivism. The sex/violence subscale significantly predicted imminent (within 45 days) sexual, violent, and any recidivism after controlling for the combined Static-99/Stable-2007 categories whereas the general recidivism Acute score only added incrementally to the prediction of violent and general recidivism. Accordingly, specific rules on how to combine static, stable, and acute factors into three priority levels were constructed by the authors. For risk communication relative risk ratios for sexual recidivism within 45 days based on combined Static-99, Stable-2007, and Acute-2007 scores are presented for the three priority levels. Recently, Babchishin (2013) investigated the temporal stability of the factor structure of the Acute-2007 and found observed changes to be attributed to true changes on risk-relevant propensities assessed by the Acute-2007, as opposed to measurement error.

Violence Risk Scale-Sexual Offender Version (VRS-SO)

The VRS-SO (Wong, Olver, Nicholaichuk, & Gordon, 2003) is a 24-item interview- and file-review-based instrument comprised of 7 static (e.g., age at release, prior sex offenses, unrelated victim) and 17 dynamic items which are scored on a 4-point Likert-type scale ranging from 0 to 3, with higher scores indicating increased risk for sexual recidivism. Factor analysis of the dynamic items generated three factors labeled sexual deviance ($\alpha = 0.87$; e.g., deviant sexual preference, offense planning, sexual compulsivity), criminality ($\alpha = 0.79$; e.g., impulsivity, substance abuse, compliance with community supervision), and treatment responsivity ($\alpha = 0.72$; e.g., insight, treatment compliance, cognitive distortions). Accordingly, the first two factors are consistent with the two major constructs related to sexual reoffending discussed above. All 24 items are used to assess recidivism risk. However, the VRS-SO was designed to integrate sex offender risk assessment and risk reduction through treatment. Therefore, the dynamic items are used to identify treatment targets and to measure change. Here, change is measured on the basis of a modified application of the key transtheoretical constructs of stages of change (SOC; Prochaska, DiClemente, & Norcross, 1992). The progression in the SOC is supposed to indicate the extent to which the offender has improved (i.e., changed). Therefore, treatment targets (i.e., dynamic items rated 2 or 3) are given a SOC rating at pre- and posttreatment and both ratings are compared to quantify change (Olver, Wong, Nicholaichuk, & Gordon, 2007).

The developers of the scale investigated the psychometric properties of the VRS-SO (Olver et al., 2007). Excellent interrater reliability has been found for the pretreatment (ICC=0.74) and posttreatment (ICC=0.79) dynamic item total score. The predictive accuracy of the VRS-SO total score was found to be high for sexual recidivism for both pretreatment (AUC=0.71) and posttreatment (AUC=0.72). Also, both the VRS-SO static and dynamic item total scores made unique contributions to the prediction of sexual recidivism after controlling for Static-99. These findings were replicated in an independent validation study (Beggs & Grace, 2010). One limitation of this research is that similar to other scales, Olver, Beggs Christofferson, and Wong (2015) have found significant variability in the recidivism rates of two samples, even after controlling for the VRS-SO pretreatment score. Such variability poses a challenge for the creation of generalizable recidivism estimates.

Importantly, therapeutic change (i.e., positive change in dynamic items) was found to be significantly related to reduction in sexual recidivism after controlling for risk and follow-up time (Beggs & Grace, 2011; Olver et al., 2007, 2014). In their most recent risk communication efforts, Olver et al. (2015) applied an intuitively useful method of conceptualizing and communicating change to the VRS-SO. Olver and colleagues used the Clinically Significant Change model, which incorporates offenders' change relative to external standards of what is "functional" and takes into account whether the change is reliable (i.e., likely accounted for by more than measurement error). Using this technique, the authors found that Clinically Significant Change provided some unique information in predicting recidivism beyond pretreatment risk scores, and they offered examples of how this approach can facilitate risk communication.

Survey Findings: What Is Used in Applied Practice?

Several surveys have been conducted to assess practical applications of risk assessment (e.g., what scales are used and how the information is incorporated). Examining 111 risk assessment reports for preventative detention hearings in Canada (intended for offenders at high risk of violent recidivism), Blais and Forth (2014) found that over 90 % of experts (appointed by either the prosecution or appointed by the court) used an actuarial risk assessment scale, compared to 53 % who used an SPJ scale. The PCL-R (Psychopathy Checklist-Revised), designed to assess the construct of psychopathy (not as a risk assessment scale), was used in over 95 % of risk assessment reports. In terms of scales designed to assess risk of recidivism, the most commonly used scale was the Static-99, used in over 60 % of cases, which is surprising given that not all candidates for preventative detention are sex offenders. The next most commonly used scales were the VRAG (Violence Risk Appraisal Guide; 48 % of reports) and the SORAG (Sex Offender Risk Appraisal Guide; 42 % of reports), both of which are actuarial. Other risk scales were used in one quarter or less of cases.

In a particularly large study, Singh and colleagues (2014) surveyed 2135 mental health professionals who had conducted at least one violence risk assessment. Half of the respondents were from Europe, followed by 21 % from North America, 5 % from Australasia, and 3 % each from South America and Asia. Among this diverse sample, over 400 different instruments were reported as being used for violence risk assessment, although roughly half had been developed specifically for personal or institutional use only. Among the 12 most frequently used risk scales, half were actuarial and half were SPJ, with the HCR-20 (Historical Clinical Risk Management 20, an SPJ scale) reported as the most commonly used, followed by the PCL-R.

Neal and Grisso (2014) surveyed 434 psychologist and psychiatrist members of various professional associations, mostly from the United States, Canada, Europe, Australia, and New Zealand, who described 868 cases they had completed. The most common types of referrals these professionals dealt with included competence to stand trial, violence risk, sex offender risk, insanity, sentencing, disability, child custody, civil commitment, child protection, and civil tort. Use of structured assessment tools (e.g., note this is broader than risk assessment tools and could include personality assessments) varied based on the type of assessment being conducted, with the lowest rates of structured tool use reported for competence to stand trial cases (58 %), disability cases (66 %), and civil tort cases (67 %). Sex offender risk cases were most likely to use structured tools (97 %), followed by child protection cases (93 %) and violence risk cases (89 %).

Among sex offender risk cases, Neal and Grisso (2014) found that the most frequently used tools were by far the Static-99/R or Static-2002/R (which were clumped together), used in 66 % of cases. The next most commonly used tools were all either designed to assess a single construct or were personality assessments — none were designed for sex offender risk assessments. These included the PCL-R (35 % of cases), Minnesota Multiphasic Personality Inventory (MMPI; 27 % of cases), Personality Assessment Inventory (PAI; 23 % of cases), and the Millon Clinical Multiaxial Inventory (MCMI; 17 % of cases). Other sex or violent risk assessment scales, such as the Sexual Violence Risk-20 (SVR-20), Risk for Sexual Violence Protocol (RSVP), Stable-2007, SORAG, and VRAG, were used in less than 15 % of cases. Note that the SVR-20 and RSVP are SPJ scales, whereas the others are actuarial. Similar results were found in a survey of American psychologists, conducted by Archer, Buffington-Vollum, Stredny, and Handel (2006). For adult sex offender risk assessments, Static-99 was still the most commonly used scale (mentioned by roughly half of participants), but with a smaller margin over other frequently used scales, which included the SVR-20, Minnesota Sex Offender Screening Tool-Revised (MnSOST-R), Rapid Risk Assessment for Sex Offense Recidivism (RRASOR), and the SORAG. Note that Stable-2007 did not exist when this survey was completed. These findings mirror survey results of sex offender civil commitment evaluators (Jackson & Hess, 2007) and sex offender treatment programs (McGrath et al., 2010) which found Static-99 to be the most commonly used risk scale, by a wide margin. Additionally, among treatment programs, dynamic risk scales were being more widely adopted, with Stable-2007 being the most frequently used (McGrath et al., 2010).

Other important findings from surveys pertain to how experts use information from risk scales. In SPJ scales, the only information available is a nominal risk category (with the exception of the SARA, which provides some percentile information, although not for the final risk judgment; Kropp & Gibas, 2010). In actuarial scales, it is possible to report absolute recidivism estimates. Additionally, some scales may also provide information on percentiles or nominal risk ratios. In their study of Canadian preventative detention hearings, Blais and Forth (2014) found that over 95 % of risk assessment reports mentioned a nominal risk level. For actuarial scales, roughly two thirds of reports mentioned a total score, 37 % reported a percentile, and over 90 % reported absolute recidivism estimates. For SPJ scales, although the intent of the scales is NOT to sum the risk factors, 24 % of reports also included a mechanical total score from the scale. In a more recent survey of 109 experts who use the Static-99R in Sexually Violent Predator evaluations in the

United States (Chevalier et al., 2014), 83 % included nominal risk categories and absolute recidivism in their reports, while 35 % included percentiles and 33 % include risk ratios. When asked to rank the importance of the various risk communication metrics, 54 % of the evaluators reported that absolute recidivism estimates provided the most important information about recidivism risk, compared to 25 % who felt the nominal risk categories provided the most important information.

Clinical Advantages to Actuarial Risk Assessment

Psychologists have been instrumental for more than a century in developing, validating, refining, and implementing scientifically rigorous procedures that have advanced our understanding of psychological constructs and our prediction of future behavior. Evidence-based practice, or the practice of providing services that have empirically demonstrated effectiveness for each client's needs, has become the standard among clinicians and within most organizations and has extended into the field of assessment. Hunsley and Mash (2010) note that evidence-based assessment "relies on research and theory to guide the selection of constructs to be assessed for a specific assessment purpose, the methods and measures to be used in the assessment, and the manner in which the assessment process unfolds" (p. 7). In the area of correctional intervention, the use of evidence-based assessment tools such as actuarial risk measures is the first step in a comprehensive evidence-based approach, which includes assessing the client, formulating a case conceptualization, determining the client's needs, deciding on and implementing a program of treatment, and monitoring and evaluating the outcome.

Evidenced Based Practice in Correctional Settings

There is extensive research into the basic principles that should be adhered to for human services to have the greatest positive impact. Within correctional work, research supports that the more risk, need, and responsivity factors a program adheres to, the more effective it is in reducing recidivism, while programs that do not incorporate these principles potentially increase recidivism (Dowden & Andrews, 2004; Flores, Russell, Latessa, & Travis, 2005; Lowenkamp, Pealer, Smith, & Latessa, 2006; Smith & Schweitzer, 2012; Wormith, Althouse, Reitzel, Fagan, & Morgan, 2007). Specifically, intervention is most effective when targeted proportionally to offender risk (risk principle), focusing on criminogenic needs (need principle), and matched to the learning style and needs of the offenders (responsivity principle).

Consequently, evidence-based assessment is a critical first component to an effective correctional intervention (i.e., identification of the first two principles: risk and need). As part of that approach, risk assessment tools can "facilitate decisions about the intensity of intervention in accordance with risk needs responsivity (RNR) principles" (Hilton, 2014, p. 88), thus maximizing intervention effectiveness. However, Andrews and Dowden (2005) note that inconsistencies or a lack of implementation integrity across providers is related to differences in program outcomes. Risk assessment tools, like any part of an evidence-based intervention, must be implemented with integrity to be maximally effective. For example, two field studies examining the real-world utility of Static-99 show remarkable variability. In Texas, Static-99 demonstrated minimal accuracy in predicting sexual recidivism (AUC=0.57; Boccaccini, Murrie, Caperton, & Hawes, 2009). In contrast, California implemented the scale with rigorous training, mentoring, and ongoing quality control policies (e.g., mandatory re-certification by users) and reported exceptionally high predictive accuracy (AUC=0.82; Hanson, Lunetta, Phenix, Neeley, & Epperson, 2014). The discrepancy in these results from two American jurisdictions highlights the importance of implementation integrity. Additionally, Hanson et al. (2014) found meaningfully higher predictive accuracy for actuarial risk scales scored by front-line staff who were more committed to the project (defined as those who completed all the requested information). For additional suggestions on best practices for quality control, see Fernandez and colleagues (2014).

In the second half of this chapter, we argue that actuarial measures form a critical part of evidence-based practice and particularly enhance program integrity by providing a standardized and structured approach to the critical first steps (assessment) of any correctional intervention. We focus on the advantages of actuarial measures as part of implementing an effective evidence-based intervention program within a clinical practice, forensic setting, or organization. Adapting Bernfeld, Blase, and Fixsen (1990) "multilevel systems perspective," the strengths and usefulness of actuarial risk assessment instruments in clinical practice are discussed across the four levels important to human service delivery: namely, the client, program, organizational, and societal levels.

The Client Level

Actuarial risk assessment has the potential for several direct advantages for the client including providing opportunities for a collaborative working relationship with the assessor, an introduction to the therapeutic relationship and to the concept of risk, identification of treatment targets, and making the best match between the client and the appropriate type of treatment. Shingler and Mann (2006) note that risk assessment offers a unique collaborative opportunity to build rapport and set the stage for subsequent intervention. The first step of their sexual offender intervention program, the Structured Assessment of Risk and Need (SARN; Webster et al., 2006), specifically integrates collaboration into the risk assessment process. Their in-house training encourages assessors to approach the risk assessment as a critical first step in the treatment process and emphasizes that the experience the offenders have during a risk assessment can heavily impact their desire to engage in treatment and the offenders' trust of the process. Offenders themselves have expressed the importance of contributing to the assessment, and getting their side represented, in their sense of fairness and confidence in the outcome of the risk assessment process (Attrill & Liell, 2007). A thorough assessment at the front end of treatment using measures that identify factors empirically related to recidivism can help to focus the client on the important issues necessary for offenders to be able to identify and cope with risk factors to reduce the risk of recidivism (Proulx, Tardiff, Lamoureeux, & Lussier, 2000), saving them both time and effort as they move through the rehabilitative process. A collaborative approach to risk assessment, particularly an approach in which risk factors are thoroughly explained and the client contributes to identification of their most relevant treatment needs, provides clients with a sense that they have some control over their assessment and subsequent treatment, in contrast to feeling that assessment and intervention are something done "to them" (Attrill & Liell, 2007; Shingler & Mann, 2006). A structured approach to matching client risk and needs to treatment level can contribute to a sense of "fairness" within risk assessment, which is another area identified as important to offenders (Attrill & Liell, 2007).

While little research has examined offenders' perceptions of risk assessment, Attrill and Leill (2007) interviewed 60 adult sexual offenders regarding their views of risk assessment. A consistent finding during these discussions was offenders' concerns about the level of skill and training of the professionals completing the assessments. The identification of relevant risk factors that are empirically related to recidivism combined with the defined weighting of those risk factors offers an advantage to actuarial measures in this respect. The structured system for weighting the items can make it clear to the client that the assessor's personal biases, level of experience, and skills do not directly influence the assessed level of risk. This is in contrast to SPJ tools that encourage professionals to rely on their experience and skills to examine the risk factors present and determine an overall risk level without a specific structure for combining risk factors (Skeem & Monahan, 2011). The structure associated with actuarial tools, however, has the potential to provide offenders with some sense of consistency, transparency, and evenhandedness to the outcome regardless of the real or perceived qualifications of the assessor.

Critics of actuarial measures note that the specified structure of actuarial tools necessarily limits the "individuality" of risk assessments; this concern was voiced by offenders themselves (Attrill & Liell, 2007). However, as noted earlier in this chapter, the move in recent years toward the integration of dynamic risk assessment with static risk factors provides room for individualization within the overall risk assessment while maintaining the consistency necessary for defensible integrity in implementation. Further, dynamic risk factors allow for more attention to some positive attributes or strengths, which may foster the therapeutic relationship and help in establishing approach rather than avoidance treatment goals (Mann, Webster, Schofield, & Marshall, 2004). As such we would argue that actuarial tools, when implemented well, have the advantage of providing the structure and consistency necessary for strong program integrity and limiting variability in assessor experience and knowledge while still allowing for individuality in the overall assessment.

The Program Level

As described in the first half of this chapter, actuarial risk assessment has evolved as an alternative to UCJ, widely recognized as less accurate, unreliable, and non-replicable. In fact, concerns about the predictive validity of clinical judgment have resulted in the mandated use of actuarial measures within some organizations (e.g., SIR-R used at intake within Correctional Services of Canada; Structured Assessment of Risk and Need, HM Prison Service) and legal jurisdictions. Critics of UCJ note that given its subjective nature, it is difficult to standardize judgments made by a single clinician over time let alone to standardize judgments made by multiple clinicians within one setting. Larger practices and organizations that employ multiple clinicians are often faced with considerable variability in terms of prior training and experience among staff. In more isolated or rural areas, clinicians may be called upon to provide assessments on rare occasions, meaning they bring limited knowledge and expertise to the assessment. The experience and knowledge required to appropriately and effectively use structured professional judgment tools may simply not exist or be realistic in these circumstances.

An advantage of actuarial measures as previously stated is they provide clear direction regarding not only the relevant factors but how to combine those factors into an assessed risk level. Within an intervention program, the detailed manuals that come with many actuarial tools contribute to consistency in application, potentially serve as a guide against which assessments can be audited, provide a training base for new employees, and can minimize program "drift" that may otherwise occur when clinicians are left to make decisions without structured direction. Not only do the manuals associated with actuarial measures provide a framework for appropriate training and skill acquisition for clinicians involved in an evidence-based program, but clinicians report enhanced confidence in their assessments based on actuarial measures (Dr. A. Schweighofer personal communication, 2014). In Neal and Grisso's (2014) survey, the second most common reason cited by psychologists and psychiatrists for using structured tools in risk assessment after ensuring an evidence-based method was "to improve the credibility of my assessment." The third most common reason was "to standardize the assessment" indicating that clinicians themselves perceive value to ensuring that risk assessments have consistent meaning across clinicians, sites, and organizations. Thus there are substantial advantages to the inclusion of actuarial tools in terms of training, consistency, and implementation integrity within evidence-based programs.

The Organizational Level

Leschied, Bernfeld, and Farrington (2001) note that there is political and sometimes philosophical opposition to "what works" in effective correctional interventions. Managerial doubts can undermine the impact and effectiveness of a program.

A good defense to this is to rely on tools with heavy empirical support and demonstrated consistency and replicability; this leaves less room for argument. Actuarial risk assessment meets four goals critical to any organization managing offenders: (1) they identify the level of risk for an individual within a group or population of individuals, (2) they identify contributing salient risk factors that are appropriate targets for intervention (assuming dynamic risk assessment is used), (3) they identify strategies that manage or minimize risk, and (4) they communicate risk information (Mills, Kroner, & Morgan, 2011).

The identification of risk level within a population, along with the contributing risk factors, appropriate treatment targets, and strategies for managing risk, has the potential to directly impact policy in relation to management and intervention of offenders within an organization. A clear management framework and consistent structure for handling offenders within an organization (based on their risk assessment results) should result in time and resource efficiencies. Additionally, a standardized approach facilitates the identification of, planning for, and streamlining of staff training needs. Good quality staff development and training along with subsequent supervision can balance inequality in prior qualifications, knowledge, and skill level among staff members (Mann, Fernandez, & Ware, 2011).

Additionally, the fourth goal of risk communication is critical to the ethical and appropriate management of offenders within an organization. Mills and Kroner (2006) found that risk judgments given using high, moderate, and low categorizations were overestimated, even when the base rate of offending was provided. They note that subjective risk categories lack "solid empirical meaning" and may cause under- or over-estimates of risk, resulting in suboptimal resource allocation to offenders managed within the organization. As noted earlier, actuarial measures typically provide multiple methods to quantify risk, including recidivism estimates, percentiles, and risk ratios along with nominal risk categories. Thus an advantage to actuarial measures is that they provide a common language for risk communication. With appropriate training risk communication will hold the same meaning for everyone within the organization, including decision makers, and directly impact resource allocation.

The Societal Level

Controversy in the use of actuarial risk assessment has focused primarily on its use for decisions related to incarceration (e.g., civil commitment) and release (e.g., parole). There is less controversy over the use of risk assessment as part of treatment planning or about the identification of treatment needs using dynamic risk assessment measures, as is primarily discussed above. There is very little empirical research on the consumption of actuarial risk estimates generally (Scurich, Monahan, & John, 2012). Identified concerns include that decision makers may be misled to think that actuarial tools are more precise than they in fact are (Campbell, 2007) and consequently overly or inappropriately influence decisions made that impact offenders' lives directly. However, this concern does not appear to be supported in recent research. For example, offenders referred for full SVP evaluations tend to have higher risk-measure scores than those who are not referred; mental health evaluators are more likely to conclude that an offender meets the criteria for civil commitment when risk scores are high; and attorneys are more likely to select cases for trial when risk measures are high (Boccaccini et al., 2009; Levenson, 2004; Murrie, Boccaccini, Rufino, & Caperton, 2012) suggesting that actuarial risk scores play an appropriate and essential role in determining who are the judges and jurors eventually (see Boccaccini, Turner, Murrie, Henderson, and Chevalier, 2013).

Once at trial, however, research suggests that mock jurors asked to make decisions in SVP cases are more likely influenced by testimony based on clinical judgment than risk assessment instruments and do not perceive actuarial testimony to be any more scientific than clinical testimony (Krauss, McCabe, & Lieberman, 2012; McCabe, Krauss, & Lieberman, 2010). Similarly, Boccaccini et al. (2013) found that risk-measure scores had little impact on real jurors surveyed after trial in Texas SVP cases. The authors posited that jurors may perceive that most offenders who are eligible for SVP commitment (most of whom are identified through actuarial measures) are "dangerous enough" or that jurors have retributive motives rather than being concerned with "protecting the public." Regardless of the explanation, it appears that the use of actuarial measures serves an important purpose at the front end of this process (i.e., helping to ensure that the most restrictive measures are applied to the higher risk offenders) while idiosyncratic features may have more influence during the actual legal proceedings. Neal and Grisso (2014) make the interesting argument that current forensic training that encourages a too flexible approach to assessment may be a liability in that it interferes with the ability of courts to appropriately use risk assessment information as they are "required to become familiar with a bewilderingly wide range of tools" (p. 1417). The authors suggest that this could be minimized if clinicians are trained to select tools that are both appropriate to the referral question and have the best psychometric properties.

As we have noted previously, to be valuable risk assessment results must be communicated in a clear and appreciable manner to consumers (Heilbrun, Dvoskin, Hart, & McNeil, 1999). A reliable and valid risk assessment is of no use and in fact may be "worse than useless" if decision makers misapprehend the results (Heilbrun et al., 1999, p. 94). Interestingly, one study found that "unpacking" actuarial violence (i.e., explicitly articulating the extent to which individual risk factors impact the overall risk) appeared to aid subjects identified as "innumerate" with interpreting the results of actuarial risk assessments and more effectively applying the group-level risk estimates to the individual case (Scurich et al., 2012). Given the stakes involved in legal dispositions, we would argue that experts have a particular ethical obligation when communicating actuarial risk assessment results in high-stakes circumstances to precede the sharing of results with appropriate education on the meaning of risk.

Conclusions

While controversy remains regarding the use of actuarial risk assessment, actuarial measures continue to provide the most accurate available information, including for legal decision-making (Heilbrun, 1997). Critics of actuarial tools argue that because actuarial tools do not account for individual differences within their schemes, clinicians are unable to modify level of risk based on mitigating factors, and therefore there is a substantial margin of error inherent in actuarial measures (Hart & Cooke, 2013; Hart, Michie, & Cooke, 2007). Please note, however, that the statistics employed by Hart and colleagues (2007) cannot be used to support their position that group data cannot meaningfully be used to support inferences about individuals (e.g., Hanson & Howard, 2010; G. T. Harris, Rice, & Quinsey, 2008; Mossman & Sellke, 2007; Scurich & John, 2012). Also, it remains to be determined if the posited limitations on individuality produce greater error than clinical overrides based on individual items as applied in SPJ. Further, individuality can be incorporated (at least to some extent) into risk assessment by adding actuarial measures of dynamic risk factors and ensuring that the risk assessment process involves collaboration with the offender. Good risk assessment should use risk estimates obtained by actuarial methods and implemented with integrity, as an "anchor" alongside other measures that include factors that would allow for risk management. Actuarial measures do not replace a clinician's integration and synthesis of information and selection and implementation of a plan of therapeutic action; rather, they can contribute to each aspect of the process. In other words, "scoring an actuarial risk tool is not a risk assessment" (Hanson, 2009, p. 174).

While some of the advantages of actuarial scales described in the present chapter are currently being realized, not all of them are necessarily being maximized by clinicians, programs, or organizations where actuarial risk measures are implemented. When asked, offenders often report a poor understanding of risk assessment, the benefits to them, and little sense of control or impact on the process (Attrill & Liell, 2007). Further, although many newer risk assessment tools include dynamic risk factors, there continues to be a lack of focus on strength or protective factors (Wilson, Desmarais, Nicholls, & Brink, 2010) in the risk assessment process. Wilson et al. note that strengths are not just the opposite of deficits, but capture unique information. This appears to be the next step in risk assessment research.

We also acknowledge that while the importance of consistency and reliability in risk assessment cannot be overemphasized, actuarial measures work best when the offender being assessed possesses characteristics similar to the development sample or validation research of the measure. Regardless of the measure chosen (whether by the clinician or as part of a standardized program or mandated by legislation), it is up to the clinician to ensure that measures used are appropriate to the client being assessed. Actuarial measures are not appropriately applied to every client, and there are circumstances where the current state of the research means that clinical judgment remains the only option. However, in the majority of cases, anchored risk assessment as part of a comprehensive "case conceptualization" should be used to inform intervention at a more individualized level. In our estimation, the integrated-actuarial approach to risk assessment, when implemented with thought and integrity, holds some valuable clinical advantages while leaving sufficient room for individualization.

References

Ægisdóttir, S., White, M. J., Spengler, P. M., Maugherman, A. S., Anderson, L. A., Cook, R. S., ... Rush, J. D. (2006). The meta-analysis of clinical judgment project: Fifty-Six years of accumulated research on clinical versus statistical prediction. *The Counseling Psychologist, 34*, 341–382. doi:10.1177/0011000005285875

Aiken, L. R. (1985). *Psychological testing and assessment* (5th ed.). Newton, MA: Allyn and Bacon.

Alexander, J., & Austin, J. (1992). *Handbook for evaluating objective prison classification systems*. San Francisco, CA: National Council on Crime and Delinquency.

Alison, L. J., & Stein, K. L. (2001). Vicious circles: Accounts of stranger sexual assault reflect abusive variants of conventional interactions. *The Journal of Forensic Psychiatry, 12*(3), 515–538. doi:10.1080/09585180127391.

Altman, D. G., Vergouwe, Y., Royston, P., & Moons, K. G. M. (2009). Prognosis and prognostic research: Validating a prognostic model. *BMJ [British Medical Journal], 338*, 1432–1435. doi:10.2307/25671796.

American Psychological Association. (2013). Specialty guidelines for forensic psychology. *American Psychologist, 68*, 7–19.

Anderson, D., & Hanson, R. K. (2010). Static-99: An actuarial tool to assess risk of sexual and violent recidivism among sexual offenders. In R. K. Otto & K. S. Douglas (Eds.), *Handbook of violence risk assessment* (pp. 251–267). New York, NY: Taylor & Francis.

Andrews, D. A., & Bonta, J. (2010). *The psychology of criminal conduct*. Cincinnati, OH: Anderson Publishing Co.

Andrews, D. A., Bonta, J., & Wormith, J. S. (2006). The recent past and near future of risk and/or need assessment. *Crime & Delinquency, 52*, 7–27. doi:10.1177/0011128705281756.

Andrews, D. A., & Dowden, C. (2005). Managing correctional treatment for reduced recidivism: A meta-analytic review of programme integrity. *Journal of Legal and Criminological Psychology, 10*, 173–187. doi:10.1348/135532505X36723.

Andrews, D. A., Zinger, I., Hoge, R. D., Bonta, J., Gendreau, P., & Cullen, F. (1990). Does correctional treatment work? A clinically relevant and psychologically informed meta-analysis. *Criminology, 28*(3), 369–404.

Archer, R. P., Buffington-Vollum, J. K., Stredny, R. V., & Handel, R. W. (2006). A survey of psychological test use patterns among forensic psychologists. *Journal of Personality Assessment, 87*, 84–94.

Association for the Treatment of Sexual Abusers. (2014). *ATSA practice guidelines for assessment, treatment interventions, and management strategies for male adult sexual abusers*. Beaverton, OR: Professional Issues Committee, ATSA.

Attrill, G., & Liell, G. (2007). Offenders' views on risk assessment. In N. Padfield (Ed.), *Who to release? Parole, fairness and criminal justice* (pp. 191–201). Cullompton, UK: Willan.

Austin, J., Johnson, K. D., & Weitzer, R. (2005). *Alternatives to the secure detention and confinement of juvenile offenders*. Washington, DC: Office of Justice Programs.

Babchishin, K. M. (2013). *Sex offenders do change on risk-relevant propensities: evidence from a longitudinal study of the ACUTE-2007* (Doctoral dissertation). Retrieved from Proquest Dissertations and Theses Global. (MR60297)

Babchishin, K. M., Hanson, R. K., & Blais, J. (2015). A brief scale for predicting violent and general recidivism among sexual offenders. *Sexual Abuse: A Journal of Research and Treatment.* Advance online publication. doi:10.1177/1079063215569544

Babchishin, K. M., Hanson, R. K., & Helmus, L. (2012a). Communicating risk for sex offenders: Risk ratios for Static-2002R. *Sexual Offender Treatment, 7*(2), 1–12.

Babchishin, K. M., Hanson, R. K., & Helmus, L. (2012b). Even highly correlated measures can add incrementally to predicting recidivism among sex offenders. *Assessment, 19*, 442–461. doi:10.1177/1073191112458312.

Babchishin, K. M., & Helmus, L. M. (2015). The influence of base rates on correlations: An evaluation of proposed alternative effect sizes with real-world dichotomous data. Behavior Research Methods. Advance online publication. doi:10.3758/s13428-015-0627-7.

Beggs, S. M., & Grace, R. C. (2010). Assessment of dynamic risk factors: An independent validation study of the Violence Risk Scale: Sexual Offender Version. *Sexual Abuse: A Journal of Research and Treatment, 22*, 234–251. doi:10.1177/1079063210369014.

Beggs, S. M., & Grace, R. C. (2011). Treatment gain for sexual offenders against children predicts reduced recidivism: A comparative validity study. *Journal of Consulting and Clinical Psychology, 79*, 182–192. doi:10.1037/a0022900.

Bennell, C., Alison, L. J., Stein, K. L., Alison, E. K., & Canter, D. V. (2001). Sexual offenses against children as the abusive exploitation of conventional adult-child relationships. *Journal of Social and Personal Relationships, 18*(2), 155–171. doi:http://dx.doi.org/10.1177/0265407501182001.

Bernfeld, G. A., Blase, K. A., & Fixsen, D. L. (1990). Towards a unified perspective on human service delivery systems: Application of the Teaching-Family Model. In R. J. McMahon & R. D. Peters (Eds.), *Behavior disorders of adolescents: Research, intervention and policy in clinical and school settings* (pp. 191–205). New York, NY: Plenum.

Blais, J., & Forth, A. E. (2014). Prosecution-retained versus court-appointed experts: Comparing and contrasting risk assessment reports in preventative detention hearings. *Law and Human Behavior, 38*, 531–543. doi:10.1037/lhb0000082.

Boccaccini, M. T., Murrie, D. C., Caperton, J. D., & Hawes, S. W. (2009). Field validity of the Static-99 and MnSOST-R among sex offenders evaluated for civil commitment as sexually violent predators. *Psychology, Public Policy, and Law, 15*, 278–314. doi:10.1037/a0017232.

Boccaccini, M. T., Turner, D. B., Murrie, D. C., Henderson, C. E., & Chevalier, C. (2013). Do scores from risk measures matter to jurors? *Psychology, Public Policy, and Law, 19*, 259–269. doi:10.1037/a0031354.

Boer, D. P., Wilson, R. J., Gauthier, C. M., & Hart, S. D. (1997). Assessing risk of sexual violence: Guidelines for clinical practice. In C. D. Webster & M. A. Jackson (Eds.), *Impulsivity: Theory, assessment, and treatment* (pp. 326–342). New York, NY: Guilford Press.

Bonta, J. (1996). Risk-needs assessment and treatment. In A. T. Harland (Ed.), *Choosing correctional options that work: Defining the demand and evaluating the supply* (pp. 18–32). Thousand Oaks, CA: Sage.

Bonta, J. (2002). Offender risk assessment: Guidelines for selection and use. *Criminal Justice & Behavior, 29*(4), 355–379.

Bonta, J., Law, M., & Hanson, R. K. (1998). The prediction of criminal and violent recidivism among mentally disordered offenders: A meta-analysis. *Psychological Bulletin, 123*, 123–142. doi:10.1037/0033-2909.123.2.123.

Bonta, J., & Motiuk, L. L. (1990). Classification to halfway houses: A quasi-experimental evaluation. *Criminology, 23*(3), 497–506.

Brouillette-Alarie, S., Babchishin, K. M., Hanson, R. K., & Helmus, L. M. (2015). Latent constructs of static risk scales for the prediction of sexual recidivism: A 3-factor solution. *Assessment.* Advance online publication. doi:10.1177/1073191114568114

Campbell, T. W. (2007). *Assessing sex offenders: Problems and pitfalls* (2nd ed.). Springfield, IL: Charles Thomas.

Canter, D. V. (1994). *Criminal shadows.* London: Harper Collins.

Canter, D. V. (2004). Offender profiling and investigative psychology. *Journal of Investigative Psychology and Offender Profiling, 1*(1), 1–15. doi:10.1002/jip.7.

Canter, D. V., Bennell, C., Alison, L. J., & Reddy, S. (2003). Differentiating sex offences: A behaviorally based thematic classification of stranger rapes. *Behavioral Sciences & the Law, 21*(2), 157–174. doi:http://dx.doi.org/10.1002/bsl.526.

Canter, D. V., & Heritage, R. (1990). A multivariate model of sexual offence behaviour: Developments in 'offender profiling'. *The Journal of Forensic Psychiatry, 1*(2), 185–212. doi:10.1080/09585189008408469.

Canter, D. V., Hughes, D., & Kirby, S. (1998). Paedophilia: Pathology, criminality, or both? The development of a multivariate model of offence behaviour in child sexual abuse. *The Journal of Forensic Psychiatry, 9*(3), 532–555. doi:10.1080/09585189808405372.

Chevalier, C., Boccaccini, M. T., Murrie, D. C., & Varela, J. G. (2014). Static-99R reporting practices in sexually violent predator cases: Does norm selection reflect adversarial allegiance? *Law and Human Behavior*. Advance online publication. doi:10.1037/lhb0000114

Cortina, J. M. (1993). What is coefficient alpha? An examination of theory and applications. *Journal of Applied Psychology, 78*, 98–104. doi:10.1037//0021-9010.78.1.98.

Crawford, J. R., & Garthwaite, P. H. (2009). Percentiles please: The case for expressing neuropsychological test scores and accompanying confidence limits as percentile ranks. *The Clinical Neuropsychologist, 23*, 193–204. doi:10.1080/13854040801968450.

Cronbach, L. J. (1951). Coefficient alpha and the internal structure of tests. *Psychometrika, 16*, 297–334. doi:10.1007/BF02310555.

Dahle, K.-P., Biedermann, J., Lehmann, R. J. B., & Gallasch-Nemitz, F. (2014). The development of the crime scene behavior risk measure for sexual offense recidivism. *Law and Human Behavior, 38*, 569–579. doi:10.1037/lhb0000088.

Dawes, R. M., Faust, D., & Meehl, P. E. (1989). Clinical versus actuarial judgment. *Science, 243*, 1668–1674. doi:10.1126/science.2648573.

Doren, D. M. (2004). Stability of the interpretative risk percentages for the RRASOR and Static-99. *Sexual Abuse: A Journal of Research and Treatment, 16*, 25–36. doi:10.1177/107906320401600102.

Dowden, D., & Andrews, D. A. (2004). The importance of staff practice in delivering effective correctional treatment: A meta-analytic review of core correctional practice. *International Journal of Offender Therapy and Comparative Criminology, 48*, 203–214. doi:10.1177/0306624X03257765.

Eher, R., Matthes, A., Schilling, F., Haubner-MacLean, T., & Rettenberger, M. (2012). Dynamic risk assessment in sexual offenders using STABLE-2000 and the STABLE-2007: An investigation of predictive and incremental validity. *Sexual Abuse: A Journal of Research and Treatment, 24*, 5–28. doi:10.1177/1079063211403164.

Elmore, J. G., & Gigerenzer, G. (2005). Benign breast disease: The risk of communicating risk. *New England Journal of Medicine, 353*, 297–299. doi:10.1056/NEJMe058111.

Farrington, D. P., & Ttofi, M. M. (2011). Protective and promotive factors in the development of offending. In T. Bliesener, A. Beelmann, & M. Stemmler (Eds.), *Antisocial behavior and crime: Contributions of developmental and evaluation research to prevention and intervention* (pp. 71–88). Cambridge, MA: Hogrefe Publishing.

Fernandez, Y. (2008, October). *An examination of the inter-rater reliability of the Static-99 and STABLE-2007*. Poster presented at the 27th Annual Conference of the Association for the Treatment of Sexual Abusers, Atlanta, GA.

Fernandez, Y., Harris, A. J. R., Hanson, R. K., & Sparks, J. (2014). *STABLE-2007 coding manual – revised 2014*. Unpublished report. Ottawa, ON: Public Safety Canada.

Flores, A. W., Russell, A. L., Latessa, E. J., & Travis, L. F. (2005). Evidence of professionalism or quackery: Measuring practitioner awareness of risk/need factors and effective treatment strategies. *Federal Probation, 69*, 9–14.

Gail, M. H., & Pfeiffer, R. M. (2005). On criteria for evaluating models of absolute risk. *Biostatistics, 6*, 227–239. doi:10.1093/biostatistics/kxi005.

Goodwill, A. M., Alison, L. J., & Beech, A. R. (2009). What works in offender profiling? A comparison of typological, thematic, and multivariate models. *Behavioral Sciences & the Law, 27*, 507–529. doi:10.1002/bsl.867.

Grove, W. M., Zald, D. H., Lebow, B. S., Snitz, B. E., & Nelson, C. (2000). Clinical versus mechanical prediction: A meta-analysis. *Psychological Assessment, 12*, 19–30. doi:10.1037//1040-3590.12.1.19.

Häkkänen, H., Lindlöf, P., & Santtila, P. (2004). Crime scene actions and offender characteristics in a sample of Finnish stranger rapes. *Journal of Investigative Psychology and Offender Profiling, 1*(1), 17–32. doi:10.1002/jip.1.

Häkkänen, H., Puolakka, P., & Santtila, P. (2004). Crime scene actions and offender characteristics in arsons. *Legal and Criminological Psychology, 9*(2), 197–214. doi:10.1348/1355325041719392.

Hanson, R. K. (2005). Twenty years of progress in violence risk assessment. *Journal of Interpersonal Violence, 20*, 212–217. doi:10.1177/0886260504267740.

Hanson, R. K. (2009). The psychological assessment of risk for crime and violence. *Canadian Psychology, 50*, 172–182. doi:10.1037/a0015726.

Hanson, R. K., Babchishin, K. M., Helmus, L., & Thornton, D. (2013). Quantifying the relative risk of sex offenders: Risk ratios for Static-99R. *Sexual Abuse: A Journal of Research and Treatment, 25*, 482–515. doi:10.1177/107906321246906.

Hanson, R. K., & Bussière, M. T. (1998). Predicting relapse: A meta-analysis of sexual offender recidivism studies. *Journal of Consulting and Clinical Psychology, 66*, 348–362. doi:10.1037/0022-006X.66.2.348.

Hanson, R. K., & Harris, A. J. R. (2000). Where should we intervene? Dynamic predictors of sexual offense recidivism. *Criminal Justice and Behavior, 27*, 6–35. doi:10.1177/0093854800 027001002.

Hanson, R. K., & Harris, A. J. R. (2013). Criminogenic needs of sexual offenders on community supervision. In L. A. Craig, L. Dixon, & T. A. Gannon (Eds.), *What works in offender rehabilitation: An evidenced-based approach to assessment and treatment* (pp. 421–435). Chichester, UK: Wiley-Blackwell.

Hanson, R. K., Harris, A. J. R., Scott, T.-L., & Helmus, L. (2007). *Assessing the risk of sexual offenders on community supervision: The Dynamic Supervision Project*. Ottawa, ON: Public Safety Canada.

Hanson, R. K., Helmus, L.-M., & Harris, A. J. R. (2015). Assessing the Risk and Needs of Supervised Sexual Offenders: A Prospective Study Using STABLE-2007, Static-99R, and Static-2002R. *Criminal Justice and Behavior, 42*(12), 1205–1224. doi:10.1177/0093854815602094.

Hanson, R. K., Helmus, L., & Thornton, D. (2010). Predicting recidivism among sexual offenders: A multi-site study of Static-2002. *Law and Human Behavior, 34*, 198–211. doi:10.1007/ s10979-009-9180-1.

Hanson, R. K., & Howard, P. D. (2010). Individual confidence intervals do not inform decision-makers about the accuracy of risk assessment evaluations. *Law and Human Behavior, 34*, 275–281. doi:10.1007/s10979-010-9227-3.

Hanson, R. K., Lloyd, C. D., Helmus, L., & Thornton, D. (2012). Developing non-arbitrary metrics for risk communication: Percentile ranks for the Static-99/R and Static-2002/R sexual offender risk tools. *International Journal of Forensic Mental Health, 11*, 9–23. doi:10.1080/14999013. 2012.667511.

Hanson, R. K., Lunetta, A., Phenix, A., Neeley, J., & Epperson, D. (2014). The field validity of Static-99/R sex offender risk assessment tool in California. *Journal of Threat Assessment and Management, 1*, 102–117. doi:10.1037/tam0000014.

Hanson, R. K., & Morton-Bourgon, K. E. (2005). The characteristics of persistent sexual offenders: A meta-analysis of recidivism studies. *Journal of Consulting and Clinical Psychology, 73*, 1154–1163. doi:10.1037/0022-006X.73.6.1154.

Hanson, R. K., & Morton-Bourgon, K. E. (2009). The accuracy of recidivism risk assessments for sexual offenders: A meta-analysis of 118 prediction studies. *Psychological Assessment, 21*, 1–21. doi:10.1037/a0014421.

Hanson, R. K., & Thornton, D. (2000). Improving risk assessments for sex offenders: A comparison of three actuarial scales. *Law and Human Behavior, 24*, 119–136. doi:10.1023/A:1005482921333.

Hanson, R. K., Thornton, D., Helmus, L., & Babchishin, K. M. (2015). What sexual recidivism rates are associated with Static-99R and Static-2002R scores? *Sexual Abuse: A Journal of Research and Treatment*. Advance online publication. doi:10.1177/1079063215574710

Hare, R. D. (2003). *The Hare Psychopathy Checklist-Revised technical manual* (2nd ed.). Toronto, ON, Canada: Multi-Health Systems.

Harris, A. J. R., & Hanson, R. K. (2010). Clinical, actuarial and dynamic risk assessment of sexual offenders: Why do things keep changing? *Journal of Sexual Aggression, 16*, 296–310. doi:10.1080/13552600.2010.494772.

Harris, A., Phenix, A., Hanson, R. K., & Thornton, D. (2003). *Static-99: Coding rules revised 2003*. Ottawa, ON: Solicitor General Canada.

Harris, G. T., & Rice, M. E. (2015). Progress in violence risk appraisal and communication: A commentary on hypotheses and evidence. *Behavioral Sciences and the Law, 33*, 128–145. doi:10.1002/bsl.2157.

Harris, G. T., Rice, M. E., Quinsey, V. L., Lalumière, M. L., Boer, D., & Lang, C. (2003). A multi-site comparison of actuarial risk instruments for sex offenders. *Psychological Assessment, 15*, 413–425.

Harris, G. T., Rice, M. E., & Quinsey, V. L. (2008). Shall evidence-based risk appraisal be abandoned? *British Journal of Psychiatry, 192*, 154. (expanded version at http://bjp.rcpsych.org/cgi/eletters/190/49/s60#5674).

Hart, S. D., & Cooke, D. J. (2013). Another look at the (im-) precision of individual risk estimates made using actuarial risk assessment instruments. *Behavioral Sciences & the Law, 31*, 81–102. doi:10.1002/bsl.2049.

Hart, S. D., Michie, C., & Cooke, D. J. (2007). Precision of actuarial risk assessment instruments: Evaluating the 'margins of error' of group v. individual predictions of violence. *The British Journal of Psychiatry, 190*, s60–s65.

Heilbrun, K. (1997). Prediction versus management models relevant to risk assessment: The importance of legal decision-making context. *Law and Human Behavior, 21*, 347–359. doi:10.1023/A:1024851017947.

Heilbrun, K., Dvoskin, J., Hart, S., & McNeil, D. (1999). Violence risk communication: Implications for research, policy, and practice. *Health, Risk & Society, 1*, 91–106.

Helmus, L., Babchishin, K. M., & Hanson, R. K. (2013). The predictive accuracy of the Risk Matrix 2000: A meta-analysis. *Sexual Offender Treatment, 8*(2), 1–24.

Helmus, L., & Hanson, R. K. (2013). *STABLE-2007: Updated recidivism rates* (includes combinations with Static-99R, Static-2002R, and Risk Matrix 2000). Unpublished report. Ottawa, ON: Public Safety Canada.

Helmus, L., Hanson, R. K., Babchishin, K. M., & Thornton, D. (2014). Sex offender risk assessment with the Risk Matrix 2000: Validation and guidelines for combining with the STABLE-2007. *Journal of Sexual Aggression*. Advance online publication. doi:10.1080/13552600.2013.870241

Helmus, L., Hanson, R. K., Thornton, D., Babchishin, K. M., & Harris, A. J. R. (2012). Absolute recidivism rates predicted by Static-99R and Static-2002R sex offender risk assessment tools vary across samples: A meta-analysis. *Criminal Justice and Behavior, 39*, 1148–1171. doi:10.1177/0093854812443648.

Helmus, L., & Thornton, D. (2014). The MATS-1 risk assessment scale: Summary of methodological concerns and an empirical validation. *Sexual Abuse: A Journal of Research and Treatment*. Advance online publication. doi:10.1177/1079063214529801

Helmus, L., Thornton, D., Hanson, R. K., & Babchishin, K. M. (2012). Improving the predictive accuracy of Static-99 and Static-2002 with older sex offenders: Revised age weights. *Sexual Abuse: A Journal of Research and Treatment, 24*, 64–101. doi:10.1177/1079063211409951.

Hilton, N. Z. (2014). Actuarial assessment in serial intimate partner violence: Comment on Cook, Murray, Amat and Hart. *Journal of Threat Assessment and Management, 1*, 87–92. doi:10.1037/tam0000013.

Hilton, N. Z., Carter, A. M., Harris, G. T., & Sharpe, A. J. (2008). Does using nonnumerical terms to describe risk aid violence risk communication? Clinician agreement and decision making. *Journal of Interpersonal Violence, 23*, 171–188.

Hilton, N. Z., Scurich, N., & Helmus, L. M. (2015). Communicating the risk of violent and offending behavior: Review and introduction to special issue. *Behavioral Sciences and the Law, 33,* 1–18. doi:10.1002/bsl.2160.

Hunsley, J. D., & Mash, E. J. (2010). The role of assessment in evidence-based practice. In M. M. Antony & D. H. Barlow (Eds.), *Handbook of assessment and treatment planning for psychological disorders* (2nd ed.). New York, NY: Guilford Press.

Hunsley, J., & Meyer, G. J. (2003). The incremental validity of psychological testing and assessment: Conceptual, methodological, and statistical issues. *Psychological Assessment, 15,* 446–455. doi:10.1037/1040-3590.15.4.446.

Interstate Commission for Adult Offender Supervision. (2007). *Sex offender assessment information survey.* (ICAOS Documents No. 4-2007).

Jackson, R. L., & Hess, D. T. (2007). Evaluation for civil commitment of sex offenders: A survey of experts. *Sexual Abuse: A Journal of Research and Treatment, 19,* 425–448. doi:10.1177/107906320701900407.

Kahneman, D. (2011). *Thinking fast and slow.* New York, NY: Macmillan.

Kahneman, D., & Klein, G. (2009). Conditions for intuitive expertise: A failure to disagree. *American Psychologist, 64,* 515–526. doi:10.1037/a0016755.

Krauss, D. A., McCabe, J., & Lieberman, J. (2012). Dangerously misunderstood: Representative jurors' reactions to expert testimony on future dangerousness in a sexual violent predator trial. *Psychology, Public Policy, and Law, 18,* 18–49.

Kropp, P. R., & Gibas, A. (2010). The Spousal Assault Risk Assessment Guide (SARA). In R. K. Otto & K. S. Douglas (Eds.), *Handbook of violence risk assessment* (pp. 227–250). New York, NY: Routledge.

Kropp, P. R., & Hart, S. D. (2000). The Spousal Assault Risk Assessment (SARA) Guide: Reliability and validity in adult male offenders. *Law and Human Behavior, 24,* 101–118. doi:10.1023/A:1005430904495.

Lehmann, R. J. B., Goodwill, A. M., Gallasch-Nemitz, F., Biedermann, J., & Dahle, K.-P. (2013). Applying crime scene analysis to the prediction of sexual recidivism in stranger rapes. *Law and Human Behavior, 37,* 241–254. doi:10.1037/lhb0000015.

Lehmann, R. J. B., Goodwill, A. M., Hanson, R. K., & Dahle, K.-P. (2014). Crime scene behaviors indicate risk-relevant propensities of child molesters. *Criminal Justice and Behavior, 41*(8), 1008–1028. doi:10.1177/0093854814521807.

Lehmann, R. J. B., Goodwill, A. M., Hanson, R. K., & Dahle, K.-P. (2015). *Acquaintance rape: Applying crime scene analysis to the prediction of sexual recidivism.* Sexual Abuse: A Journal of Research and Treatment. Advance online publication. doi:10.1177/1079063215569542.

Lehmann, R. J. B., Hanson, R. K., Babchishin, K. M., Gallasch-Nemitz, F., Biedermann, J., & Dahle, K.-P. (2013). Interpreting multiple risk scales for sex offenders: Evidence for averaging. *Psychological Assessment, 25,* 1019–1024. doi:10.1037/a0033098.

Lehmann, R. J. B., Thornton, D., Helmus, L. M., & Hanson, R. K. (2015). *Developing non-arbitrary metrics for risk communication: Norms for the Risk Matrix 2000.* Unpublished manuscript.

Leschied, A. W., Bernfeld, G. A., & Farrington, D. P. (2001). Implementation issues. In G. A. Bernfeld, D. P. Farrington, & A. W. Leschied (Eds.), *Offender rehabilitation in practice: Implementing and evaluating effective programs* (pp. 3–24). Chichester, UK: Wiley.

Levenson, J. S. (2004). Sexual predator civil commitment: A comparison of selected and released offenders. *International Journal of Offender Therapy and Comparative Criminology, 48,* 638–648. doi:10.1177/0306624X04265089.

Lösel, F., & Farrington, D. P. (2012). Direct protective and buffering protective factors in the development of youth violence. *American Journal of Preventive Medicine, 43*(suppl 1), S8–S23. doi:10.1016/j.amepre.2012.04.029.

Lowenkamp, C., Pealer, J., Smith, P., & Latessa, E. J. (2006). Adhering to the risk and need principles: Does it matter for supervision-based programs? *Federal Probation, 70,* 3–8.

Mann, R., Fernandez, Y., & Ware, J. (2011, November). *Managing sex offender treatment programmes: A professional development workshop for managers and supervisors.* Full day pre-conference workshop presented at the Association for the Treatment of Sexual Abusers, 30th Annual Research and Treatment Conference, Toronto, ON, Canada.

Mann, R. E., Hanson, R. K., & Thornton, D. (2010). Assessing risk for sexual recidivism: Some proposals on the nature of psychologically meaningful risk factors. *Sexual Abuse: A Journal of Research and Treatment, 22,* 191–217. doi:10.1177/1079063210366039.

Mann, R. E., Webster, S. D., Schofield, C., & Marshall, W. L. (2004). Approach versus avoidance goals in relapse prevention with sexual offenders. *Sexual Abuse: A Journal of Research and Treatment, 16,* 65–75. doi:10.1023/B:SEBU.0000006285.73534.57.

McCabe, J., Krauss, D. A., & Lieberman, J. (2010). Reality check: A comparison of college students and community samples of mock jurors in a simulated sexual violent predator civil commitment. *Behavioral Sciences & the Law, 28,* 730–750. doi:10.1002/bsl.902.

McGrath, R. J., Cumming, G. F., Burchard, B. L., Zeoli, S., & Ellerby, E. (2010). *Current practices and emerging trends in sexual abuser management: The Safer Society 2009 North American Survey.* Brandon, VT: Safer Society Press.

Meehl, P. E. (1954). *Clinical versus statistical prediction: A theoretical analysis and a review of the evidence.* Minneapolis, MN: University of Minnesota Press.

Mills, J. F., Jones, M. N., & Kroner, D. G. (2005). An examination of the generalizability of the LSI-R and VRAG probability bins. *Criminal Justice and Behavior, 32,* 565–585. doi:10.1177/0093854805278417.

Mills, J. F., & Kroner, D. G. (2006). The effect of base-rate information on the perception of risk for reoffense. *American journal of forensic psychology, 24*(3), 45–56.

Mills, J. F., Kroner, D. G., & Morgan, R. D. (2011). *Clinician's guide to violence risk assessment.* New York, NY: Guildford Press.

Mokros, A. (2007). *Die Struktur der Zusammenhänge von Tatbegehungsmerkmalen und Persönlichkeitseigenschaßen bei Sexualstraftätem* [The structure of the relationship between crime scene actions and personality characteristics in sex offenders]. Frankfurt: Verlag für Polizeiwissenschaft.

Monahan, J., & Silver, E. (2003). Judicial decision thresholds for violence risk management. *International Journal of Forensic Mental Health, 2*(1), 1–6.

Mossman, D. (1994). Assessing predictions of violence: Being accurate about accuracy. *Journal of Consulting and Clinical Psychology, 62,* 783–792. doi:10.1037/0022-006X.62.4.783.

Mossman, D. & Sellke, T. (2007). Avoiding errors about "margin of error." *British Journal of Psychiatry;* Electronic letter in response to Hart, Michie, & Cooke, 2007.

Murrie, D. C., Boccaccini, M. T., Rufino, K., & Caperton, J. (2012). Field validity of the Psychopathy Checklist-Revised in sex offender risk assessment. *Psychological Assessment, 24,* 524–529. doi:10.1037/a0026015.

National Policing Improvement Agency. (2010). *Guidance on protecting the public: Managing sexual offenders and violent offenders.* Retrieved from http://www.acpo.police.uk/documents/crime/2010/20110301%20CBA%20ACPO%20%282010%29%20Guidance%20on%20Protecting%20the%20Public%20v2%20main%20version.pdf.

Neal, T. M. S., & Grisso, T. (2014). Assessment practices and expert judgment methods in forensic psychology and psychiatry: An international snapshot. *Criminal Justice and Behavior, 41,* 1406–1421. doi:10.1177/0093854814548449.

Olver, M. E., Beggs Christofferson, S. M., Grace, R. C., & Wong, S. C. P. (2014). Incorporating change information into sexual offender risk assessments using the Violence Risk Scale – Sexual Offender version. *Sexual Abuse: A Journal of Research and Treatment, 26,* 472–499. doi:10.1177/1079063213502679.

Olver, M. E., Beggs Christofferson, S. M., & Wong, S. C. P. (2015). Evaluation and applications of the Clinically Significant Change method with the Violence Risk Scale - Sexual Offender version: Implications for risk-change communication. *Behavioral Sciences and the Law, 33,* 92–110. doi:10.1002/bsl.2159.

Olver, M. E., Wong, S. C. P., Nicholaichuk, T. P., & Gordon, A. (2007). The validity and reliability of the Violence Risk Scale-Sexual Offender version: Assessing sex offender risk and evaluating therapeutic change. *Psychological Assessment, 19,* 318–329. doi:10.1037/1040-3590.19.3.318.

Pedneault, A. (2014). *Linking crime scene behaviors and propensities in child molesters: A replication*. Paper presented at the Annual Research and Treatment Conference of the Association for the Treatment of Sexual Abusers (ATSA), San Diego, CA.

Phenix, A., & Epperson, D. (2015). Overview of the development, reliability, validity, scoring, and uses of the Static-99, Static-99R, Static-2002, and Static-2002R. In A. Phenix & H. M. Hoberman (Eds.), *Sexual offending: Predisposing conditions, assessments, and management*. Springer.

Phenix, A., Helmus, L., & Hanson, R. K. (2015). *Static-99R & Static-2002R evaluator's workbook*. Retrieved from http://www.static99.org/pdfdocs/Static-99RandStatic-2002R_Evaluators Workbook2012-07-26.pdf.

Prochaska, J. O., DiClemente, C. C., & Norcross, J. C. (1992). In search of how people change: Applications to addictive behaviors. *American Psychologist, 47*, 1102–1114. doi:10.1037/0003-066X.47.9.1102.

Proulx, J., Tardiff, M., Lamoureeux, B., & Lussier, P. (2000). How does recidivism risk assessment predict survival? In D. R. Laws, S. M. Hudson, & T. Ward (Eds.), *Remaking relapse prevention with sex offenders: A sourcebook*. Thousand Oaks, CA: Sage Publications.

Quesada, S. P., Calkins, C., & Jeglic, E. L. (2013). An examination of the interrater reliability between practitioners and researchers on the Static-99. *International Journal of Offender Therapy and Comparative Criminology, 58*, 1364–1375. doi:10.1177/0306624X13495504.

Quinsey, V. L., Harris, G. T., Rice, M. E., & Cormier, C. A. (2006). *Violent offenders: Appraising and managing risk* (2nd ed.). Washington, DC: American Psychological Association.

Rockhill, B., Byrne, C., Rosner, B., Louie, M. M., & Colditz, G. (2003). Breast cancer risk prediction with a log-incidence model: Evaluation of accuracy. *Journal of Clinical Epidemiology, 56*, 856–861. doi:10.1016/S0895-4356(03)00124-0.

Santtila, P., Häkkänen, H., Canter, D., & Elfgren, T. (2003). Classifying homicide offenders and predicting their characteristics from crime scene behavior. *Scandinavian Journal of Psychology, 44*(2), 107–118. doi:10.1111/1467-9450.00328.

Scurich, N., & John, R. S. (2012). A Bayesian approach to the group versus individual prediction controversy in actuarial risk assessment. *Law and Human Behavior, 36*, 237–246. doi:10.1037/h0093973.

Scurich, N., Monahan, J., & John, R. S. (2012). Innumeracy and unpacking: Bridging the nomothetic/idiographic divide in violence risk assessment. *Law and Human Behavior, 36*, 548–554. doi:10.1037/h0093994.

Shanteau, J. (1992). Competence in experts: The role of task characteristics. *Organizational Behavior and Human Decision Processes, 53*, 252–262. doi:10.1016/0749-5978(92)90064-E.

Shingler, J., & Mann, R. E. (2006). Collaboration in clinical work with sexual offenders: Treatment and assessment. In W. L. Marshall, Y. Fernandez, L. Marshall, & G. Serran (Eds.), *Sexual offender treatment: Controversial issues*. London: Wiley & Sons, Ltd.

Singh, J. P., Desmarais, S. L., Hurducas, C., Arbach-Lucioni, K., Condemarin, C., Dean, K., … Otto, R. K. (2014). International perspectives on the practical application of violence risk assessment: A global survey of 44 countries. *International Journal of Forensic Mental Health, 13*, 193–206. doi:10.1080/14999013.2014.922141

Skeem, J. L., & Monahan, J. (2011). Current directions in violence risk assessment. *Current Directions in Psychological Science, 20*, 38–42. doi:10.1177/0963721410397271.

Smith, P., & Schweitzer, M. (2012). The therapeutic prison. *Journal of Contemporary Criminal Justice, 28*, 7–22. doi:10.1177/1043986211432201.

Snowden, R. J., Gray, N. S., Taylor, J., & MacCulloch, M. J. (2007). Actuarial prediction of violent recidivism in mentally disordered offenders. *Psychological Medicine, 37*, 1539–1549. doi:10.1017/S0033291707000876.

Social Work Inspection Agency, HM Inspectorate of Constabulary for Scotland, and HM Inspectorate of Prisons. (2009). *Multi-agency inspection: Assessing and managing offenders who present a high risk of serious harm 2009*. Retrieved from http://www.scotland.gov.uk/Resource/Doc/275852/0082871.pdf

Swets, J. A., Dawes, R. M., & Monahan, J. (2000). Psychological science can improve diagnostic decisions. *Psychological Science in the Public Interest, 1*(1), 1–26. doi:10.1111/1529-1006.001.

Thornton, D., Mann, R., Webster, S., Blud, L., Travers, R., Friendship, C., & Erikson, M. (2003). Distinguishing and combining risks for sexual and violent recidivism. *Annals of the New York Academy of Sciences, 989*(1), 225–235. doi:http://dx.doi.org/10.1111/j.1749-6632.2003.tb07308.x

Varela, J. G., Boccaccini, M. T., Cuervo, V. A., Murrie, D. C., & Clark, J. W. (2014). Same score, different message: Perceptions of offender risk depend on Static-99R risk communication format. *Law and Human Behavior, 38*, 418–427. doi:10.1037/lhb0000073.

Viallon, V., Ragusa, S., Clavel-Chapelon, F., & Bénichou, J. (2009). How to evaluate the calibration of a disease risk prediction tool. *Statistics in Medicine, 28*, 901–916. doi:10.1002/sim.3517.

Ward, T., Polaschek, D. L. L., & Beech, A. R. (2005). *Theories of sexual offending*. Chichester, England: Wiley.

Webster, C. D., Douglas, K. S., Eaves, D., & Hart, S. D. (1997). Assessing risk of violence to others. In C. D. Webster & M. A. Jackson (Eds.), *Impulsivity: Theory, assessment, and treatment* (pp. 251–277). New York, NY: Guilford Press.

Webster, S. D., Mann, R. E., Carter, A. J., Long, J., Milner, R. J., O'Brien, M. D., … & Ray, N. (2006). Inter-rater reliability of dynamic risk assessment with sexual offenders. *Psychology, Crime, & Law, 12*, 439–452.

Welsh, J. L., Schmidt, F., McKinnon, L., Chattha, H. K., & Meyers, J. R. (2008). A comparative study of adolescent risk assessment instruments predictive and incremental validity. *Assessment, 15*, 104–115.

Wilson, C. M., Desmarais, S. L., Nicholls, T. L., & Brink, J. (2010). The role of client strengths in assessments of short-term violence risk. *International Journal of Forensic Mental Health Services, 9*, 282–293.

Wilson, M. A., & Leith, S. (2001). Acquaintances, lovers, and friends: Rape within relationships. *Journal of Applied Social Psychology, 31*(8), 1709–1726. doi:10.1111/j.1559-1816.2001.tb02747.x.

Wong, S. C. P., Olver, M. E., Nicholaichuk, T. P., & Gordon, A. (2003). *The Violence Risk Scale: Sexual Offender version (VRS: SO)*. Saskatoon, Saskatchewan, Canada: Regional Psychiatric Centre and University of Saskatchewan.

Wormith, J. S., Althouse, M. S., Reitzel, L. R., Fagan, T. J., & Morgan, R. D. (2007). The rehabilitation and reintegration of offenders: The current landscape and some future directions for correctional psychology. *Criminal Justice and Behaviour, 34*, 879–892. doi:10.1177/0093854807301552.

Wormith, J. S., Hogg, S., & Guzzo, L. (2012). The predictive validity of a general risk/needs assessment inventory on sexual offender recidivism and an exploration of the professional override. *Criminal Justice and Behavior, 39*, 1511–1538. doi:10.1177/0093854812455741.

Chapter 4
Risk Formulation: The New Frontier in Risk Assessment and Management

Caroline Logan

Introduction

This chapter focuses on the structured professional judgement (SPJ) approach to the clinical risk assessment and management of men and women whose sexual behaviour is harmful to others. The SPJ approach promotes the use of clinical guidelines—such as the *Risk for Sexual Violence Protocol* (RSVP; Hart et al., 2003)—to help practitioners appraise the relevance of risk factors to the individual client and to create an understanding of that person's risk potential, on the basis of which comprehensive and proportionate risk management plans can be prepared, implemented, evaluated, and repeatedly updated towards managed risk. This chapter makes the case that the most important part of the clinical risk assessment and management process using the SPJ approach is risk formulation—the process of generating an understanding of harmful behaviour that directly links assessment findings to management actions.

Individuals who are not well understood—whose actions challenge our understanding—may not be risk managed with focus, clarity of objectives, or confidence (Hart & Logan, 2011; Logan, Nathan, & Brown, 2011; Reid & Thorne, 2007). For example, the behaviour of men and women who have in the past committed one single act of serious harm (e.g. sexual assault or homicide) in the context of a relatively managed lifestyle can often be a problem to risk assess because past behaviour was not part of a pattern from which the form of possible future acts can be extrapolated. Also challenging is the assessment and management of the risks posed by clients who cannot or who outright refuse to cooperate with evaluations

C. Logan (✉)
Greater Manchester West Mental Health NHS Foundation Trust, Prestwich Hospital, Bury New Road, Prestwich, Manchester M25 3BL, UK

University of Manchester, Manchester, UK
e-mail: caroline.logan@gmw.nhs.uk

© Springer International Publishing Switzerland 2016
D.R. Laws, W. O'Donohue (eds.), *Treatment of Sex Offenders*,
DOI 10.1007/978-3-319-25868-3_4

for whatever reason or who deny any involvement in the offences of which they have been accused. In such cases, restrictive interventions may be more likely to prevail as a consequence of the assessor's ignorance or uncertainty about the origins and circumstances of past and therefore future possible offending behaviour. However, in such cases and similar others, the process of risk formulation offers a means by which as broad and relevant an understanding as possible may be acquired in a systematic way; formulation links empirically based risk assessment to practical risk management and outlines the practitioner's current understanding of the underlying mechanism of an individual's harm potential in order to develop hypotheses about action to facilitate change (embodied in the risk management plan). Therefore, because of its utility to the complex and challenging cases that are a feature of the caseloads of so many practitioners working with sexual offenders, this chapter will describe the SPJ process with particular focus on risk formulation.

Formulation is an essential clinical activity for practitioners in mental health settings (e.g. Eells, 2007; Tarrier, 2006) and especially in forensic mental health and corrections (Hart, Sturmey, Logan, & McMurran, 2011; Sturmey & McMurran, 2011). What is discussed here will not be unfamiliar to anyone who is a practitioner. What *is* more novel, however, is the focus on formulation practice as it applies to risk and, on the discussion that follows, on determining the quality of formulations. Because it is only when practitioners and researchers have a sound basis for telling a good formulation from a poor one that we can really move forward in terms of demonstrating that formulation has a role to play in risk management — and clinical practice more generally — and defining what that role is (Bieling & Kuyken, 2003; Hart et al., 2011). Consequently, this chapter will also describe ongoing work towards determining the efficacy of risk formulation and how it might be possible to tell good formulations from poor, and effective formulations from those that contribute little to risk management. This chapter will conclude with a review of the key issues and learning points and a set of good practice recommendations.

The SPJ Approach to Clinical Risk Assessment and Management

In the last two decades, research and practice in the risk assessment field has been informed by the publication of a variety of instruments, tools, and guidelines structuring the assessment process and — though much less frequently — risk management. These guidelines have emerged from a broad range of research studies seeking to characterise and identify the individual and contextual variables that are most strongly or commonly associated with the harmful outcome that is of interest to the practitioner and which he or she is motivated to prevent (Logan & Johnstone, 2013; Otto & Douglas, 2010). For example, it is a well-established fact that a history of deviant sexual arousal is strongly associated with sexual violence recidivism (e.g. Hanson & Morton-Bourgon, 2009). Therefore, it follows that deviant sexual arousal is a risk factor for sexual violence in a number of risk assessment guides focused on sexual violence as a specific harmful outcome (e.g. the RSVP). The risk assessment guidelines currently available to practitioners vary in content—that is, they vary in the range of risk factors described and, in some cases, the weight of each factor in the final judgement about risk. Such variance among guidelines is justified because the different outcomes—such as non-sexual violence, intimate partner violence, suicide, as well as sexual violence, and so on—emerge from sometimes quite different developmental pathways, which the guidance seeks to capture. Guidelines assist the practitioner in their examination of individual clients against all the risk factors described in the specific risk assessment guide they have chosen to use and to denote through a rating whether each factor is present or not and, if present, the extent to which each is present (e.g. definitely or partially). What happens next depends on whether the guidance stipulates a discretionary or non-discretionary approach to the development of final judgements or conclusions about risk (e.g. Hart & Logan, 2011; Meehl, 1954/1996; Mossman, 2006).

Non-discretionary approaches, which may be described as actuarial or statistical, guide decision-making about risk according to the application of a set of predetermined, explicit, and fixed rules. The outcome of the application of such approaches, as exemplified by, for example, the *Static-99R* and the *Static-2002R* (e.g. Brouillette-Alarie & Proulx, 2013; Hanson, Babchishin, Helmus, & Thornton, 2013; Phenix, Helmus, & Hanson, 2012), the *Violence Risk Appraisal Guide-Revised* (VRAG-R; Rice, Harris, & Lang, 2013), and the *Sex Offender Risk Appraisal Guide* (Harris, Rice, Quinsey, & Cormier, 2015), is a finding about level or volume of risk over a specific time frame. Such non-discretionary approaches offer no clear support to decision-making about the optimal nature of risk management or the conditions in which nature and level of risk may alter. In addition, non-discretionary approaches support judgements about risk at the group rather than individual level (Hart, Michie, & Cooke, 2007, but see also Mossman, 2015). There is no place for risk formulation in the use of such guides—understanding the individual's past harmful behaviour is not a factor in measuring or managing its risk of recurrence. Non-discretionary approaches are commonly used in research and in court hearings and practice settings where a simple quantification of risk is all that is required, such as to guide sentencing or level of supervision.

On the other hand, discretionary approaches to risk assessment permit assessors to exercise a degree of professional judgement in their decision-making about risk, in relation to the weighing and combination of risk-relevant information (Hart & Logan, 2011); guidelines provide either very little structure (as in unaided clinical judgement) or a considerable degree of structure (as in the SPJ approach). Structured discretionary approaches promote the use of formulation as the essential bridge between risk assessment and risk management (e.g. Logan, 2014). Further, discretionary approaches support the development of risk management plans based specifically on the risk formulation, that is, the assessors understanding of the client's risk potential. Such approaches have applications in cases where risk management and prevented harm are the objectives, making them more attractive to practitioners in correctional and forensic mental health settings required to manage over the medium to long term those with a history of harmful behaviour. Examples of such discretionary risk assessment guidelines include the RSVP and the *Historical-Clinical-Risk Management-20* (HCR-20 version 3 (HCR-20[V3]); Douglas, Hart, Webster, & Belfrage, 2013).

Operationalising SPJ in Risk Assessment and Management

The SPJ approach is operationalised by clinical guidelines developed for practitioners to apply with professional discretion to clients whose risk potential they are attempting to understand and manage. SPJ guidelines are presented in the form of a manual and accompanying worksheet. The assessor proceeds through the worksheet with the aid of the manual, which offers guidance on the collection of relevant information, decision-making about its relevance to the risk to be prevented, the combination of relevant information in formulation, scenario planning, risk management decision-making, and case prioritisation. In general, practitioners commence assessments without a clear understanding of the risks posed by their client or the most optimal risk management strategies to prevent or at least limit harmful outcomes, and the evaluation process should enable them to derive both in a systematic, evidence-based, and transparent way.

SPJ guidelines for risk assessment and management require the practitioner to work through six distinct evaluation stages or steps. In the first step, relevant information is gathered from a variety of key sources, including the client, if he or she chooses to collaborate with the assessment and to the extent to which he or she can be encouraged to do so willingly and honestly (Logan, 2013). Under some circumstances, it is possible and indeed necessary to undertake assessments of clients who refuse to engage with the assessor (e.g. Heilbrun, 2001). For example, if a client is reasonably thought to be at risk of engaging in a harmful act yet he or she refuses to be assessed by a concerned practitioner, it would be ethical to proceed with a risk assessment in order to protect the client and others via the application of an informed risk management plan (e.g. British Psychological Society, 2009). The information gathered at this step, whether the client collaborates or not, will pertain to his or her history of harmful behaviour and the circumstances in which it occurred previously and to evidence relating to the possible recurrence of such harmful conduct (e.g. the existence of plans or feasible preparations). Practitioners are prompted to collect specific types of information by the risk factors contained within the guidelines chosen for use.

In the second step of the SPJ process and based on all the information collected, the practitioner makes a judgement as to whether each of the risk factors identified in the guidance is *present* and to what degree (not at all, partially, definitely). In the RSVP, there is an additional consideration — recent change — that also features in the SVR-20 although not in the HCR-20^{V3}. In the third and very important step of the SPJ process, practitioners determine whether and the extent to which in their opinion those risk factors that are present are also *relevant* to the client's potential to be harmful again in the future, where relevance is defined in terms of the factor's role in the direct occurrence of harmful incidents or to future risk management. To illustrate, one client may have identified the past victims of his sexual assaults directly through his employment (e.g. as a postal delivery worker, which gave him the opportunity to identify women living alone whom he could safely burglarise and assault). This fact would make employment problems both present and directly relevant to his future offending—he uses purposeful activity to hunt for potential victims. However, another client may struggle to gain employment because of learning difficulties or limited opportunities, but his sexual offending is not related in any way to his employment status or specific job. In this latter case, problems with employment may be present but they are not in any way relevant to his future potential. Therefore, a risk factor can be present in a client's history but not relevant to his or her future sexual offending behaviour. As with presence ratings, the relevance of individual risk factors is rated on a three-point scale—that is, not relevant, somewhat or partially relevant, or definitely relevant.

In the fourth step, the important formulation step, the risk factors identified as relevant are added to with clinical judgements about potential protective factors of importance to the individual case. Protective factors may be defined as those characteristics of the individual and his or her environment that appear to limit the severity or frequency of harmful behaviour by moderating the effect of one or more risk factors (e.g. positive attitudes towards treatment and risk management, which maximise engagement and permit close supervision and monitoring). All of the information most relevant to the risk of sexual violence in the client is then organised. This is in order to understand the range and operation—the codependency—of vulnerability factors, triggers, maintenance, and protective factors. Once organised, consideration is given to what would appear to be the key motivational drivers for sexually harmful behaviour in that individual, based on what is understood about the person and his or her past conduct, and the decisions that would appear to have been made then and on what basis (Hart & Logan, 2011). Future scenarios are then detailed—at least two—and used to elaborate on what is understood (Chermack & Lynham, 2002; van der Heijden, 1994), in particular, about triggers and protective factors.

Scenario planning 'is a process of positing several informed, plausible and imagined alternative future environments in which decisions about the future may be played out, for the purpose of changing current thinking, improving decision-making, enhancing human and organization learning and improving performance' (Chermack & Lynham, 2002, p. 366). It is a particularly useful technique to use in situations in which there is uncertainty yet a strong need to prepare for all or the most serious eventualities (van der Heijden, 1994). For example, scenario planning is used extensively in military operations where the consequences of inadequate preparation and anticipation of problems could be measured in lives lost and serious injuries sustained. Scenarios are descriptions of possible futures; in the case of sexual violence, possible ways in which a particular client might be sexually harmful again in the future given what is known about his or her past and current situation and decision-making processes. Therefore, scenarios are not predictions. Instead they are forecasts based on what and the evaluator's understanding of why the client has acted in a similar way in the past. As a consequence of their uniqueness to the client's personal circumstances, preferences, and decision-making, only a limited number of scenarios are likely to be plausible. And it is these scenarios, with their origins laid bare by the evidence-based risk assessment and formulation process, which underpin risk management.

On the basis of the work undertaken at this important scenario-planning step, it is then possible to start preparing the actual formulation—a narrative statement of understanding about the client's sexual violence risk, which will explain why they are at risk and under what circumstances and why that potential may become realised. Due to such an exposé of the individual's risk, it is possible to design action—risk management—that is based directly upon what matters most to the individual. Risk formulation will be described in a little more detail shortly.

Specific risk management actions or strategies are then elaborated upon in the fifth step of the SPJ process. Strategies are hypotheses for action intended to influence the operation of relevant risk and protective factors on overall risk potential, thus minimising or preventing future harmful conduct on the part of the client. This leads to the sixth and final step wherein summary judgements are made regarding the urgency of risk management action (case prioritisation), the identification of any risks that exist in other areas (e.g. self-harm or suicide, non-sexual violence, and so on), any immediate preventative action required, and the date for next case review including reassessment of risk.

These six steps are the SPJ process in a nutshell. Figure 4.1 illustrates each of its component parts and how they are linked together.

Focus on Risk Management

Risk management is the collection of actions taken to prevent potentially harmful outcomes, where the nature of those potential outcomes has been speculated about in some detail during in the formulation and scenario-planning step (step four above). Therefore, risk management should be based directly on the practitioner's explanation—or understanding—of the client's harm potential. Risk management strategies for sexual offenders include direct *treatment* interventions for offending behaviour and conditions linked to offending (e.g. mental health problems, substance misuse, relationship problems), *supervision* strategies such as limited opportunities to access potential victims through the imposition of curfews or indefinite detention, the active

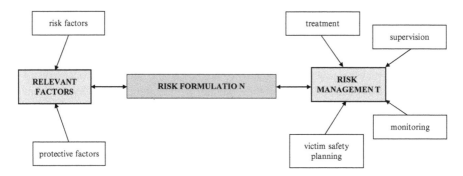

Fig. 4.1 Structured professional judgement in a nutshell

monitoring of risk factors through their surveillance in the course of supervisory and other supportive contacts, and *victim safety planning* in the event that a previous victim may be re-victimised or new potential victims become identifiable. Risk management per se has not been subject to a great deal of research (re. Heilbrun, 2001), certainly nothing commensurate with the research carried out into risk assessment. This is unfortunate. While it is the case that, on the whole, interventions with sexual offenders have had a positive impact on the frequency and severity of offending (e.g. Kim, Benekos, & Merlo, 2015), it remains unclear what combination of strategies works best for whom under what circumstances to prevent the recurrence of harmful sexual behaviour. The potential for risk management to exceed the risks presented by the individual cannot be overlooked or minimised, certainly in Europe in the age of the *European Convention on Human Rights* and the requirement for demonstrably proportionate legal sanctioning. This situation as regards evidence is only likely to change when the link between risk assessment and risk management processes is better conceptualised, which is why risk formulation has assumed such importance in the last few years. Each risk management option will now be discussed in more detail before we turn to risk formulation.

Treatment

Treatment strategies oriented towards managed risk are those proactive interventions that are intended to repair or restore deficits in functioning linked to sexual violence risk. Therefore, treatment strategies are intended to diminish the potency of risk factors most relevant to the sexually harmful conduct of the client. Treatment strategies include but are not limited to psychological and psychosocial interventions for the range of interpersonal, cognitive, emotional, and social deficits experienced by many sexual offenders and that are often encapsulated in a sexual offender treatment programme (e.g. Marshall, Fernandez, Hudson, & Ward, 2013). In addition, interventions for substance misuse problems that can co-occur with sexually harmful behaviour (e.g. Kraanen & Emmelkamp, 2011) and, where indicated, medication for the symptoms of the mental disorders that disinhibit the client (Kingston, Olver, Harris, Wong, & Bradford, 2015) are also common treatment strategies. Treatment strategies may also be directed towards the enhancement of protective factors in order to make them more effective in moderating or mediating risk factors. For example, individual or couple therapy may help to improve a client's self-awareness and capacity to utilise and benefit from close social support, thus weakening the link between stress and loneliness and sexual offending. Very broadly, treatment strategies for sexual offenders will include psychological therapies (e.g. cognitive behaviour therapy for mood problems, cognitive behavioural interventions for criminogenic needs), psychopharmacological interventions (e.g. antipsychotic medication, mood stabilisers, anti-libidinals), and psychosocial interventions (e.g. detention in a therapeutic community or in a setting offering neurocognitive rehabilitation or compensation) delivered one-to-one or in groups, in institutions, or in the community, where compliance is voluntary or required by legal order (e.g. Marshall et al., 2013).

Supervision

Supervision strategies target the environment or the setting in which the client is based now or likely to be based in the future in order to limit the power of risk factors and improve the effectiveness of protective factors, thus diminishing risk potential overall. Supervision strategies can be applied in two different ways. First, supervision may involve the imposition of restrictions on the client's activities, movements, associations, or communications, which is intended to limit his or her access or exposure to the circumstances that could trigger one (or more) of the hypothesised risk scenarios (Hart et al., 2003). Examples of supervisory risk management strategies would include denial of unsupervised—or any—access to preferred victim groups, such as children, a ban on drinking alcohol or drug-taking, non-association lists as part of conditional release requirements, and imprisonment, which serves the joint purpose of punishment and the restriction of access to potential victims. Second, supervisory strategies also include those adjustments—or enhancements—to the individual's lifestyle that are intended to improve the performance of protective strategies. Examples of such supervisory strategies may include training and support to secure and maintain suitable paid employment offering routine, purpose, financial reward, and an opportunity for positive self-regard, in addition to regular contact with an understanding person or organisation sensitive to the needs of sexual offenders, such as through involvement with Circles of Support and Accountability (Elliott & Beech, 2013; McCartan et al., 2014). Supervision strategies are particularly important in cases where the client denies involvement in sexual offending, thus severely limiting treatment options.

Monitoring

Monitoring in risk management terms is the identification of early warning signs of a relapse to sexually harmful behaviour (e.g. an increasing level of sexual preoccupation, watching or even following preferred victim types in public places), ideally derived from the client through their engagement with treatment and supervision. However, monitoring also refers to the collaborative preparation of plans to be implemented when evidence is provided for the presence of such early warning signs. Such plans would include the actions to be taken to prevent early warning signs from evolving into new offences, like the ones mapped out in the formulation and scenario-planning stage, and might include recall to prison or an increase in the frequency of meetings with a supervisor. Monitoring strategies are intended to be implemented by the client and by others (e.g. probation officers, managers of approved premises, etc.), where others will be relied upon more if the client's insight into his or her offending behaviour is limited or motivation to engage is only partial or wavering. In risk management terms, monitoring differs from supervision because monitoring focuses on surveillance rather than on controlling or managing the client's activities. This makes monitoring a much less intrusive risk management strategy although just as essential as all the others.

Victim Safety Planning

Finally, victim safety planning refers to the action that might be recommended to a past or possible future victim of the client—and his or her carers or guardians—in order to keep them safe. The client may have targeted a potential future victim previously (e.g. their child), but contact is nonetheless possible and desired by the parties involved (e.g. both parents, who choose to stay in some kind of contact with one another because they have several children together). A potential victim could also be an as yet unknown partner (e.g. a future boyfriend or girlfriend) or provider of treatment or supervision (e.g. a social worker or probation officer, a psychologist) who may become victimised when, for example, they make demands of the client or endeavour to enforce the limitations that were an agreed requirement of conditional release. Victim safety plans should include provision of emergency safety procedures, personal alarms, prohibition of unaccompanied meetings, communication strategies, and so on, all of which are intended to make victimisation either less likely to happen or less damaging in its effects.

Concluding Comments

In this section, the SPJ process has been described in some detail. SPJ should be regarded as evidence-based guidelines for risk assessment and management that are tailored to the needs of individual clients, to the practitioners who work with them over lengthy periods of time, and to the harmful conduct to be prevented. The SPJ approach to risk assessment and management is most applicable to practice settings in which convicted sexual offenders are subject to long-term treatment and supervision, in institutions or in the community (such as correctional or forensic mental health facilities), and in legal contexts where risk management is a primary consideration (e.g. parole board hearings). However, assessment is not understanding, and risk management that is not based on an understanding of the problems experienced by the client in trying to manage his or her own behaviour is at risk of being poorly designed and executed. It is therefore to risk formulation that we will now turn.

Risk Formulation

Formulation is the process in clinical and forensic practice whereby an organisational framework is applied to our current knowledge of a client in order to produce an explanation for the underlying mechanism of his or her presenting problems and thereby generate linked hypotheses for action that will facilitate positive and progressive change (e.g. Johnstone & Dallos, 2013; Persons, 1989; Sturmey & McMurran, 2011; Tarrier, 2006). The knowledge to which the formulation process is applied is the collection of that gleaned from clinical interviews and direct observations of the client (if available); relevant information from collateral sources, both professional and personal (e.g. family members); and data derived from the application of formal structured assessments (e.g. a set of guidelines for the assessment of risk factors, such as the RSVP or the HCR-20^{V3}). It is acceptable to formulate risk on less than this ideal collection of information (re. Heilbrun, 2001), as when a risk assessment has to proceed for public safety reasons. In which case, the formulation would be described as preliminary and would be updated as soon as additional relevant information is received.

A formulation is a length of narrative text—perhaps between one and several paragraphs in length—in which the presenting problems are described, explanations in the form of hypotheses offered for their occurrence, origins, and potential recurrence (usually underpinned by one or more theoretical models relevant to the nature of the problem), and options for comprehensive action thereby proposed (e.g. Hart & Logan, 2011; Logan & Hird, 2014). The formulation should be accessible to the reader, including the client. Further, the formulation should be the product of collaboration between the assessor and the client—or if not the client then between the assessor and a key other person, such as the client's main carer, or their probation or prison officer, or their forensic mental health nurse. A theory relevant to the problem of interest will underpin the formulation (e.g. a theory of sexual offending), thus enabling or facilitating connections between relevant pieces of information. Over time, the formulation becomes the basis for determining the nature and quality of change achieved in the period until the client is next reviewed and the changes detected used to determine whether the original formulation was correct and any adjustments required to the explanation provided therein. Thus, the formulation remains a 'live' document—a statement of current understanding, which is updated regularly with new information and insights—and the driver of progressive action based on an evolving understanding of the person and their behaviour.

The formulation process may be applied to one specific problem or a range of linked problems. For example, the process can be used to understand harmful behaviour as a specific problem—such as sexual or non-sexual violence towards others, or harm directed towards the self, or all of these potential outcomes in the same complex person. Such formulations—risk formulations—when prepared will tend to have a narrow focus and are often comparatively short (one or maybe two pages of text). However, the formulation process may also be applied to the whole person, or 'case'. Case formulations, by virtue of the need to describe the developmental origins of the range of current problems and how they interconnect, will be much broader in focus and consequently lengthier (maybe two to four pages of text).

What Is the Purpose of Formulation?

Whatever the focus—on one or more specific problems such as risk of sexual violence, or the whole case, the journey taken by the sexually harmful person to reach the point where they are at now—a formulation must by definition go beyond the findings of individual structured assessments or diagnoses to provide a rational and evidence-based theory of the client and the matter or matters of concern (Eells, Kendjelic, & Lucas, 1998; Hart et al., 2011; Nezu & Nezu, 1989; Persons, 1989; Tarrier, 2006). Numbers—such as summary test scores—or diagnoses are not in themselves explanatory and reduce a person to a banal abstraction that will bear little relationship to the lived experience of the client and of who he or she is and the problems they experience. For people with complex problems to be understood, they need to be considered as fully as possible, and formulation is a clinically meaningful process for achieving that outcome (Persons, 1989). Further, for complex problems and damaging people to be managed safely, they ought to be explained and understood if rational and proportionate action is to follow with at least some degree of cooperation from the client (Hart & Logan, 2011; Logan et al., 2011; Reid & Thorne, 2007).

The primary purpose of formulation is to organise and make systematic what is known about the client (Hart & Logan, 2011). A number of organisational models have been proposed for this purpose (e.g. the 4Ps model of Weerasekera (1996) or generating a comprehensive timeline), which are intended to highlight to the evaluator what is known and not known about the client, as a prompt to further and more targeted information gathering around the problem (or problems) of concern. The secondary purpose of formulation is to make connections between relevant pieces of information in order to create a psychological explanation of the client and his or her problems (Hart & Logan, 2011)—to link the biological, psychological, and social characteristics and experiences to one another in a rational explanation for past and possible future outcomes. The application of a relevant theoretical model assists with making these connections. The outcome of this endeavour should be an answer to the following questions: *Why has this person been sexually harmful in the past, and why might she or he decide to do so again in the future and under what circumstances?*

Its third purpose relates to the essential collaborative nature of its generation; formulation should be an explanatory narrative generated by the labour of the evaluator working alongside others, principally the client. In this way, collaborative formulation gives the process a role to play in both explaining the client and in motivating him or her to become involved in understanding the need for change and what is required; by contributing to the formulation, the client is encouraged to invest in it and change. However, a mutually agreed understanding between the client and the evaluator is not always possible—or desirable—as when an evaluator is supporting practitioners such as probation officers to work effectively with complex clients that the evaluator may never meet. Formulation through the process of consultation then becomes like a route map for such a practitioner, encouraging a more psychologically informed way of working.

Fourth, hypotheses for action to facilitate change emerge from the formulation because of its expression of the underlying mechanism of the presenting problems, making action linked directly to understanding. Indeed, a formulation cannot be described as such unless the understanding communicated is paired with proposals for action. Finally, the finished product, the explanatory narrative, becomes the focus of communicating and engaging with others, including the client (Hart & Logan, 2011). A challenge to write, and write well, the formulation is and should always be the most meaningful and interesting part of any report, and the emphasis on the relatively brief length of this part of the work is in order to ensure it is read and regarded as such. Formulations of 20 or 200 pages or more may be very interesting indeed. However, they are unlikely to engage the reader, including the client, which is the essential final purpose of formulation, and an unread formulation is no formulation at all.

How Is a Risk Formulation Prepared?

Risk formulations may be prepared in one of two ways. First, a risk formulation may be prepared in collaboration with the client. Such a formulation will draw from several sources of information, as suggested above, including the client (Logan, 2014). The client may be engaged in a general assessment of sexual violence risk and relevant other variables, such as substance misuse, deviant sexual arousal, psychopathy, and so on. Once these assessments have been completed, the assessor may then sit with the client and the formulation process commences. The assessor might begin by summarising the findings of the assessments completed: 'Let me go over what I have observed about you from the time we have spent together', an opening statement that offers the assessor the opportunity to determine the extent to which the formulation can be prepared collaboratively based on the client's response to feedback. In the event that some degree of collaboration appears possible, the assessor may then say something like the following: 'What I would like to do now is to prepare a paragraph or two that describe what we agree on about your risk of being sexually harmful again in the future—and what we all need to do to manage that risk and prevent any such harm from occurring. I'd like what we write to represent what we disagree on too. Are you okay with that?' Were the client denies all or part of the offending behaviour of which he or she has been accused or already convicted, the focus could instead be on their risk of being accused again. Such an approach offers more opportunities for fruitful discussion than does the prospect of an argument over whether the client was truly guilty or not. The assessor can then start to write something there in the room with the client: for example, 'This risk formulation describes what we understand about Mr Smith's risk of being sexually harmful again in the future. Mr Smith has helped me to understand that he has carried out sexually motivated assaults on women who are strangers to him because he is attracted to them but anticipates that if he approached them, they would reject him. When Mr Smith sees a woman he is attracted to, he can visualise her rejection—this makes him angry with her before he has even spoken to her, and then he attacks and humiliates her with a sexualised assault as a way of punishing her for what he believes she would have done. Mr Smith told me about his early experiences with women' … and so on. The assessor would take the lead with the writing, and the client would be encouraged to help, and at the end of the meeting, there would be a rough draft of a formulation that could be prepared in typed form for the next meeting, where it would be edited and eventually completed.

A slightly different approach would be for the assessor to agree to prepare such a narrative for their next meeting and to bring a copy then for the assessor and client to go through together. This approach is generally quicker, but it offers the client less control. The alternative approach, that of preparing the formulation together in session, may be more helpful with clients for whom having some control is important—because they generally feel powerless yet want to have a say or because feeling less in control will make them agitate to obtain more. The potential gain from such a collaborative approach to risk formulation is the investment it signals in collaborative risk management; keeping clients involved offers more opportunities to monitor risk.

A second way of preparing a risk formulation on a client is to do so through a third party, such as a probation officer, a forensic mental health nurse, a prison officer working closely with the client in a special prison unit, or a whole multidisciplinary team. The assessor may not be able or available to work directly with the client (e.g. because there is one assessor and dozens of clients), or perhaps the purpose of the service is to enhance psychological ways of working by all practitioners in the facility and not just by the assessor. In whichever case, the assessor takes the information he or she can gain about the client directly from the practitioner (or the multidisciplinary team), and working together they prepare a formulation of the client. Assisting the practitioner (or team) to understand the client's behaviour and risks is intended to help the practitioner think more psychologically about the client and to generate more compassion for challenging individuals with whom it can often be hard to establish and maintain rapport (Johnstone, 2013; Minoudis et al., 2013; Minoudis, Shaw, & Craissati, 2012).

Concluding Comments

Risk formulation is a theory about a particular client's sexual harm potential based on what we understand to be the most relevant risk and protective factors related to this particular outcome. Risk assessment guidelines can help assessors select information most important to this outcome. Risk formulation is the stage where all that relevant information is woven together into an account that will help assessors, those with whom they must communicate (e.g. the courts, the parole board), and their clients understand and agree on the circumstances in which sexually harmful behaviour may happen again and why and what has to change in order to prevent such an outcome. However, preparing risk formulations is a very intense undertaking, with huge individual variation in style, content, theoretical orientation, and presentation. And assessors can easily disagree with their colleagues about the value of alternative formulations—an often time-wasting process of competitive formulation—because there is little agreement about what a good formulation looks like. So, what are the essential component parts of acceptable formulations, and how might we tell a good risk formulation from a poor one?

Evaluating the Quality of Risk Formulations

The ultimate measure of the quality of a risk formulation is that it has a direct and positive impact on managed risk, which would not have been achieved at all, as effectively, or as quickly, in its absence. How might we test this? We can undertake studies in which we compare sexual offenders whose risk management has and has not been informed by a formulation in order to examine whether the simple presence of a formulation is associated with positive outcomes. Alternatively, we can devise standards against which the quality of individual risk formulations can be measured. Such standards would allow us to explore the difference to risk management made by good formulations as opposed to any old piece of writing that calls itself by this name. But what might these standards be? By what qualities should we differentiate good from indifferent from poor risk formulations?

In 2011, Professors Peter Sturmey of the City University of New York and Mary McMurran of the University of Nottingham in England published an edited book entitled *Forensic Case Formulation* (Sturmey & McMurran, 2011). While much has been written about formulation before this publication, this particular work set in motion the first real effort to identify the basic definition of formulation in forensic practice, the essential features of formulations, and evaluative criteria or standards by which the quality of formulations could start to be determined in forensic settings—all as a basis for moving this essential clinical practice from something of an art form into the realm of scientific endeavour. A subsequent publication (Hart et al., 2011) consolidated their work in this book and suggested ten standards by which formulations may be judged. The focus of this paper was on wider case formulations, but the ten standards set down are a starting point for the consideration of risk formulations also. A later publication by McMurran and Bruford (2016), following research with focus groups evaluating the standards themselves, has refined and simplified the definitions originally described, which are presented below:

1. The formulation should be a *narrative*—therefore, risk formulations should be presented in text (as opposed to a drawing subject to ambiguous or inconsistent interpretations), written in everyday language (as opposed to numbers or lists of facts or diagnoses), which tells a coherent, ordered, and meaningful story about the risks posed by the client.
2. The formulation should have *external coherence*—therefore, a risk formulation should be explicitly consistent with (or anchored by) an empirically supported psychosocial theory of problematic behaviour, such as sexual offending or decision-making, which provides both (a) essential guidance to the assessor in determining which facts are noteworthy or identifying which explanations are legitimate and (b) a critical evidence base to the process.
3. The formulation should have *factual foundation*—therefore, risk formulations should be based on information about the client that is relevant to risk and adequate in terms of its quality and quantity, and any limitations in this requirement are clearly indicated and the risk formulation identified as preliminary if so.

4. The formulation should have *internal coherence*—therefore, risk formulations should rest on propositions or make assumptions about the client's behaviour that are compatible or noncontradictory, cogent, and consistent.

5. The formulation should exercise a high degree of *completeness*—therefore, risk formulations should have explanatory breadth; they should account for a substantial amount of the critical evidence (the information anchors) and have a plot that ties together as much as possible all the information relevant to the reason why the risk formulation has been prepared.

6. The formulation represents *events that are understood by the way they relate over time*—that is, the risk formulation ties together information about the past, the present, and the future; it describes the developmental trajectory of risk from the past into the possible future and accounts for the critical vulnerability factors, triggers, maintenance, and protective factors.

7. The formulation should be *simple*—that is, it should be free from unnecessary, overly complex, or superfluous details, propositions, and assumptions.

8. The formulation should be *predictive*—that is, a risk formulation should go beyond mere description, statement of factor, or classification, to generate a new or more developed understanding about individual risk, in particular, to make detailed and testable forecasts about outcomes in the event of the implementation of specific treatment and management strategies.

9. The formulation should be *action oriented*—that is, risk formulations should be tied to action; they should assist with the planning and, importantly, the prioritisation of a range of management interventions over the period of time until next review.

10. Finally, the formulation should demonstrate a degree of *overall quality*—that is, risk formulations should be comprehensive, logical, coherent, focused, informative, acceptable, and useful to those who are required to make use of them.

Minoudis et al. (2013) examined the statistical properties of the above standards—compiled as the McMurran *Case Formulation Quality Checklist* (McMurran, Logan, & Hart, 2012)—in a study involving probation officers in the London area. The inter-rater reliability, the test-retest reliability, and the internal consistency of the checklist were all calculated from the scores derived from randomised formulations generated by a sample of 64 probation officers from fictitious case vignettes. The study found that all the statistical properties of the checklist were acceptable—inter-rater agreement was judged to be moderate to good, test-retest reliability was excellent, and internal validity was also excellent—all suggesting that the checklist is an appropriate tool for evaluating the construct of formulation. More recently, McMurran and Bruford (2016), in attempting to evolve the original standards proposed in 2011, have sought to improve its overall validity and reliability as well as to firmly establish in the literature the expectation that risk formulations can and should be evaluated. Work will and should continue to develop this and indeed other frameworks for determining the quality of formulations in order to standardise this essential area of practice and overall raise its quality.

Risk Formulation in Practice: An Example

In order to demonstrate risk formulation, an example will now be offered—
Mr Smith, who was referred to in a previous section. This example is necessarily
brief, but it will offer an opportunity to demonstrate what a risk formulation could
look like, something of the value it adds to assessment findings, and how the
evaluative criteria listed above may be applied.

Mr Smith

Mr Smith is a 47-year-old man, who is approaching the end of an 8-year prison
sentence for grievous bodily harm with intent to rape. His victim was Ms Cooper, a
28-year-old woman, whom he followed from a nightclub and attacked while she
was walking from there to her home in the small hours of a Saturday morning.
Ms Cooper reported that Mr Smith had approached her twice while she was in the
nightclub sitting with friends, asking her to dance and to allow him to buy her a
drink. However, she was wary of him because he appeared too demanding and
aggressive—and also intoxicated—and so she refused him on both occasions. She
had not seen him leave the nightclub, and when she left for home, she assumed that
she was making the short journey alone and in safety. Ms Cooper had consumed
some alcohol in the course of the evening but she was not intoxicated. When
approached again by Mr Smith while walking home, she understood the danger she
was in immediately and tried to attract the attention of neighbours by shouting for
help. Mr Smith immediately struck her repeatedly with a hammer causing injuries
to her head, face, shoulders, and arms. However, the attack was stopped quite
quickly when two neighbours intervened and wrestled Mr Smith to the ground.
When the police arrived and arrested Mr Smith, they found in his possession a
length of rope, adhesive tape, and a long and very sharp boning knife. When questioned, Mr Smith indicated that he had been greatly angered by Ms Cooper's rejec-
tions of him during the course of the evening—he stated to interviewing officers that
she had no right to treat him that way. When he saw the victim prepare to leave the
nightclub, Mr Smith left immediately and fetched the rope, tape, knife, and hammer
from the boot of his nearby car. He watched her depart and her route of travel, and
he followed her till the point at which he attacked her. As he did so, Ms Cooper
recalls—and witnesses confirm—that he called her a variety of obscene and deroga-
tory names in an angry manner.

Mr Smith has eight previous convictions, all for violent offences, all of which
targeted adult women who were strangers to him. A sexual motive has been assumed
in all these prior offences, but his convictions are variously for assault, burglary,
grievous bodily harm, indecent assault, and rape. His first offence—burglary (of the
home of a single female occupant)—was committed when he was 17 years of age.
His first conviction for an explicit sexual offence was when he was 23 years of

age—indecent assault, against a 19-year-old student in a railway underpass. When he was 32 years of age, Mr Smith was convicted of the rape of a 17-year-old school-girl on a train. Since the age of 17 years, Mr Smith has spent a total of 16 years in prison and 8 years subject to various community licence conditions and sexual offence prevention orders. His most recent offence that against Ms Cooper was committed when he was 41 years of age and just over 2 years following his release from his previous conviction for indecent assault. Mr Smith was living alone at the time of the offence and working as a forklift truck driver in a builder's yard. Mr Smith has no current partner although he has had long-term relationships with women in the past. He has two now adult children with whom he has no contact.

While in prison on his current sentence, Mr Smith undertook the sexual offender treatment programme. He has completed this programme on two occasions before, during previous prison sentences. He has also undertaken treatment programmes relating to violent offending generally and thinking skills. While he has engaged with these programmes, reports suggest that his engagement has been superficial at best. He has been subject to various assessments, the conclusions of which indicate that he is a man with no acute mental health problems, but with a long-standing diagnosis of narcissistic personality disorder with paranoid traits (as assessed using the *International Personality Disorder Examination*; Loranger, 1999), in addition to prominent traits of psychopathy (as assessed by the *Psychopathy Checklist-Revised*; Hare, 2003; total score of 26 where an arrogant and deceitful interpersonal style and deficient affective experience are especially pronounced). Mr Smith has behaved reasonably well while he has been in prison—he has been subject to occasional punishment relating to bullying activity only—and he is due to be released on licence during the next 6 months. An evaluation of risk has been prepared by a forensic psychologist using the RSVP. The purpose of this evaluation is to inform the conditions of Mr Smith's licence.

In brief, the risk assessment clarified that Mr Smith demonstrates a chronic and escalating pattern of violent sexually motivated offending against adult women involving high levels of physical (and no psychological) coercion. Personality pathology is a critical factor, and his presentation suggests significant traits of antagonism, dominance, deceitfulness, lack of emotional depth, self-centredness, sense of entitlement, and a detached and unempathic style of relating to others. These traits are especially pronounced in his relations with women. Deviant sexual arousal is suspected—specifically, sexual sadism—but it has not been formally assessed. Mr Smith's discussions of his offending behaviour suggest a pattern of minimisation and either a lack of or a reluctance to develop any real degree of self-awareness. Problems with treatment response and supervision were also noted.

Mr Smith was broadly cooperative with the assessment; he appeared to see it as a necessary evil. He flirted with the female psychologist at the beginning of the assessment, but, when he realised that her professional stance was unwavering and that she was achieving some success in exposing aspects of himself that he would prefer remained hidden, his attitude towards her became dismissive and at times hostile. However, he completed the assessment, and he provided quite a lot of infor-mation the psychologist could use alongside credible collateral information.

Following the assessment phase, the psychologist would have preferred to write the formulation together with Mr Smith. However, he was not interested in doing this and told her to write it herself. He did wish to see it, however, and he brought a red pen to the session during which they were to discuss its contents as he anticipated that much would be wrong with it. The psychologist prepared the following text, which she went through with Mr Smith line by line, changing very little in response to Mr Smith's feedback.

This risk formulation describes what we understand about Mr Smith's risk of being sexually harmful to women again in the future. During the course of five meetings over approximately 7 h, and following a review of his records, Mr Smith has helped me to understand that he has carried out sexually motivated assaults on adult women who are strangers to him because he is attracted to them—but he anticipates that if he approached them, they would reject him. When Mr Smith sees a woman he is attracted to, he can visualise a perfect relationship between them. However, very quickly, he can also visualise her rejection of him. The belief that she will reject him floods him with anger and resentment, which motivates him to act towards the woman as if she really had rejected him. Therefore, Mr Smith explains his attacks on women as if they were reasonable punishments for their very rude, unkind, and unjust treatment of him. Mr Smith's stance in describing what he has done is that of victim—and his attitude towards his incarceration that it is unfair and undeserved. Mr Smith believes himself to have been justified in attacking his victims as viciously as he has because of the very dreadful pain and humiliation he felt they caused him by their imagined rejection—thus, his actions were in his view proportionate to the pain he believes they caused him.

Mr Smith told me about his early experiences with women. His mother was a single parent of Mr Smith and his two siblings—an older brother and a younger sister. His mother worked very hard to raise money for the family, but she was frequently depressed and drank alcohol most days to numb her pain. Therefore, it was often the case that she was not there physically while Mr Smith was growing up, or she was there in body but not available to him emotionally. It seems that Mr Smith, who had always been a strong willed and self-centred child, spent large parts of his childhood imagining what it would be like to be really cared for and at the centre of a really loving family—the most favoured, the most beloved son. And he grew resentful of his mother for not providing this for him. As he grew into adolescence, Mr Smith spent more and more time fantasising about perfect relationships with teachers and friends and, increasingly, with perfect young women in order to make himself feel better. However, such a pattern of coping evolved at the same time as an increasing problem with controlling his anger when frustrated, and increasing dependence on alcohol—and all his coping strategies became fused.

Mr Smith's offending behaviour was primarily motivated by anger at his victims for not being the perfect, loving and accepting women he wanted them to be; over time, his resentment at the role women have played in his incarceration when he is at least as much a victim as they are, has at least maintained if not increased both his anger and his risk of reoffending. Therefore, the key to managing Mr Smith's risk of harm to women in the future is to impose both restrictions on his movements through strict and extended licence conditions *and* to attempt to modify his attitudes towards women. Mr Smith accepts that the licence conditions imposed on him will be comprehensive. However, he has expressed an interest in considering the possibility of making more deep-rooted changes to his attitudes towards women. Why now? Because Mr Smith wishes not to return to prison. He understands that it is his beliefs about women and what he thinks they owe him that are major factors in having him act such that he is returned to prison over and over. Therefore, Mr Smith is interested in trying to understand himself more so that he might not return to prison again. If such a process enables him to understand the experience of those whom he has attacked, that would be okay although this is not his primary consideration—and it may be hard for him to do this because of the kind of personality he has. However, behaviour change in order to stay out of prison is possible, he thinks, and such change would limit if not prevent his victimisation of others, and that would be a very good outcome indeed.

Mr Smith found it quite hard to go through this formulation with me—he has protected himself from feelings of shame and loneliness for so long with beliefs about his right to be angry towards women and to humiliate them as he feels they humiliate him. However, his wish not to return to prison is very strong now because there is so much that he would really like to see and to do in the community while he is still young enough to enjoy them—for example, he used to love fishing when he was a child and he loves to go to soccer matches, both with his older brother who has stood by him through all his prison sentences. Therefore, although working on this formulation together has been hard, it has enabled us to agree on a future pathway for Mr Smith. Now we can begin plotting the different supports we have to put in place to help him to get and to stay there, and to keep others safe from him.

Mr Smith and I have agreed that we will review this formulation again in 5 months time once we have all our plans in place to manage his risk of reoffending in the community. At that meeting, we will add to this formulation with more details on how he will try to manage situations that put him at risk of re-offending and we will review all the measures that will be taken to prevent him from actually doing so.

Comment on Mr Smith's Formulation

In terms of quality, the above formulation demonstrates most key requirements, albeit very briefly. The text states clearly what it is attempting to explain—Mr Smith's risk of sexual violence towards adult women who are strangers to him—and gives an indication of the range of information on which the opinions have been based (it has *factual foundation*). The formulation goes into some detail on the developmental origins of his harmful behaviour (*events are understood over time*), and it offers a psychological explanation for Mr Smith's harmfulness in which his behaviour is linked to possible motivational drivers consistent with accepted theories of sexually violent behaviour (e.g. Baumeister, Catanese, & Wallace, 2002; Malamuth, 1996; Marshall, 1989; Marchall & Barbaree, 1990; it attempts to achieve *external coherence*). As a consequence of such a psychological explanation, it is possible to develop hypotheses for action that will facilitate change, whether generated from within Mr Smith or directed by the range of services likely to be supervising him in the months and years to come (the formulation is *action oriented*). Also, the formulation has been written in a style that tries to avoid the use of jargon and that is intended to be readable, comprehensible, interesting, and engaging (the formulation has a *narrative* and is of reasonable *overall quality*). Finally, it offers a coherent summary of Mr Smith's situation now (it has *internal coherence*), containing information relevant only to his risk of sexual harm (the formulation demonstrates *completeness* and *simplicity*). Subsequent follow-ups of Mr Smith, in which risk management and change are reviewed, will allow the veracity of the formulation to be tested (the formulation is *predictive*).

Conclusions and Good Practice Recommendations

This chapter has focused on the SPJ approach to the clinical risk assessment and management of men and women whose sexual behaviour is harmful to others. In this chapter, the case has been made that the most important part of the risk assessment and management process using the SPJ approach is risk formulation—the process of generating an understanding of harmful behaviour that directly links assessment findings to management actions. As such, risk formulation offers a means by which as broad and as relevant an understanding as possible may be acquired in a systematic way such that a practitioner's current understanding of the underlying mechanism of an individual's harm potential may be used to develop hypotheses about action to facilitate change. This chapter has also given attention to recent work attempting to establish quality standards for formulation, a process intended to generate thought and research in order to improve both the frequency with which formulation is a part of risk evaluations and the confidence with which practitioners prepare, communicate, and evolve them over time in a collaborative way. It is only when we have such a means of determining efficacy that we will move from the art to the science of formulation practice (Bieling & Kuyken, 2003).

So, what are the good practice recommendations emerging from the work reviewed in this chapter? Two are proposed as follows:

1. Risk formulation should be an essential part of sexual violence risk assessment and management—in fact, in clinical risk assessment and management in all areas. Assessment findings need to be explained with relevance to the subject of the evaluation, and risk management has to be linked directly to that explanation in order to be acceptable, proportionate, and effective, especially in complex cases. This is specially the case for those practitioners whose job is to manage clients with a history of sexually harmful behaviour as oppose to offer a judgement about the likelihood of reoffending. The latter application of risk assessment technology has dominated the field for much of the last 20 years. Risk formulation is the new frontier in *clinical* risk assessment and management

because once identified as at risk of sexual reoffending, it is formulation that offers the best hope of maintaining over time the focus, interest, and engagement of this most challenging of client groups.

2. Risk formulation is a challenging task—in part because, while core business for most practitioners, it is not clear what are the essential component parts of a formulation whatever its theoretical underpinnings and how we can know a good formulation from a poor one. This chapter has proposed one quality assurance framework for formulation—others are sure to be prepared. Research on their application, and the demonstration that formulations judged to be good are effective in managing risk, is strongly recommended in order to improve the quality and the confidence with which this most important endeavour is discharged.

References

Baumeister, R. F., Catanese, K. R., & Wallace, H. M. (2002). Conquest by force: A narcissistic reactance theory of rape and sexual coercion. *Review of General Psychology, 6*, 92–135.

Bieling, P. J., & Kuyken, W. (2003). Is cognitive case formulation science or science fiction? *Clinical Psychology: Science and Practice, 10*, 52–69. doi:10.1093/clipsy.10.1.52.

British Psychological Society. (2009). *Code of ethics and conduct*. Leicester: The British Psychological Society.

Brouillette-Alarie, S., & Proulx, J. (2013). Predictive validity of the Static-99R and its dimensions. *Journal of Sexual Aggression, 19*, 311–328.

Chermack, T. J., & Lynham, S. A. (2002). Definitions and outcome variables of resource planning. *Human Resource Development Review, 1*, 366–383.

Douglas, K. S., Hart, S. D., Webster, C. D., & Belfrage, H. (2013). *HCR-20: Assessing risk for violence* (3rd ed.). Vancouver, BC: Mental Health, Law and Policy Institute, Simon Fraser University.

Eells, T. D. (2007). Psychotherapy case formulation: History and current status. In T. D. Eells (Ed.), *Handbook of psychotherapy case formulation* (2nd ed., pp. 3–32). New York, NY: Guilford Press.

Eells, T. D., Kendjelic, E. M., & Lucas, C. P. (1998). What is a case formulation? Development and use of a content coding manual. *Journal of Psychotherapy Practice and Research, 7*, 144–153.

Elliott, I. A., & Beech, A. R. (2013). A UK cost-benefit analysis of Circles of Support and Accountability interventions. *Sexual Abuse, 25*, 211–229.

Hanson, R. K., Babchishin, K. M., Helmus, L., & Thornton, D. (2013). Quantifying the relative risk of sex offenders risk ratios for Static-99R. *Sexual Abuse, 25*, 482–515.

Hanson, R. K., & Morton-Bourgon, K. E. (2009). The accuracy of recidivism risk assessments for sexual offenders: A meta-analysis. *Psychological Assessment, 21*, 1–21.

Hare, R. D. (2003). *Hare psychopathy checklist-revised: Technical manual* (2nd ed.). Toronto, ON: Multi-Health Systems.

Harris, G. T., Rice, M. E., Quinsey, V. L., & Cormier, C. A. (2015). *Violent offenders: Appraising and managing risk*. Washington, DC: American Psychological Association.

Hart, S. D., & Logan, C. (2011). Formulation of violence risk using evidence-based assessments: The structured professional judgment approach. In P. Sturmey & M. McMurran (Eds.), *Forensic case formulation* (pp. 83–106). Chichester: Wiley-Blackwell.

Hart, S. D., Michie, C., & Cooke, D. J. (2007). Precision of actuarial risk assessment instruments: Evaluating the 'margins of error' of group vs individual predictions of violence. *British Journal of Psychiatry, 190*, 60–65.

Hart, S. D., Sturmey, P., Logan, C., & McMurran, M. M. (2011). Forensic case formulation. *International Journal of Forensic Mental Health, 10*, 118–126.

Heilbrun, K. (2001). Risk *assessment and risk management: Towards an integration.* Plenary session delivered at the International Conference, Violence Risk Assessment and Management: Bringing Science and Practice Closer Together. Sundsvall, Sweden.

Johnstone, L. (2013). Using formulation in teams. In L. Johnstone & R. Dallos (Eds.), *Formulation in psychology and psychotherapy: Making sense of people's problems* (2nd ed.). London: Routledge.

Johnstone, L., & Dallos, R. (Eds.). (2013). *Formulation in psychology and psychotherapy: Making sense of people's problems* (2nd ed.). London: Routledge.

Kim, B., Benekos, P. J., & Merlo, A. V. (2015). Sex offender recidivism revisited: Review of recent meta-analyses on the effects of sex offender treatment. *Trauma, Violence, & Abuse, 17*, 105–117.

Kingston, D. A., Olver, M. E., Harris, M., Wong, S. C., & Bradford, J. M. (2015). The relationship between mental disorder and recidivism in sexual offenders. *International Journal of Forensic Mental Health, 14*, 10–22.

Kraanen, F. L., & Emmelkamp, P. M. (2011). Substance misuse and substance use disorders in sex offenders: A review. *Clinical Psychology Review, 31*, 478–489.

Logan, C. (2013). Risk assessment: Specialist interviewing skills for forensic practitioners. In C. Logan & L. Johnstone (Eds.), *Managing clinical risk: A guide to effective practice.* Oxford: Routledge.

Logan, C. (2014). The HCR-20 Version 3: A case study in risk formulation. *International Journal of Forensic Mental Health, 13*, 172–180.

Logan, C., & Johnstone, L. (2013). (Eds.), *Managing clinical risk: A guide to effective practice.* Oxford: Routledge.

Logan, C., & Hird, J. (2014). Psychopathy and sexual offending. In D. T. Wilcox, T. Garrett, & L. Harkins (Eds.), *Sex offender treatment: A case study approach to issues and interventions.* Chichester: Wiley Blackwell.

Logan, C., Nathan, R., & Brown, A. (2011). Formulation in clinical risk assessment and management. In R. W. Whittington & C. Logan (Eds.), *Self-harm and Violence: Towards best practice in managing risk* (pp. 187–204). Chichester: Wiley-Blackwell.

Loranger, A. (1999). *International personality disorder examination manual: DSM-IV module.* Washington, DC: American Psychiatric Press.

Malamuth, N. M. (1996). The confluence model of sexual aggression: Feminist and evolutionary perspectives. In D. M. Buss & N. M. Malamuth (Eds.), *Sex, power, conflict: Evolutionary and feminist perspectives* (pp. 269–295). New York, NY: Oxford University Press.

Marchall, W. L., & Barbaree, H. E. (1990). An integrated theory of the etiology of sexual offending. In W. L. Marshall, D. R. Laws, & H. E. Barbaree (Eds.), *Handbook or sexual assault: Issues, theories, and treatment of the offender* (pp. 257–275). New York, NY: Plenum Press.

Marshall, W. L. (1989). Invited essay: Intimacy, loneliness and sexual offenders. *Behaviour Research and Therapy, 27*, 491–503.

Marshall, W. L., Fernandez, Y. M., Hudson, S. M., & Ward, T. (Eds.). (2013). *Sourcebook of treatment programs for sexual offenders.* New York, NY: Springer Science & Business Media.

McCartan, K., Kemshall, H., Westwood, S., Solle, J., MacKenzie, G., Cattel, J., & Pollard, A., (2014). *Circles of support and accountability (CoSA): A case file review of two pilots.* Project Report. England: Ministry of Justice.

McMurran, M.M., & Bruford, S., (2016). Case formulation quality checklist: A revision based upon clinicians' views. *Journal of Forensic Practice.*

McMurran, M., Logan, C., & Hart, S. (2012). *Case formulation quality checklist.* Nottingham: Institute of Mental Health.

Meehl, P. E. (1996). *Clinical versus statistical prediction: A theoretical analysis and a review of the literature.* Northvale, NJ: Jason Aronson (Original work published in 1954.).

Minoudis, P., Craissati, J., Shaw, J., McMurran, M. M., Freestone, M., Chuan, S. J., & Leonard, A., (2013). An evaluation of case formulation training and consultation with probation officers. *Criminal Behaviour and Mental Health, 23*, 252–262.

Minoudis, P., Shaw, J., & Craissati, J. (2012). The London Pathways Project: Evaluating the effectiveness of a consultation model for personality disordered offenders. *Criminal Behaviour and Mental Health, 22,* 218–232.

Mossman, D. (2006). Critique of pure risk assessment or, Kant meets Tarasoff. *University of Cincinnati Law Review, 75,* 523–609.

Mossman, D. (2015). From group data to useful probabilities: The relevance of actuarial risk assessment in individual instances. *Journal of the American Academy of Psychiatry and the Law Online, 43,* 93–102.

Nezu, A. M., & Nezu, C. M. (Eds.). (1989). *Clinical decision-making in behavior therapy: A problem-solving perspective.* Champaign, IL: Research Press.

Otto, R. K., & Douglas, K. S. (Eds.). (2010). *Handbook of violence risk assessment tools.* Milton Park: Routledge.

Persons, J. B. (1989). *Cognitive therapy in practice: A case formulation approach.* New York, NY: W.W. Norton & Company.

Phenix, A., Helmus, L., & Hanson, R. K. (2012). *Static-99R & Static-2002R evaluators' workbook.* Retrieved from http://www.static99.org/pdfdocs/Static-99RandStatic-2002R_EvaluatorsWorkbook-Jan2015.pdf.

Reid, W. H., & Thorne, S. A. (2007). Personality disorders and violence potential. *Journal of Psychiatric Practice, 13,* 261–268.

Rice, M. E., Harris, G. T., & Lang, C. (2013). Validation of and revision to the VRAG and SORAG: The violence risk appraisal guide—Revised (VRAG-R). *Psychological Assessment, 25,* 951.

Sturmey, P., & McMurran, M. (Eds.). (2011). *Forensic case formulation.* Chichester: Wiley-Blackwell.

Tarrier, N. (2006). *Case formulation in cognitive behaviour therapy: The treatment of challenging and complex cases.* London: Routledge.

van der Heijden, K. (1994). Probabilistic planning and scenario planning. In G. Wright & P. Ayton (Eds.), *Subjective probability* (pp. 549–572). Chichester: Wiley.

Weerasekera, P. (1996). *Multiperspective case formulation: A step toward treatment integration.* Malabar, FL: Krieger.

Chapter 5
Measurement of Male Sexual Arousal and Interest Using Penile Plethysmography and Viewing Time

Robin J. Wilson and Michael H. Miner

Introduction

The precise reasons why some people engage in sexually inappropriate conduct are unknown; although many theories exist. Some suggest sexual interests and preferences are learned (Bem, 1996) while others question whether people might be born with certain sexual interests or preferences (Seto, 2008, 2012). While this distinction may have implications for larger discussions regarding sexual orientation, there are also implications for professionals working in sexual violence prevention. Research has shown that people who have sexually offended are at higher risk to do so again if they experience inappropriate sexual arousal (Hanson & Bussière, 1998; Hanson & Morton-Bourgon, 2005). Therefore, knowing about a client's sexual interests and preferences is an important part of the assessment and risk management process. However, in talking to clients during forensic psychosexual evaluations, it is often difficult to ensure truthful responding due to the consequences associated with being labeled sexually deviant or a risk to others. Some people in trouble for sexually inappropriate conduct will openly admit to having strong sexual interest in or even a sexual preference for abnormal targets (e.g., children, animals, fetish items) or behaviors (e.g., exposing, peeping, bondage, and discipline), but this is by no means commonplace.

R.J. Wilson, Ph.D., A.B.P.P. (✉)
Wilson Psychological Services LLC, 4047 Bee Ridge Road, Suite C, Sarasota, FL 34233, USA

Department of Psychiatry & Behavioural Neurosciences, McMaster University,
Hamilton, ON, Canada
e-mail: dr.wilsonrj@verizon.net

M.H. Miner, Ph.D.
Program in Human Sexuality, Department of Family Medicine and Community Health,
University of Minnesota, 1300 So. Second Street, Suite 180, Minneapolis, MN 55454, USA
e-mail: miner001@umn.edu

© Springer International Publishing Switzerland 2016   107
D.R. Laws, W. O'Donohue (eds.), *Treatment of Sex Offenders*,
DOI 10.1007/978-3-319-25868-3_5

Conventional wisdom would suggest that those people who engage in inappropriate sexual conduct because they like or prefer it are at higher risk to reengage in such behaviors than those who do so for other reasons (e.g., poor boundaries, poor sexual problem-solving, or deficient sexual self-regulation). The fifth edition of the *Diagnostic and Statistical Manual of Mental Disorders* (DSM-5, American Psychiatric Association, 2013) lists a number of paraphilic presentations, including pedophilia, exhibitionism, fetishism, and sexual sadism. Presumably, those diagnosed with a paraphilia or paraphilic disorder would be among those at higher risk, and meta-analytic findings (e.g., Hanson & Bussière, 1998; Hanson & Morton-Bourgon, 2005) have indicated that sexual offenders with sexually deviant interests (as measured by penile plethysmography—see below) are more likely to recidivate.

However, the broader literature has been somewhat inconsistent in regard to the correlation of deviant interests and engagement in sexually inappropriate conduct. For example, two groups of researchers (Kingston, Firestone, Moulden, & Bradford, 2007; Moulden, Firestone, Kingston, & Bradford, 2009; Wilson, Abracen, Looman, Picheca, & Ferguson, 2011) independently found that a DSM diagnosis of pedophilia was not a particularly good predictor of future pedophilic behavior. Regarding sexual sadism, much has been written about the inability of clinicians to agree on what the diagnostic criteria should be (e.g., Marshall, Kennedy, Yates, & Serran, 2002) and the failure of DSM criteria to adequately predict engagement in sexually sadistic conduct (see Kingston, Seto, Firestone, & Bradford, 2010). Therefore, if the most commonly used diagnostic tome is unable to help distinguish those persons with entrenched and/or preferential deviant interests from those who engage in deviant behavior without necessarily having the attendant problematic interests or preferences, what should clinicians do? One possible answer to this question would require the use of methods that objectively measure sexual interests or preferences.

Objective Measurement of Male Sexual Arousal and Interests

At present, there are two major methods for measuring male sexual arousal or interest: penile plethysmography (PPG) and viewing time (VT). The first of these takes direct measurements of penile physiology during presentation of audiovisual stimuli intended to cause some differential degree of sexual arousal. The second method requires test takers to view pictures of models of varying ages and gender while measurements are taken of the differential length of time the individual looks at each picture. Those stimulus categories to which individuals show most sexual arousal (via PPG) are assumed to be of strong interest or preference to the individual, while those photos that the test taker lingers on the longest (during VT assessment) are assumed to represent the age and gender category in which he has greatest sexual interest.

PPG and VT each have their defenders and detractors; however, the literature does not often provide comparative information. In this chapter, we will describe each method, listing its strengths and weaknesses, and then we will draw some comparative conclusions as to the relative utility of the methods.

Penile Plethysmography

In their seminal text, *Human Sexual Response*, Masters and Johnson (1966) suggested that the best way to tell if a man is sexually aroused is to look at what is happening with his penis. Accordingly, a basic assumption would be that those stimuli resulting in greater penile tumescence likely represent the individual's sexual interests or preferences. However, are there reliable and valid means by which to measure differential penile tumescence; that is, methods that are reliable and valid enough to be used for diagnostic and risk management purposes?

Czech psychiatrist Kurt Freund (1957; Freund, Diamant, & Pinkava, 1958; see history in Wilson & Freund-Mathon, 2007) has been widely touted as the "inventor" of the penile plethysmograph (PPG), sometimes referred to as the phallometric test. This is, however, not entirely true. Although Freund was certainly the pioneer of the modern phallometric method, as used in forensic and sexological research and clinical contexts over the past 60 years, he cannot be credited with being the first to use such methods in studying sexual arousal. Bayliss (1908) is believed to be the first to use a plethysmograph to study sexual response; in his case, sexual arousal patterns in dogs. Use of PPG technology to study human sexuality did not occur until nearly 30 years later (Hynie, 1934). Subsequently, Ohlmeyer, Brilmayer, and Hullstrung (1944) devised a crude circumferential device to aid in their investigations of nocturnal erections. However, the Ohlmeyer et al. device was only an "on/off" sensor and was not designed to measure gradations of sexual arousal.

Volumetric Phallometry

Freund devised a volumetric transducer and originally used it as a means of discriminating gender preference, ostensibly, as a way to check the veracity of homosexuality claims made by Czech men attempting to avoid compulsory military service. He subsequently surmised that the PPG had applications beyond this original purpose, and that the method could be expanded to assess patterns of sexually deviant behavior eventually known as paraphilias (APA, 2013).

In Freund's method, the penis is inserted through an inflatable ring (fashioned from a prophylactic) and then into a glass cylinder. When the ring is inflated, an airtight seal is created between the penis and cylinder such that changes in air volume result in pressure differentials that can be converted to electrical output for further processing by an analog-to-digital converter. The digitized data are then stored and can be regenerated in analog form and subsequently scored, plotted, edited of artifact, rescored, and finally evaluated for diagnostic or research purposes (see Blanchard, Klassen, Dickey, Kuban, & Blak, 2001; Freund & Blanchard, 1989; Freund & Watson, 1991). The stimulus category to which the client demonstrated the highest average level of arousal is assumed to represent his erotic preference.

Circumferential Phallometry

Subsequent to Freund's introduction of the volumetric phallometer (which measures the penis as a three-dimensional object), Fisher, Gross, and Zuch (1965) fashioned a circumferential device based on a mercury-in-rubber strain gauge described by Whitney (1949) in his study of nocturnal erections and impotence. Fisher et al.'s device was then modified slightly by Bancroft and associates (1966), and it is the Bancroft-style device that is most widely used today. Another circumferential device was later devised by Barlow and associates (1970), but it has proven to be less popular.

Bancroft's circumferential method employs a simple strain gauge comprised of a length of silicon tubing filled with mercury (or, more recently, indium-gallium) and fitted with an adjustable electrode at either end (Bancroft et al., 1966). When made into a ring, it is placed around the penis midway along the shaft. As with the volumetric device, analog signals (resulting from stretching of the tube) are converted to digital data that can be used to assess differential levels of arousal, with the same assumptions in place (i.e., highest arousal equals most preferred age-gender group).

Strengths and Weaknesses of the Methods

Each technique has its pros and cons. A clear advantage the strain gauge has over the volumetric device is that it is simpler, less expensive (at least initially), and commercially available (e.g., Behavioral Technology [Monarch]; Limestone Industries). Because there is no commercially available version, Freund's volumetric method requires production of both specialized equipment and software; however, once all the equipment is assembled, the ongoing costs are actually quite small. Although it has been suggested that Freund's device is more cumbersome and awkward (Bancroft et al., 1966; Barlow et al., 1970), which may be true initially, experience (of author RJW) has shown that the client becomes quickly accustomed to the apparatus.

One particular positive aspect of the volumetric method is that it is more precise and sensitive than the strain gauge device (Clark, 1972; Freund, Langevin, & Barlow, 1974; Kuban, Barbaree, & Blanchard, 1999; McConaghy, 1974a). This superiority in precision and sensitivity is likely because the volumetric device measures three-dimensional changes in the penis, not just circumference. In the first few seconds of arousal, penile volume is known to increase while circumference decreases (McConaghy, 1974a), meaning that volumetric devices register a *positive* change in size/arousal while a strain gauge would actually show a *decrease* in circumference. The strain gauge appears to be a good indicator of gross sexual arousal; however, volumetric phallometry allows for accurate discrimination of exceptionally small responses (Freund, Langevin, et al., 1974), which is particularly helpful in combating test taker interference (e.g., faking—see Freund, 1971; Freund, Watson, & Rienzo, 1988; Wilson, 1998—see also below). Overall, output measured concurrently by the two methods has been shown to be highly correlated, with the strength of the correlation increasing proportionally with the degree of arousal (Kuban et al., 1999). A possible limitation of the increased sensitivity of volumetric phallometry is that it is arguably more sensitive to extraneous movement artifact than circumferential methods.

Use of the PPG in Clinical Practice

Phallometric testing is presently used for diagnostic, treatment planning, and risk management purposes in a variety of international jurisdictions. However, despite the relatively widespread use of phallometric procedures, there have been only a few comprehensive critical evaluations of the method's sensitivity and specificity, and standardization remains elusive. Regarding standardization, surprisingly little has been published regarding ideal stimulus sets and methods to ensure accuracy (Marshall & Fernandez, 2003). Two major suppliers exist for purchase of and training on circumferential PPG equipment, but how buyers ultimately use the technology is subject to a degree of site-specific idiosyncrasy. Each of those suppliers provides stimulus sets for use during testing; however, users are not necessary required to use them and are able to devise sets of their own. This potentially contributes to greater disparity in the approaches used by individual sites, even though the basic equipment may be very similar.

Stimuli

Almost 60 years after the adaptation of the PPG for use in paraphilia diagnosis, certain problems still exist. One of those problems concerns which types of stimulus materials are likely to produce the most objective and effective results. Great differences may be observed from country to country, as well as state to state (or province) within those countries. Over time, the world has become less tolerant of images of nude children and other sexually abusive media, regardless of their purpose. In Canada and Europe, many phallometric laboratories use visual stimuli including nudes. However, many US jurisdictions have made use of phallometry difficult, owing to conservative views and policies regarding sexually explicit materials—visual or auditory. The social climate has changed so dramatically over the past 45 years that materials relatively easily obtained or produced in the late 1960s and early 1970s are now socially and legally problematic. Some have suggested the use of computer-generated images (e.g., Konopasky & Konopasky, 2000; see also Renaud et al., 2009); however, it remains an open research question as to whether such images will elicit sexual responding in the same way that "real" pictures do. And the same concerns remain regarding the perception of computer-generated stimulus materials as child pornography and other illegal materials (e.g., depictions of rape or sexual sadism).

Visual stimuli are likely to assist in maximizing test specificity, due to their lack of ambiguity (see Miner, West, & Day, 1995); however, the addition of audio descriptions of activities engaged in by or with the person depicted appears to increase the degree of responding (Freund & Watson, 1991). Still photographs and motion pictures have been compared by both Freund, Langevin, and Zajac (1974) and McConaghy (1974b), with motion picture stimuli being better than still photography. This is presumably because of the more lifelike qualities inherent in motion pictures.

In attempting to establish which stimulus form might be best, one must consider the variety of sexually deviant interests and preferences that the examiner may be attempting to identify. The means by which you would stimulate an age/partner preference offender (e.g., pedophilia, hebephilia—sexual interest in children or early adolescents, respectively) may be different from the way you would stimulate an activity preference offender (e.g., rape, sadism, courtship disorders—Freund & Watson, 1991). In the former, one might conjecture that body shape is more important, requiring use of visual stimuli; whereas, activity preference issues may require more descriptiveness ultimately better served by audiotaped narratives.

Scoring and Interpretation

There is currently no standardized way to score or interpret phallometric outcome data; however, the literature provides guidance (e.g., Her Majesty's Prison Service, 2007; Lalumière & Harris, 1998; Marshall & Fernandez, 2003). Presumably, diagnosticians make inferences about erotic preferences and risk for recidivism based on the client's differential responses to the various categories of stimuli. In this, people with histories of sexually inappropriate conduct who demonstrate deviant arousal are more likely to be both paraphilic and at risk for future illegal sexual conduct (Freund & Blanchard, 1989); however, it is important to remember that this is not always the case.

No matter which method is used, volumetric or circumferential, change scores are calculated representing the level of arousal achieved during presentation of the stimuli. In the case of volumetric processes, change scores are often represented as an aggregate of the degree of arousal demonstrated along with the speed with which that arousal was achieved. In circumferential phallometry, the most common change score recorded is percentage of full arousal (with full arousal being established at the beginning of the test procedure). Most researchers agree that these change scores are ultimately best translated to standard scores (i.e., z-scores) because they facilitate interpretation (see Freund & Blanchard, 1989; Lalumière & Harris, 1998). As most phallometric procedures include multiple presentations of individual stimulus categories, it is common for final scores to be an average of multiple presentations across the category. This gives a more reliable indication of client interest or preference in a particular category than a single presentation alone (see Freund & Watson, 1991; Lalumière & Quinsey, 1994).

Psychometric Properties

Despite its widespread use, it is surprising that standardization remains phallometry's greatest challenge. Calls for greater standardization have been made by such esteemed groups as the Association for the Treatment of Sexual Abusers (ATSA, 2005), and there are individual laboratories that have standardized their own PPG procedures; however, standardization across sites remains less than optimal (Marshall & Fernandez, 2003). Currently, most laboratories in Canada and the USA likely purchase their equipment and stimuli from one of two main companies—Behavioral Technology or Limestone Technologies, which has no doubt led to at least some greater degree of standardization. However, the general lack of standardization extends beyond simply using the same equipment and stimuli to methods of scoring and interpretation (Her Majesty's Prison Service, 2007; Marshall & Fernandez, 2003).

Overall, the phallometric method has not enjoyed strong support in regard to reliability—the degree to which a test provides consistent findings. Acceptable levels of internal consistency have been achieved by increasing the number of stimuli per category (e.g., children, pubescent, adults—see Lalumière & Quinsey, 1994) and by attempting to standardize stimulus sets. Regarding test-retest reliability, evaluations of offenders against either adults or children have produced only minimal agreement (see Marshall & Fernandez, 2003). A principal reason for low reliability in phallometric testing is likely its susceptibility to learning and faking (see Marshall & Fernandez, 2003; Wilson, 1998). As is common throughout psychological testing, the more familiar one becomes with the methods and intent of a given procedure, the more control one can exert over the outcome. PPG testing includes a high degree of social desirability regarding demonstration of "nondeviant" responses, and it comes as no great surprise that clients are highly motivated to control the outcome of the test (Freund et al., 1988; Orne, 1962; Wilson, 1998).

Specificity refers to the method's propensity to give true-negative results; that is, how often does the test indicate nondeviant arousal in someone who actually is not arousal by the "deviant" stimulus categories? Freund and Watson (1991) reported a specificity rate of 97 %, meaning that only three of every 100 persons without sexual interest in minors would show arousal to minors (i.e., a 3 % false-positive rate). To achieve this high degree of specificity, however, Freund and Watson had to establish a control group consisting of sexual offenders against adults who professed no sexual interest in children. Surprisingly, nearly 20 % of paid community volunteers (mostly college students and job placement clients) in their study became sexually aroused to stimuli depicting children, leading to a belief that these subjects' test-taking attitudes were not equivalent to child molester clients regarding demand situation (e.g., people behave differently depending on what they perceive are the relative pros and cons depending on the situation—see Orne, 1962).

Overall, specificity does not seem to be a major problem for the phallometric test, with most studies reporting rates in the 95 % range (e.g., Barsetti, Earls, Lalumière, & Belanger, 1998; Chaplin, Rice, & Harris, 1995; Marshall, Barbaree, & Christophe, 1986). Blanchard and associates (2001), who found a specificity rate of 96 %, showed that the degree to which a test subject could be assumed to be gynephilic (a sexual preference for female adults, as demonstrated by number of female adult partners) was positively correlated with increased specificity.

Notwithstanding issues with respect to reliability, the most important question regarding use of PPG testing relates to how sensitive the test is to deviant sexual arousal in those who actually have such interests. It is important to acknowledge that not all sexual offenders have sexually deviant preferences and not all persons with sexually deviant preferences are sexual offenders. In establishing the validity of the method, we first must establish how often the method gives true positive results (sensitivity); that is, how often does the phallometric test for pedophilia identify arousal to children in persons who are truly pedophilic? Sensitivity levels reported in the research have varied, with Marshall and associates (1986) reporting 40 % sensitivity in their child molester clients, while Malcolm, Andrews, and Quinsey (1993) reported 41 % and Barsetti et al. (1998) reported 68 % for intrafamilial child molesters and 65 % for extrafamilial child molesters. Blanchard and associates (2001) reported sensitivity of 61 % for "men with the most offenses against children." Each of these studies reported approximately 95 % specificity in their (supposedly) nondeviant comparison samples.

In their 1991 study of the specificity and sensitivity of the volumetric method, Freund and Watson demonstrated that degree of sensitivity varies depending on the target gender and number of victims. In clients with at least two victims, sensitivity was 78.2 % for those who targeted girls and 88.6 % for those who targeted boys. Of those offenders with only one victim, sensitivity was 44.5 % for those with a female victim versus 86.7 % for those with a male victim. Freund, Watson, and Dickey (1991) showed additionally that pedophilic arousal on phallometric testing could be predicted by both number of victims and whether victims were solicited from outside familial contexts.

Accurate and reliable appraisal of deviant sexual arousal is an important aspect of the evaluation, treatment, and risk management continuum. Once identified, how does deviant sexual arousal respond to interventions and to what degree does such arousal potentially exacerbate efforts to manage risk in the community? Simply put, do people demonstrating deviant sexual arousal represent ongoing problems in these domains (i.e., does the PPG demonstrate predictive validity)? If one subscribes to the adage "the best predictor of future behavior is past behavior," then it makes some sense that persons who demonstrate deviant arousal and who have acted on it should be more likely to engage additional such conduct. In two influential meta-analyses of the predictors of sexual reoffending (Hanson & Bussière, 1998; Hanson & Morton-Bourgon, 2005), a pedophilia index derived from phallometric testing was the most robust predictor of future sexual offending against children. This finding was also established in research by Kingston et al. (2007; see also Moulden et al., 2009) and Wilson et al. (2011). Each of these research groups found that deviant arousal on phallometric testing was predictive of future offending against children. Others have suggested that the phallometric test can be used to reliably diagnose sexual dangerousness (e.g., Lalumière, Quinsey, Harris, Rice, & Trautrimas, 2003); however, the degree of diagnostic power in that domain remains well below that enjoyed by the phallometric protocol for age and gender preferences.

Interference, Faking, and Other Problems with Phallometric Testing

A major concern in using the PPG (and many other psychophysiological methods) is the degree of conscious control that a subject may exert on the body function being measured (e.g., sexual arousal). It is well known that phallometric responses can be faked, which presents very real difficulties for clinicians and researchers—especially those working in forensic circumstances where issues of risk and reintegration are considered.

As early as 1969, Laws and Rubin were aware that subjects could manipulate their sexual arousal when instructed to do so, using such techniques of suppression such as reciting poetry, counting, and other methods. Laws and Rubin showed that subjects in their research could effectively suppress their arousal by as much as 50 %, while Card and Farrall (1990) found that suppression was easier to achieve than enhancement. Others (Smith & Over, 1987; Wilson, 1998) have shown that by fantasizing about preferred stimuli, clients can effectively increase their levels of arousal to non-preferred stimulus categories. Regarding the circumferential method, Malcolm and associates (1993) showed that clients achieving arousal levels of 50 % of full erection or greater were easily able to exert control over their responses.

Freund and associates (1988; see also Wilson, 1998) studied the degree to which community volunteers could control their sexual arousal. These researchers were looking for patterns in the faked responses that could then be used to identify invalid test protocols or to thwart client attempts at dissimulation. Freund et al. (1988) found that some test subjects engaged in "pumping"—voluntary perineal muscle contractions with the intent of increasing response to a particular category (see also Fisher et al., 1965; Quinsey & Bergersen, 1976) while others showed greatest mean responses to sexually neutral stimuli (e.g., images of landscapes)—a sign of suppression. Otherwise, it is likely that low responding in either volumetric or circumferential testing may indicate response suppression (Freund, 1977), especially for younger men.

Currently, no method of identifying or thwarting faking works perfectly. Quinsey and Chaplin (1987) described a semantic tracking task in which the subject was required to listen for verbal cues in audiotaped stimuli and then press buttons appropriately as a means to ensure that clients were paying attention. Others have attempted to address faking by maximizing stimulus intensity, ostensibly in an attempt to "flood" the subject, so that he is unable to "escape" from the stimuli. Virtual reality visors are available for purchase from both of the well-established PPG suppliers. Further, some sexual offender programs require concurrent use of polygraph testing to help verify adherence to test expectations (see Kaine & Mersereau, 1986). However, it is important to stress again that although these attempts to identify and diminish the effects of faking may help, they have not eliminated the problem.

Viewing Time

Due to concerns about the sensitivity of PPG, the degree to which individuals could affect their arousal responses, and the invasiveness of the procedure, clinicians have looked for other objective measures of deviant sexual interest. This leads to the development of methods for inferring sexual interest through measures of viewing time (VT).

There are several mechanisms that underlie the use of viewing time as a measure of sexual interest. One is that individuals will look longer at pictures they find sexually attractive and that a summary profile of their viewing times will show this attractiveness/unattractiveness differential (Laws & Gress, 2004). This conceptualization dates to work by Rosenweig (1942) who discovered that psychiatric patients who were rated by staff as more sexually preoccupied looked longer at sexually explicit stimuli than those rated by staff as less sexually preoccupied. Further investigation indicated that sexual interest could be determined through length of viewing time. Early investigations found that heterosexual men had longer viewing times for pictures of nude women than homosexual males, and that homosexual men had longer viewing times for pictures of nude men than did heterosexual men (Zamanski, 1956).

A second possible underlying mechanism is sexual content-induced delay (SCID: Greer & Bellard, 1996; Greer & Melton, 1997). SCID has a longer latency in responding when sexual content is introduced into a cognitive task. SCID has been found in word recognition tasks (Greer & Bellard, 1996) and in Stroop-type tasks (Price & Hanson, 2007; Smith & Waterman, 2004; Williams & Broadbent, 1986). SCID might account for the longer VT found for preferred stimuli, which would have sexual content for the participant, when there is some type of task, such as rating the attractiveness of the presented stimuli.

The final explanation is that the major factors driving the longer latencies seen in attractive vs. non-attractive stimuli are the task demands. That is, denying sexual attraction is a fast rejection process, while affirming sexual attraction requires a more complex evaluation of the stimulus (Imhoff, Schmidt, Wei, Young, & Banse, 2012). That would mean that VT is not related to the attention-grabbing aspect of the stimuli but is related to the task-adequate response, that is, the determination and evaluation of attractiveness or sexual interest (Larue et al., 2014).

As noted above, there are at least three explanations for what mechanism underlies the VT measure used to assess sexual interest. Which mechanism is being measured depends on the methodology of the assessment technique, and more specifically, when the VT is measured. For instance, some procedures involve two exposures to the testing stimuli. In the first exposure, the testee is asked to familiarize themselves with the slides, while in the second exposure, they are asked to rate the slides either in attractiveness or sexual interest (procedures will be described in more detail later). If the VT is measured during the first exposure, it would appear to be assessing the degree to which the stimulus attracts the testee's attention, while if the VT is measured during the second exposure, it is likely assessing either the SCID or the complexity of the attraction assessment process.

Bourke and Gormley (2012) is the only study identified by these writers that explored the above possible mechanisms. As part of a comparison between VT and a pictorial Stroop task, Bourke and Gormley (2012) presented participants with two sets of trials, one where the task was to browse the images because they would be asked questions about them when the task was completed (VT1), and a second where they were asked to rate the image on a scale from extremely sexually unattractive to extremely sexually attractive (VT2). VT was measured during both tasks. Participants were 35 non-offending males, 11 of whom identified as homosexual and 24 who identified as heterosexual. The authors found that for VT1, heterosexual men viewed adult female images significantly longer than did homosexual participants and that homosexual participants viewed adult male images longer than the heterosexual participants. In general, homosexual men also had longer VTs to adolescent male images than did the heterosexual participants. Interesting, the impact of gender was only significant at the adult age level for heterosexual participants, while the impact of gender was significant at the adult and adolescent level, but not the child level, for homosexual participants. Also, the effect of age was only significant for female stimuli for the heterosexual males, and only for males in homosexual participants. For VT2, the effect of gender was significant at both the adult and adolescent levels for heterosexual males, whereas the effect of age was significant for both male and female images. For homosexual participants, there was no impact of gender for any age category and the impact of age was significant only for the male images. As for VT1, homosexual participants had longer VT then heterosexual participants in the VT2 condition.

Thus, it appears that there are many similarities between the results whether or not one includes a task as part of the VT measure, but there are also important differences. In determining how to measure viewing time, it appears that sexual orientation is important. That is, the pattern of findings differed with respect to sexual orientation, with heterosexual men showing an effect for age in both male and female images when there is a rating task present, but only for female images if such a task is not included, while homosexual participants showed the same effect of age across both VT measures. For homosexual males, the inclusion of the rating task changed the impact of gender across age category, where when no task was present, homosexual men showed a gender effect in adults and adolescents, where when the task was added, this effect was no longer present, and the homosexual participants showed no gender effect at any age level. Thus, selection of a VT method must consider the population being tested, at least with respect to sexual orientation, and the purpose of the assessment. That is, if the interest is in both age and gender of sexual interest, an attraction rating task is necessary for heterosexual men, but neither format is superior for homosexual men, in that it each case, the age effect is only present in male images.

The Validity of VT as a Measure of Sexual Interest

VT as a general construct has shown usefulness as a measure of sexual interest in sex offender populations, but its discriminative power has often been found to be of smaller magnitude than other measures. Harris, Rice, Quinsey, and Chaplin (1996) compared the ability of VT measures and PPG to discriminate between male child sex offenders ($n=26$) and heterosexual male community controls ($n=25$). They found that VT provided strong discrimination between child sex offenders and controls ($d=1.0$), but that PPG showed higher discriminatory power ($d=2.1$). Gress, Anderson, and Laws (2013) found that VT measures showed good sensitivity and specificity in distinguishing between adult sex offenders, nonsexual juvenile offenders, and college students. However, while adequate, the authors opined that the levels of sensitivity and specificity were not sufficient to recommend the use of VT for clinical purposes. Babchishin, Nunes, and Kessous (2014) also showed that VT reliably distinguishes between sexual offenders whose offenses were against children and other groups of sexual and nonsexual offenders.

In a study designed to assess how well indirect measures of sexual interest can identify those with a sadistic and/or masochistic interest, Larue and associates (2014) found that longer VT to violent stimuli than erotic stimuli was indicative of sadistic interest, but not masochistic interest, but that VT did not differentiate between consensual and nonconsensual forms of sadism. Thus, not only can VT discriminate between age and gender preference; this study provides some preliminary evidence of the use of VT to determine sadistic preference.

Commercially Available VT Assessments

There are currently two commercially available procedures for assessing sexual interest using VT: the Abel Assessment for Sexual Interest (Abel Screening, Inc., 2004) and the Affinity (Glasgow, Osborne, & Croxen, 2003). Each tool is similar in that they involve the exposure of the testee to images of males and females in bathing suits in age ranges that reflect young children, prepubescent children, adolescents, and adults.

Abel Assessment for Sexual Interest (AASI)

The VT measure used in the AASI, which has been described as a 16-measure suite of tests (Gray, Abel, Jordan, Garby, Wiegel, & Harlow, 2015), has been labeled Visual Reaction Time™. VRT is described in a recent publication (Gray et al., 2015) as one of several commercially produced variations on reaction time "with its specific scoring algorithm and its unique set of images" (p. 174). In this recent publication and on the Abel Screening website (www.abelscreening.com), it is emphasized that VRT is not a stand-alone measure but is combined with 15 other measures. However, how the measures of the AASI are combined to produce the outcomes reported, or what the "specific algorithm" is that is used to compute VRT was not described in Gray et al. (2015), the Abel Screening Website, nor any previous publication by this group.

The VT aspect of the AASI is conducted on a laptop or desktop computer. It includes 22 stimulus categories with seven exemplars in each category. For males and females there are four age categories including adults (21 or older), teenagers (14–17), grade-school children (6–13), and preschool children (5 and younger). Each category has an equal representation of Caucasian and African American stimuli. There are also slides depicting exhibitionism, voyeurism, frottage, a female suffering, a male suffering, two males hugging, two females hugging, a male and female hugging, and neutral landscapes. The pictures of individuals present a full frontal view with the subject clad in a swimsuit. The stimulus set is presented twice. In the first trial, testees are told to familiarize themselves with the pictures. In the second trial, testees are asked to rate their sexual arousal to each slide on a 1–7 scale where 1 is highly arousing and 7 is highly disgusting. VRT is measured during the second trial, that is, it reflects the time taken to view the stimulus and make the rating.

There have been four published studies, three in peer-reviewed journals, conducted by investigators independent of the developers of the AASI (the third of the peer-reviewed articles is not discussed here because it provides no useful information for this discussion). Letourneau (2002) if probably the most objective and independent of these studies. Using a sample of 57 volunteers from a military prison, VRT was compared with penile plethysmography (PPG) using the ATSA audiotaped stimuli. This study is unique in those assessing the validity of VRT in that the author was given access to the raw VT data and was not reliant on scores that had been manipulated through the unknown algorithm used to compute the VRT™ measure reported out by Abel Screening, Inc. to those using the AASI. Using the raw data, the author was able to explore the effects of outliers by using both trimmed and untrimmed VRT data. The VRT showed convergent validity in that the untrimmed measures were significantly associated with PPG arousal in the three female categories in which the two methods shared exemplars, while the trimmed measures were associated with two of the three categories, those depicting female children and those depicting male children. The significant correlation coefficients ranged from 0.277 to 0.607.

The other peer-reviewed paper published by an author not affiliated with the instrument's designer compared VRT to PPG in an outpatient setting. This study included 39 participants and used VRT data from clinically administered AASI's. Thus the authors were working from the summary reports provided by Abel Screening, Inc. and with ipsative rather than raw data. This study specifically explored the ability of each measure to correctly classify individual's sexual interest as indicated by their DSM-IV diagnosis. All participants met diagnostic criteria for pedophilia. The results indicate that overall, VRT showed a higher correct classification rate than PPG. However, this improvement over PPG was for those who the authors rated as not attempting to dissimilate, and with those rated as attempting to dissimilate, the PPG was actually better at classification than VRT, although the rate for PPG was only 55 % (Gray & Plaud, 2005). Both of these studies share a common limitation besides small samples. In both cases, PPG was performed using audio stimuli and not visual stimuli. The audio stimuli used does not distinguish between age or Tanner stage in the child stimuli, and research has shown that both sensitivity and specificity of PPG measures are increased by inclusion of visual stimuli (Miner et al., 1995). Thus, the above two studies may have failed to use the most accurate PPG procedure to assess the differences in classification rates across the two procedures.

There have been a number of studies over the years conducted by various individuals involved with the AASI or who have collaborated with Dr. Abel to conduct research on the AASI. These studies have involved large samples, due to access to the network of clinicians using the AASI. The major problem with all of these studies is that the methods of data reduction are not clearly described, since the algorithms are proprietary. That aside, studies of various versions of the AASI indicate that it is significant, although modestly associated with PPG, that the measures derived can correctly classify sexual offenders with respect to the age and gender of their victims and that it can distinguish between those who have been apprehended for sexual offending behavior and non-offenders (Abel, 1995; Abel et al., 2004; Abel, Huffman, Warberg, & Holland, 1998; Abel, Jordan, Hand, Holland, & Phipps, 2001; Abel, Lawry, Karlstrom, Osborn, & Gillespie, 1994; Abel & Wiegel, 2009).

In a recently published study, Gray and associates (2015) explored predictive validity of VRT with respect to sex offense recidivism. There sample included 621 men collected from two sites and they identified 22 individuals who had been arrested or charged with a new sex crime. Subjects were followed for a maximum of 15 years. The authors calculated a mean VRT measure by dividing the mean VRT for the eight categories of child stimuli by the mean VRT for the eight categories of adolescent and adult stimuli. This mean VRT measure was found to be significantly higher in reoffenders (0.80) than in those who did not reoffend (0.66). It should be noted, however, that even in the reoffenders, the ratio of child VRT to adolescent/adult VRT was less than 1.0, indicating more of an adult than child preference. The authors conducted a number of different assessments to look at the predictive validity of the child VRT as a predictor of sex reoffending. They provide evidence for the predictive validity of VRT and also found that this validity was not affected by whether the subject admitted to sexual abuse behavior or to some other form of deviant sexual behavior (Gray, et al., 2015). This study is the first that this author could find that assessed the predictive validity of VT. This is a critical link in that the argument for assessment of sexual interest is that sexual deviance, especially sexual arousal or interest in children has been found to be the single best predictor of sexual reoffending (Hanson & Mouton-Bourgon, 2009). Most of the research in the Hanson and Mouton-Bourgon (2009) meta-analysis used PPG to measure sexual arousal and no VT measures were included.

In summary, there is evidence that VRT, or the measures provided by the AASI, which are in some way derived from VRT, is a valid measure of sexual interest. It has a modest association with PPG, can adequately discriminate between groups of sexual offenders, although its sensitivity and specificity for female adolescents are poor, and has some evidence of predictive validity. The major concerns about VRT and the AASI are the lack of independent replication of the author's findings and the lack of transparency in their algorithms for computation of their various measures, including VRT™ which is presented as something more than VT.

Affinity

Affinity was developed for use with developmentally and cognitively delayed sexual offenders (Glasgow, 2009; Glasgow et al., 2003) and began as a method for gaining self-reported sexual interest from individuals whose intellectual disabilities limited existing interview and self-report procedures. A description of the development of Affinity is available in Glasgow (2009) and so that will not be attempted here. However, in the process of instrument development, the expansion of target population beyond those with intellectual disabilities began, and subsequent iterations of Affinity have moved away from its use as a self-report measure to a focus on the VT element of the instrument.

Affinity is a computer-based assessment, much like the AASI. It uses 80 photographs (40 images of females and 40 images of males) that are depicted fully clothed in frontal poses, within natural surrounds. The images include ten per age/gender category including small children (5 or younger), pre-juveniles (6–10), juveniles (11–15), and adults (18 and older). The images are presented in random order and upon onset of each image, the testee is asked to indicate whether he or she regards the person depicted as sexually attractive. This rating is done on a visual analog scale ranging from unattractive to attractive. In the original description of the method, two VT measures were calculated: on-task latency (OTL) was the time between onset of the stimulus and recording of the testee's rating and post-task latency (PTL) was the time from when the testee made their rating to when they clicked the "next image" button (Glasgow et al. 2003). Some investigators appear to have used the two measures (i.e., Mackaronis, Byrne, & Strassberg, 2014), while others have just used the OTL (i.e., Mokros et al., 2013).

Affinity is a newer tool than the AASI, and thus, it appears that it has been subjected to much less empirical validation. As with the AASI, most of the research available has been conducted either by the test developers or another group (Pacific Psychological Behavioural Assessment) who has taken on the commercial development and marketing of Affinity. In a study designed to assess the reliability and validity of Affinity 2.5, Mokros et al. (2013) tested 164 men, who included men convicted of hands-on sexual offenses against children who acknowledged their offenses, forensic psychiatric patients with no history of sexual offenses and no paraphilia diagnosis, and patients and visitors at a general (nonpsychiatric) hospital. The authors found that the VT measure, which was limited to OTL, had good to excellent reliability as measured by internal consistency and split half and that the image ratings had excellent reliability as measured by internal consistency and split half. The authors, however, conclude that the reliability is "insufficient for single-case diagnostics, at least as far as most of the viewing time variables are concerned" (Mokros et al., 2013, p. 247). Further, while the child sexual abusers differed significantly from the community controls on VT on all age categories and not the nonsexual offenders, the converse was true for the ratings. That is, the child sexual abusers differed from the non-sex offenders, but not from the community controls across all age categories. The authors also found that, within the child sexual abusers, there were significant effects for age, such that VT was different between pre-juvenile and adult and between juvenile and adult categories. Groups differed on the VT to juveniles, pre-juveniles, and small children, but not to adults, with child sexual abusers showing longer VT. Also, while significant correlations were found between VT and ratings in all age/gender categories except female adults, none of the correlations indicated a substantial amount of shared variance (r^2 ranged from 0.04 to 0.15).

An earlier study, designed to test the validity of Affinity with adolescent sex offenders tested 78 males aged 12–18 years from sex offender treatment centers in a Midwestern U.S. state and the Greater Toronto Area (Worling, 2006). The majority (78 %) had committed a sexual offense against at least on child (under 12 years of age and 4 or more years younger than the adolescent at the time of the offense), with the remainder offending against peers or adults. Worling (2006) found that the reliability of the ratings were consistently higher (all α's > 0.90) than the reliability of the OTL (α's range from 0.62 for female adolescents to 0.82 for female toddlers and male adolescents). Further, the author found that a deviance index derived from the OTL was only able to discriminate adolescents who had a male victim from those who did not. The ratings were able to distinguish between those adolescents with single child victims, multiple child victims, or male child victims. The correlations between the ratings and the OTL were higher than that found by Morkos, et al. (2012), ranging from 0.24 to 0.67, except for the female adult category where Worling (2006) found a significant negative association ($r = -0.26$).

In another study of adolescent males, Mackaronis et al. (2014) compared 16 adolescent males who had sexually offended using the MONARCH 21™ PPG system with the Affinity (either Affinity 2.0 or 2.5). Unlike the previous studies of Affinity, this study included both the OTL and the PTL viewing time measures and found, while both were significantly associated with the sexual attractiveness ratings, the relationship between OTL and the ratings ($r = 0.51$) was substantially higher than the relationship between the PTL and the ratings ($r = 0.22$). Further, the authors found that PPG and viewing time data (OTL) were significantly positively correlated with each other, but only when comparing raw scores rather than ipsative scores.

The empirical support for the Affinity system is rather mixed, with some measures showing validity, while others seem problematic. The only study, to date, that compares Affinity with PPG appears to be consistent with earlier studies of the AASI and other VT methods, in that the associations are significant, but modest. It is interesting that, although the Affinity was developed to assess sexual interest in cognitively challenged individuals (Glasgow, 2009; Glasgow et al., 2003), none of the subsequently published validation studies have been done with this population. Additionally, the results of the three studies here appear to indicate that the attraction ratings are better discriminators of sexual interest than the VT measure (On Task Latency). This may be an important distinction between the Affinity and the AASI. That is, the VT aspect of the Affinity was designed to be a validity check on the self-reported ratings, not as a direct measure of sexual interest (Glasgow, 2009; Glasgow et al., 2003).

Conclusions and Future Directions

In general, while the accumulating research seems to support the use of VT as an indirect measure of sexual interest, there are many problems with the research to date. The most serious problem with almost all of the studies reviewed for this chapter is that they have very small samples. While the significant discriminant validity found in most of the studies may be impressive, given the limited power in most of the research, the sample size makes it difficult to interpret the lack of associations found in some studies, when they were found in others.

Another interesting aspect of the research is that the methods tend to be inconsistent, and the available tools, the AASI and Affinity, are not always consistent with the findings, even those findings in their initial development. For example, Gress (2001 as cited in Laws & Gress, 2004) found that group discrimination was maximized by the use of both nude and clothed stimuli and early studies of VT with sex offenders (Harris et al., 1996; Quinsey et al. 1996) used only nude stimuli. Yet, neither of the commercially available methods use nude stimuli, in fact, the lack of such stimuli is used by AASI as an important selling point.

The actual VT procedure also differs across studies. Some studies only expose participants to the stimuli once, while others use one trial to familiarize the participant with the stimuli and a second trial where they make some type of rating as they look at the images, and it is at that point that VT is measured. This difference may affect the validity of the procedure for some populations (Bourke & Gormley, 2012). The two commercially available procedures differ in the ratings they ask participants to make. That is, the AASI asks participants to rate each image on how sexually arousing it is, from sexually disgusting to very sexually arousing, while the Affinity asks participants to rate each image on a scale from not sexually attractive to sexually attractive. These two tasks are fundamentally different. The AASI is asking for a rating on an emotional response, disgusted to aroused, while the Affinity is asking for a rating on a cognitive appraisal, from unattractive to attractive. Conceptually, one might expect longer VT at both ends of the AASI continuum, since both have high emotional content and both require complex appraisal, while one might only expect longer VT at the high end of the Affinity scale, either because of a SCID effect or the appraisal complexity difference between an unattractive rating and an attractive rating. Additionally, there is evidence, at least in anxious individuals, that emotional content increases VT (Bar-Haim, Lamy, Pergamin, Bakermans-Kranenburg, & van Ijzendoorn, 2007).

Thus, at the current time, it is not clear that VT is a major improvement over any of the existing measures of sexual interest. It certainly holds promise, in that there is evidence for an ability to discriminate between those whose sexual crimes were against children and other populations. It is not, at this time, clear that the fine discriminations between age and gender groups can be reliably done using available VT techniques, nor is it clear to what extent the currently available VT techniques predict future risk. There is also, to date, no evidence that whatever algorithm is used by Abel Assessment, Inc. is necessary for the reliability or validity of a VT measure.

In the studies reviewed here, the VRT™ performed no better or worse than the more straightforward VT measures. In fact, Babchishin et al. (2013) found that a combined measure using multiple indirect measures showed no better predictive accuracy than VT alone.

A final concern with the clinical application of VT measures is that none of the studies of its use within the context of sex offender assessment, including the many studies conducted by Abel and his colleagues, have considered that increased VT may be influenced by factors other than sexual interest. As noted earlier, anxiety has been shown to increase VT to stimuli that elicit this emotional reaction (Bar-Haim et al., 2007), and given the stakes in most sex offender assessments, it is likely that certain classes of stimuli might lead to increased anxiety in individuals being assessed for sexual interest. Research has also shown a positive association between fear of failure and VT for failure pictures (Duley, Conroy, Morris, Wiley, & Janelle, 2005). Fear of failure, again, is not uncommon for sexual offenders, and this could confound the VT measures and limit the degree to which longer VT can be assumed to be a function of sexual interest.

It is difficult to compare many of the studies due to methodological differences, including the nature of the questions used as a distractor task, whether participants are exposed to multiple trials within the task, and the data reduction. One study showed that the use of ipsative scores, while possibly useful for clinical purposes, may mask associations and effects when exposed to group-level statistical analyses (Mackaronis et al., 2014). Affinity seems much more available for independent validation than does the AASI. At this point, both instruments are limited in terms of independent replication. In addition, there is a need for more information on how sexual interest based on VT informs future risk for sexual offending behavior. Currently, it is likely that VT as measured either by the AASI, Affinity, or some other procedure, can provide an indication of sexual interest, at least in broad categories such as deviance or child interest ratios.

Summary and Conclusions

In this chapter, we have described two quite different methods used to infer what men like when it comes to sexual behavior—both in terms of targets (to whom or what should their sexual energies be directed) and behaviors (how will they express their sexual energies). First and foremost, it is important to acknowledge that although the two methods should be at least moderately correlated, they actually measure different things. The penile plethysmograph measures sexual arousal as ultimately suggested by Masters and Johnson (1966), whereas measures of viewing time focus on sexual interest. Though perhaps subtle, this is an important distinction.

The introduction of the phallometric method in the mid-twentieth century represented a big step forward in the understanding of male sexual arousal and preferences, particularly in regard to forensic applications. However, as demonstrated above, phallometry is not without its problems and detractors. Real questions remain regarding reliability and validity, and the situation is certainly not helped by an ongoing lack of standardization from site to site. Perhaps, the greatest limitation of the phallometric methods is related to its high rating on the "ick" factor. Specifically, PPG testing requires clients to place an apparatus over their penis, which raises issues of invasiveness and civil rights in an area already facing many challenges. Further, stimuli used to elicit sexual arousal must be sufficiently explicit to actually do so, leading to ethical questions regarding the exposure of potentially sexually dangerous persons to deviant stimuli, whether they be visual, auditory, or some combination thereof.

In spite of meta-analytic findings showing that deviant sexual preferences are robust predictors of reoffending (Hanson & Bussière, 1998) and phallometry's demonstrated ability to predict reoffending (Kingston et al., 2007; Wilson et al., 2011), there are no easy answers to these social and ethical dilemmas. With the advent of viewing time measures, some of these issues became less problematic. No longer would clients have to attach sensors to their genitalia, and depiction of children as objects for potential sexual interest was no longer necessary. But do VT measures represent a suitable or acceptable analog for phallometry?

In directly comparing PPG and VT as methods of deducing problematic sexual propensities in men who have engaged in sexually abusive conduct, there are a number of things to note. Although VT has demonstrated utility as a measure of sexual interest regarding problems related to both target choice and activity, its ability to discriminate between offenders and comparison subjects has generally been much less than that shown by the PPG (Harris et al., 1996). Along the same lines, Gress et al. (2013; see also Mokros et al., 2013) found that VT had good sensitivity and specificity overall, but ultimately advised against using such methods for clinical purposes (e.g., individual diagnosis).

Although there are other VT procedures (e.g., Affinity), there is no question that the most commonly used version is the Abel Assessment for Sexual Interest (see Gray et al., 2015). Unlike both the Affinity and the PPG, the Abel Screening group has maintained proprietary secrecy with respect to how clients are assessed as having inappropriate sexual interests. This has led to a good deal of criticism of the AASI, including within legal circumstances. In the only study (Letourneau, 2002) in which a researcher not associated with the Abel Screening group was allowed to access raw VT data, Visual Reaction Time showed convergent validity with PPG-assessed sexual arousal. In another study conducted by researchers (Gray & Plaud, 2005) not associated with the Abel Screening group, ipsative VRT data showed a higher overall correct classification rate than PPG; however, only when applied to subjects the authors assessed as not attempting to dissimilate. Overall, the single greatest limitation regarding the AASI is that the methods of data reduction are not clearly described because the algorithms are proprietary.

Problems regarding proprietary elements do not apply to other VT measures, such as the Affinity; however, other issues are evident. In their study comparing the Affinity and PPG, Mackaronis et al. (2014) found that the two methods were significantly positively correlated with one another, but only when using raw scores and not ipsative scores. Overall, empirical support for the Affinity is mixed, and some of the data seem to suggest that attraction ratings may be better discriminators of sexual interest than the viewing time task itself (Mackaronis et al., 2014; Mokros et al., 2013; Worling, 2006).

It is apparent to these authors that efforts to reliably measure male sexual arousal and interest continue to face challenges on many fronts. It would appear that deviant sexual arousal is a better proxy for risk for recidivism in sexual offenders than is sexual interest as measured by VT; however, the degree to which that deviant sexual arousal can be accurately assessed remains unclear. There are very real issues remaining regarding standardization, and thus, it is unclear how the range of stimuli, measurement techniques, and data reduction procedures affect the predictive and discriminant validity of PPG procedures. In addition, there are important ethical considerations when presenting sexually explicit materials (even within clinical contexts) to clients with demonstrated histories of engaging in sexually problematic behavior. Our humble suggestion is that an organization with international scope (like the Association for the Treatment of Sexual Abusers [ATSA] or the International Association for the Treatment of Sexual Offenders [IATSO]) would be well advised to sponsor a working group to set (at least) a set of governing principles regarding these issues.

The last point we would like to raise centers on the practical use of PPG/VT methods going forward. Specifically, we have some concerns about the capabilities of these methods to achieve the sorts of purposes for which they are being used. Freund's longstanding perspective was that the phallometric test was a diagnostic test to be used in identifying or confirming erotic preferences. Sexual interests via viewing time measures serve an analogous purpose, and, regardless of which method one uses, erotic preferences/interests are helpful in informing a clinical and risk management process in which client sexual health is addressed through treatment and prosocial lifestyle change, while efforts to maximize sexual violence prevention are advanced through comprehensive case management (see Wilson, Cortoni, Picheca, Stirpe, & Nunes, 2009) and public education (Tabachnick & Klein, 2011).

Our concern lies in assessing the potential use of PPG or VT in evaluating treatment efficacy. Notwithstanding the issues both methods face regarding standardization, reliability, and validity, we are moderately supportive of the use of such testing methods in the identification of problematic sexual arousal and interests. However, in our minds, using PPG or VT to evaluate the relative success of treatment endeavors stretches the utility of these methods. As noted earlier, these testing procedures are susceptible to test taker interference, and there are considerable concerns regarding social desirability bias, in that it does not take the test subject very long to figure out how he should be responding. Furthermore, most psychological tests are subject to a learning curve, in which the more often you take the test the more likely it is that you will achieve the "correct" answer (or at least what would be considered the socially acceptable answer).

Most treatment programs for people engaging in problematic sexual behavior focus on identifying and managing inappropriate sexual thoughts, fantasies, and urges. It would be our contention that the sorts of cognitive and behavioral approaches clients are encouraged to use when dealing with these thoughts, fantasies, and urges (e.g., thought stopping, distraction tasks, looking away) are precisely the sorts of methods identified in the literature as most successful in faking (see Freund et al., 1988; Wilson, 1998).

As such, it may be practically impossible to ascertain whether clients in treatment are showing less deviant arousal/interest because they have actually changed or because they were successful in faking the test. Using PPG or VT as an indicator of decreased risk via treatment may therefore represent an erroneous conclusion that could place the public at greater risk. We are not suggesting that treatment is unrelated to risk reduction (see Hanson, Bourgon, Helmus, & Hodgson, 2009; although the true efficacy of treatment for sexual offenders remains an open question); we are suggesting that using PPG or VT to establish treatment success comes with some peril.

In closing, we remind readers that many or most people who engage in sexually inappropriate conduct do so not because they are strongly sexually interested in or preferentially aroused by the sorts of people they victimize (children) or the behaviors in which they engage (exposing, peeping). There are a multitude of other factors (e.g., alcohol/substance abuse, intimacy deficits, poor self-regulation, poor sexual self-regulation, general antisociality—see Hanson & Yates, 2013) contributing to why some people engagement in sexually abusive conduct. As such, the utility of measures like PPG or VT will be limited to the identification of problematic arousal and interests—helpful information but, ultimately, only one slice of the comprehensive assessment and risk management pie.

Acknowledgements The authors would like to thank David Prescott for his helpful comments and suggestions on a draft of this chapter.

References

Abel, G. G. (1995). *The Abel assessment for sexual interest-2 (AASI-2)*. Atlanta, GA: Abel Screening.

Abel, G. G., Huffman, J., Warberg, B., & Holland, C. L. (1998). Visual reaction time and plethysmography as measures of sexual interest in child molesters. *Sexual Abuse: A Journal of Research & Treatment, 10*, 81–96.

Abel, G. G., Jordan, A. D., Hand, C. G., Holland, L. A., & Phipps, A. (2001). Classification models of child molesters utilizing the Abel Assessment for Sexual Interest. *Child Abuse & Neglect, 25*, 703–718.

Abel, G. G., Jordan, A., Rouleau, J.-L., Emerick, R., Barboza-Whitehead, S., & Osborn, C. (2004). Use of visual reaction time to assess male adolescents who molest children. *Sexual Abuse: A Journal of Research & Treatment, 16*, 255–265.

Abel, G. G., & Wiegel, M. (2009). Visual reaction time: Development, theory, empirical evidence and beyond. In F. Saleh, A. Grudzinskas, J. M. Bradford, & D. Brodsky (Eds.), *Sex offenders: Identification, risk assessment, treatment, and legal issues* (pp.101–118). Oxford, UK: Oxford University Press.

Abel, G. G., Lawry, S. S., Karlstrom, E. M., Osborn, C. A., & Gillespie, C. F. (1994). Screening tests for pedophilia. *Criminal Justice and Behavior, 21*, 115–131.

American Psychiatric Association. (2013). *Diagnostic and statistical manual of mental disorders* (5th ed.). Washington, DC: Author.

Association for the Treatment of Sexual Abusers. (2005). *Practice standards and guidelines for members of the association of for the treatment of sexual abusers*. Beaverton, OR: Author.

Babchishin, K. M., Nunes, K. L., & Kessous, N. (2014). A multimodal examination of sexual interest in children: A comparison of sex offenders and nonsex offenders. *Sexual Abuse: A Journal of Research & Treatment, 26*, 343–374.

Babchishin, K. M., Nunes, K. L., & Hermann, C. (2013). The validity of Implicit Association Test (IAT) measures of sexual attraction to children: A meta-analysis. *Archives of Sexual Behavior, 42*, 487–499.

Bancroft, J., Jones, H., & Pullan, G. (1966). A simple transducer for measuring penile erection, with comments on its use in the treatment of sexual offenders. *Behaviour Research & Therapy, 4*, 239–241.

Bar-Haim, Y., Lamy, D., Pergamin, L., Bakermans-Kranenburg, M. J., & van Ijzendoorn, M. H. (2007). Threat-related attentional bias in anxious and nonanxious individuals: A meta-analytic study. *Psychological Bulletin, 133*, 1–24.

Barlow, D., Becker, J., Leitenberg, H., & Agras, W. (1970). Technical note: A mechanical strain gauge for recording penile circumference change. *Journal of Applied Behavior Analysis, 3*, 73–76.

Barsetti, I., Earls, C. M., Lalumière, M. L., & Belanger, N. (1998). The differentiation of intrafamilial and extrafamilial heterosexual child molesters. *Journal of Interpersonal Violence, 13*, 275–286.

Bayliss, W. (1908). On reciprocal innervation in vaso-motor reflexes and the action of strychnine and chloroform thereon. *Proceedings of the Royal Society B: Biological Sciences, 80*, 339–375. Cited in K. Freund, Assessment of sexual dysfunction and deviation. In: M. Hersen, & A. Bellack (Eds.), *Behavioral assessment: A practical handbook*, 2nd Edition. New York, NY: Pergamon Press, 1981, pp. 427–455.

Bem, D. J. (1996). Exotic becomes erotic: A developmental theory of sexual orientation. *Psychological Review, 103*, 320–335.

Blanchard, R., Klassen, P., Dickey, R., Kuban, M. E., & Blak, T. (2001). Sensitivity and specificity of the phallometric test for pedophilia in nonadmitting sex offenders. *Psychological Assessment, 13*, 118–126.

Bourke, A. B., & Gormley, M. J. (2012). Comparing a pictorial stroop task and viewing time measures of sexual interest. *Sexual Abuse: A Journal of Research & Treatment, 24*, 479–500.

Card, R. D., & Farrall, W. R. (1990). Detecting faked responses to erotic stimuli: A comparison of stimulus conditions and response measures. *Annals of Sex Research, 3*, 381–396.

Chaplin, T. C., Rice, M. E., & Harris, G. T. (1995). Salient victim suffering and the sexual responses of child molesters. *Journal of Consulting and Clinical Psychology, 163*, 249–255.

Clark, T. O. (1972). Penile volume responses, sexual orientation and conditioning performance. *British Journal of Psychiatry, 120*, 554.

Duley, A. R., Conroy, D. E., Morris, K., Wiley, J., & Janelle, C. A. (2005). Fear of failure biases affective and attentional responses to lexical and pictorial stimuli. *Motivation and Emotion, 29*, 1–17.

Fisher, C., Gross, J., & Zuch, J. (1965). Cycle of penile erection synchronous with dreaming (REM) sleep. *Archives of General Psychiatry, 12*, 29–45.

Freund, K. (1957). Diagnostika homosexuality u muzu [Diagnosing homosexuality in men]. *Czech Psychiatry, 53*, 382–393.

Freund, K. (1971). A note on the use of the phallometric method of measuring mild sexual arousal in the male. *Behavior Therapy, 2*, 223–228.

Freund, K. (1977). Psycho-physiological assessment of change in erotic preference. *Behaviour Research and Therapy, 15*, 297–301.

Freund, K., & Blanchard, R. (1989). Phallometric diagnosis of pedophilia. *Journal of Consulting and Clinical Psychology, 57*, 1–6.

Freund, K., Diamant, J., & Pinkava, V. (1958). On the validity and reliability of the phalloplethysmographic diagnosis of some sexual deviations. *Review of Czechoslovak Medicine, 4*, 145–151.

Freund, K., Langevin, R., & Barlow, D. (1974). Comparison of two penile measures of erotic arousal. *Behaviour Research & Therapy, 12*, 355–359.

Freund, K., Langevin, R., & Zajac, Y. (1974). A note on the erotic arousal value of moving and stationary forms. *Behaviour Research and Therapy, 12*, 117–119.

Freund, K., & Watson, R. (1991). Assessment of the sensitivity and specificity of a phallometric test: An update of "Phallometric diagnosis of pedophilia". *Psychological Assessment, 3*, 254–260.

Freund, K., Watson, R., & Dickey, R. (1991). Sex offenses against female children perpetrated by men who are not pedophiles. *Journal of Sex Research, 28*, 409–423.

Freund, K., Watson, R., & Rienzo, D. (1988). Signs of feigning in the phallometric test. *Behaviour Research and Therapy, 26*, 105–112.

Glasgow, D. V. (2009). Affinity: The development of a self-report assessment of paedophile sexual interest incorporating a viewing time validity measure. In D. Thornton & D. R. Laws (Eds.), *Cognitive approaches to the assessment of sexual interest in sexual offenders* (pp. 59–84). New York, NY: Wiley.

Glasgow, D. V., Osborne, A., & Croxen, J. (2003). An assessment tool for investigating paedophile sexual interest using viewing time: An application of a single case methodology. *British Journal of Learning Disabilities, 31*, 96–102.

Gray, S. R., & Plaud, J. J. (2005). A comparison of the Abel Assessment for Sexual Interest and penile plethysmography in an outpatient sample of sexual offenders. *Journal of Sexual Offender Civil Commitment, Science and the Law, 1*, 1–10.

Gray, S. R., Abel, G. G., Jordan, A., Garby, T., Wiegel, M., & Harlow, N. (2015). Visual reaction TimeTM as a predictor of sexual offense recidivism. *Sexual Abuse: A Journal of Research and Treatment, 27*, 173–188.

Greer, J. H., & Bellard, H. S. (1996). Sexual content induced delays in unprimed lexical decisions: Gender and context effects. *Archives of Sexual Behavior, 25*, 379–395.

Greer, J. H., & Melton, J. S. (1997). Sexual content-induced delay with double-entendre words. *Archives of Sexual Behavior, 26*, 295–316.

Gress, C. L. Z. (2001). *An evaluation of a sexual interest assessment tool*. Unpublished manuscript.

Gress, C. L. Z., Anderson, J. O., & Laws, D. R. (2013). Delays in attentional processing when viewing sexual imagery: The development and comparison of two measures. *Legal and Criminological Psychology, 18*, 66–82.

Hanson, R. K., Bourgon, G., Helmus, L., & Hodgson, S. (2009). The principles of effective correctional treatment also apply to sexual offenders: A meta-analysis. *Criminal Justice and Behavior, 36*, 865–891.

Hanson, R. K., & Bussière, M. T. (1998). Predicting relapse: A meta-analysis of sexual offender recidivism studies. *Journal of Consulting and Clinical Psychology, 66*, 348–362.

Hanson, R. K., & Morton-Bourgon, K. E. (2005). The characteristics of persistent sexual offenders: A meta-analysis of recidivism studies. *Journal of Consulting and Clinical Psychology, 73*, 1154–1163.

Hanson, R. K., & Mouton-Bourgon, K. (2009). The accuracy of recidivism risk assessments for sexual offenders: A meta-analysis of 118 prediction studies. *Psychological Assessment, 21*, 1–21.

Hanson, R. K., & Yates, P. M. (2013). Psychological treatment of sex offenders. *Current Psychiatry Reports, 15*, 348.

Harris, G. T., Rice, M. E., Quinsey, V. T., & Chaplin, T. C. (1996). Viewing time as a measure of sexual interest among child molesters and normal heterosexual men. *Behaviour Research and Therapy, 34*, 389–394.

Her Majesty's Prison Service. (2007). *Penile plethysmograph (PPG): Interpretation guidelines*. London: Author.

Hynie, J. (1934). Nova objektivni metoda vysetrovani muszke sexualni potence [A new objective method of investigation of male sexual potency]. *Cslky Lekarsky Easopis, 73*, 34–39. Cited in K. Freund, Assessment of sexual dysfunction and deviation. In: M. Hersen, & A. Bellack (Eds.), *Behavioral assessment: A practical handbook*, 2nd Edition. New York, NY: Pergamon Press, 1981, pp. 427–455.

Imhoff, R., Schmidt, A. F., Wei, S., Young, A. W., & Banse, R. (2012). Vicarious viewing time: Prolonged response latencies for sexually attractive targets as a function of task—Or stimulus specific processing. *Archives of Sexual Behavior, 41*, 1389–1401.

Kaine, A., & Mersereau, G. (1986). *Lie detection and plethysmography: Their uses and limitation in offender assessment*. Ottawa, ON: Solicitor General Canada.

Kingston, D. A., Firestone, P., Moulden, H. M., & Bradford, J. M. (2007). The utility of the diagnosis of pedophilia. A comparison of various classification procedures. *Archives of Sexual Behavior, 36*, 423–436.

Kingston, D. A., Seto, M. C., Firestone, P., & Bradford, J. M. (2010). Comparing indicators of sexual sadism as predictors of recidivism among adult male sexual offenders. *Journal of Consulting and Clinical Psychology, 78*, 574–584.

Konopasky, R. J., & Konopasky, A. W. B. (2000). Remaking penile plethysmography. In D. L. Laws, S. M. Hudson, & T. Ward (Eds.), *Remaking relapse prevention with sex offenders: A sourcebook* (pp. 257–284). Thousand Oaks, CA: Sage Publications.

Kuban, M., Barbaree, H. E., & Blanchard, R. (1999). A comparison of volume and circumference phallometry: Response magnitude and method agreement. *Archives of Sexual Behavior, 28*, 345–359.

Lalumière, M. L., & Harris, G. T. (1998). Common questions regarding the use of phallometric testing with sexual offenders. *Sexual Abuse: A Journal of Research & Treatment, 10*, 227–237.

Lalumière, M. L., & Quinsey, V. L. (1994). The discriminability of rapists from non-sex offenders using phallometric measures: A meta-analysis. *Criminal Justice and Behavior, 21*, 150–175.

Lalumière, M. L., Quinsey, V. L., Harris, G. T., Rice, M. E., & Trautrimas, C. (2003). Are rapists differentially aroused by coercive sex in phallometric assessments? In R. A. Prentky, E. Janus, & M. Seto (Eds.), *Sexual coercion: Understanding and management* (pp. 211–224). New York, NY: New York Academy of Sciences.

Larue, D., Schmidt, A. F., Imhoff, R., Eggers, K., Schönbrodt, F. D., & Banse, R. (2014). Validation of direct and indirect measures of preference for sexualized violence. *Psychological Assessment, 26*, 1173–1183.

Laws, D. R., & Gress, C. L. Z. (2004). Seeing things differently: The viewing time alternative to penile plethysmography. *Legal and Criminological Psychology, 9*, 183–196.

Laws, D. R., & Rubin, H. (1969). Instructional control of autonomic sexual response. *Journal of Applied Behavioral Analysis, 2*, 93–99.

Letourneau, E. J. (2002). A comparison of objective measures of sexual arousal and interest: Visual reaction time and penile plethysmography. *Sexual Abuse: A Journal of Research & Treatment, 14*, 207–223.

Mackaronis, J. E., Byrne, P. M., & Strassberg, D. S. (2014). Assessing sexual interest in adolescents who have sexually offended. *Sexual Abuse: A Journal of Research & Treatment*. DOI: 10.1177/1079063214535818.

Malcolm, P. B., Andrews, D. A., & Quinsey, V. L. (1993). Discriminant and predictive validity of phallometrically measured sexual age and gender preference. *Journal of Interpersonal Violence, 8*, 486–501.

Marshall, W., Barbaree, H., & Christophe, D. (1986). Sexual offenders against female children: Sexual preferences for age of victims and type of behaviour. *Canadian Journal of Behavioural Science, 18*, 424–439.

Marshall, W. L., & Fernandez, Y. M. (2003). *Phallometric testing with sexual offenders: Theory, research and practice*. Brandon, VT: Safer Society Press.

Marshall, W. L., Kennedy, P., Yates, P. M., & Serran, G. A. (2002). Diagnosing sexual sadism in sexual offenders: Reliability across diagnosticians. *International Journal of Offender Therapy and Comparative Criminology, 46*, 668–676.

Masters, W., & Johnson, V. (1966). *Human sexual response*. New York, NY: Bantam Books.

McConaghy, N. (1974a). Measurements of change in penile dimensions. *Archives of Sexual Behavior, 3*, 381–388.

McConaghy, N. (1974b). Penile volume responses to moving and still pictures of male and female nudes. *Archives of Sexual Behavior, 3*, 565–570.

Miner, M. H., West, M. A., & Day, D. M. (1995). Sexual preference for child and aggressive stimuli: Comparison of rapists and child molesters using auditory and visual stimuli. *Behavior Research & Therapy, 33*, 545–551.

Mokros, A., Gebhard, M., Heinz, V., Marschall, R. W., Nitschke, J., Glasgow, D. V., … Laws, D. R. (2013). Computerized assessment of pedophilic sexual interest through self-report and viewing time: Reliability, validity, and classification accuracy of the Affinity program. *Sexual Abuse: A Journal of Research and Treatment, 25*, 230–258.

Moulden, H. M., Firestone, P., Kingston, D., & Bradford, J. (2009). Recidivism in pedophiles: An investigation using different diagnostic methods. *Journal of Forensic Psychiatry & Psychology, 20*, 680–701.

Ohlmeyer, P., Brilmayer, H., & Hullstrung, H. (1944). Periodische vorgange im schlaf [Periodical events in sleep]. *Pflügers Archiv, 248*, 559–560. Cited in K. Freund, Assessment of sexual dysfunction and deviation. In: M. Hersen, & A. Bellack (eds.), *Behavioral assessment: A practical handbook*, 2nd Edition. New York, NY: Pergamon Press, 1981, pp. 427–455.

Orne, M. (1962). On the social psychology of the psychological experiment: With particular reference to demand characteristics and their implications. *American Psychologist, 17*, 776–783.

Price, S., & Hanson, R. K. (2007). A modified Stroop task with sexual offenders: Replication of a study. *Journal of Sexual Aggression, 13*, 203–216.

Quinsey, V., & Bergersen, S. (1976). Instructional control of penile circumference assessments of sexual preference. *Behavior Therapy, 7*, 489–493.

Quinsey, V. L., Ketsetzis, M., Earls, C., & Karamanoukian, A. (1996). Viewing time as a measure of sexual interest. *Ethology and Sociobiology, 17*, 341–354.

Quinsey, V., & Chaplin, T. (1987). *Preventing faking in phallometric assessments of sexual preference*. Paper presented at the New York Academy of Sciences Conference on Human Sexual Aggression, January 7–9, 1987.

Renaud, P., Chartier, S., Rouleau, J. -L., Proulx, J., Décarie, J., Trottier, D., ... Bouchard, S. (2009). Gaze behavior nonlinear dynamics assess in virtual immersion as a diagnostic index of sexual deviancy: Preliminary results. *Journal of Virtual Reality and Broadcasting, 6*, 10 pp.

Rosenweig, S. (1942). The photoscope as an objective device for evaluating sexual interest. *Psychosomatic Medicine, 4*, 150–158.

Seto, M. C. (2008). *Pedophilia and sexual offending against children: Theory, assessment, and intervention*. Washington, DC: American Psychological Association.

Seto, M. C. (2012). Is pedophilia a sexual orientation? *Archives of Sexual Behavior, 41*, 231–236.

Smith, D., & Over, R. (1987). Male sexual arousal as a function of the content and the vividness of erotic fantasy. *Psychophysiology, 24*, 334–339.

Smith, P., & Waterman, M. G. (2004). Processing bias for sexual material: The emotional Stroop and sexual offenders. *Sexual Abuse: A Journal of Research & Treatment, 16*, 163–171.

Tabachnick, J., & Klein, A. (2011). *A reasoned approach: Reshaping sex offender policy to prevent child sexual abuse*. Beaverton, OR: Association for the Treatment of Sexual Abusers.

Whitney, P. (1949). The measurement of changes in human limb volume by means of a mercury-in-rubber strain gauge. *Journal of Psychology, 109*, 5.

Williams, J. M. G., & Broadbent, K. (1986). Distraction by emotional stimuli – Use of a Stroop task with suicide attempters. *British Journal of Clinical Psychology, 25*, 101–110.

Wilson, R. J. (1998). Psychophysiological indicators of faking in the phallometric test. *Sexual Abuse: A Journal of Research & Treatment, 10*, 113–126.

Wilson, R. J., Abracen, J., Looman, J., Picheca, J. E., & Ferguson, M. (2011). Pedophilia: An evaluation of diagnostic and risk management methods. *Sexual Abuse: A Journal of Research & Treatment, 23*, 260–274.

Wilson, R. J., Cortoni, F., Picheca, J. E., Stirpe, T. S., & Nunes, K. (2009). *Community-based sexual offender maintenance treatment programming: An evaluation* ([Research report R-188]). Ottawa, ON: Correctional Service of Canada.

Wilson, R. J., & Freund-Mathon, H. (2007). Looking backward to inform the future: Remembering Kurt Freund, 1914-1996. In D. Prescott (Ed.), *Knowledge and practice: Practical applications in the treatment and supervision of sexual abusers*. Oklahoma City, OK: Wood 'n' Barnes.

Worling, J. R. (2006). Assessing sexual arousal with adolescent males who have offended sexually: Self-report and unobtrusively measure viewing time. *Sexual Abuse: A Journal of Research & Treatment, 18*, 383–400.

Zamanski, H. (1956). A technique for measuring homosexual tendencies. *Journal of Personality, 24*, 436–448.

Chapter 6
Polygraph Testing of Sex Offenders

Don Grubin

Introduction

From tentative beginnings in the 1990s, postconviction sex offender testing (PCSOT) has become increasingly incorporated into sex offender treatment and supervision in both the United States and United Kingdom. McGrath, Cumming, Burchard, Zeoli, and Ellerby (2010), for example, reported that nearly 80 % of community adult sex offender programs in the United States and over half of residential ones make use of polygraph testing to inform treatment or supervision, while in the United Kingdom, mandatory testing of high-risk sex offenders on parole was introduced in 2014 after a number of trials. Its spread to other countries is likely, with a number of jurisdictions actively considering its use.

The growing influence of PCSOT, however, is not without controversy. The speed with which it has been embraced by programs has tended to outpace evidence, with much of its impetus coming from clinical experience supported by a research base of limited robustness. Only recently have more well-designed studies been carried out. Although this is not unusual when new procedures are introduced, PCSOT carries with it significant baggage associated with polygraph testing more generally. Thus, while proponents claim that PCSOT makes important contributions to sex offender treatment and management by bringing to attention changes in risk, facilitating disclosures, and perhaps encouraging offenders to modify their behavior (Grubin, 2008; Levenson, 2009), others are more skeptical. Commentators, for example, have argued that the type of polygraph test used in PCSOT lacks

D. Grubin, M.D., F.R.C.Psych. (✉)
Institute of Neuroscience, Newcastle University, Gosforth,
Newcastle upon Tyne NE3 3XT, UK

Northumberland, Tyne and Wear NHS Trust, St Nicholas Hospital,
Gosforth, Newcastle upon Tyne NE3 3XT, UK
e-mail: don.grubin@ncl.ac.uk

© Springer International Publishing Switzerland 2016
D.R. Laws, W. O'Donohue (eds.), *Treatment of Sex Offenders*,
DOI 10.1007/978-3-319-25868-3_6

validation, is unscientific, and is potentially dangerous (Ben-Shakhar, 2008; Iacono, 2008); polygraph testing may adversely affect the therapeutic alliance between the offender and therapist or supervisor (McGrath et al., 2010; Vess, 2011); the entire process is based on manipulation or intimidation and potentially breaches a number of basic ethical principles relating to autonomy and non-malfeasance (Chaffin, 2011; Cross & Saxe, 2001; Meijer, Verschuere, Merckelbach, & Crombez, 2008); and, common to all critical commentaries, there is an absence of research to show that it is effective (Rosky, 2013).

To what extent, then, does PCSOT make a positive contribution to sex offender treatment and management, a question sometimes simplified to, "does it work?" As a first consideration, it must be able to differentiate truth telling from deception reliably, and it should facilitate the disclosure of clinically relevant information. If it meets these requirements, it then needs to be demonstrated that in doing so it has a beneficial impact on treatment and/or management. But even if PCSOT does "work" in this way, if in the process it crosses ethical or legal red lines, then it would be hard to justify continued reliance on it.

Polygraph Testing

As indicated above, there are two primary outputs from a polygraph test, each of which complements the other.

The first, and what people usually associate with polygraph testing, is test outcome, that is, whether an examinee "passes" or "fails" the test. Although the focus is typically on "lie detection," determination of truthfulness is equally important. In order to shift attention away from the polygraph as a "lie detector," therefore, many practitioners now refer to it as a means of "credibility assessment" (Raskin, Honts, & Kircher, 2014). The fundamental questions here, of course, are how accurate polygraphy is in detecting deception and confirming honesty and whether that level of accuracy is sufficient for the setting in which it is being used. Unfortunately, this second question is often overlooked, an important oversight when translating research findings regarding accuracy into practice—what may not be accurate enough in a national security context or in a court of law may be sufficient for investigating crime or when used postconviction.

The second output of a polygraph test is disclosure. Numerous studies have reported that individuals report information during a polygraph examination they would otherwise have kept to themselves. Critics sometimes dismiss this effect as being a "bogus pipeline to the truth" as they say it depends on an examinee believing that the polygraph "works" and that disclosures would not occur if examinees did not hold this belief. This assertion, however, begs two questions: the extent to which disclosures are in fact dependent on a belief in the accuracy of the polygraph test and, if they are, the level of accuracy required to trigger this effect. As will be discussed later in this chapter, while many social psychology studies have demonstrated that disclosures do increase when subjects believe they are attached to a "lie detector," the strength of this effect is unclear. A third more philosophical consideration also arises in respect of this issue—if disclosures are a function of a belief in polygraph accuracy, but polygraphy is shown to meet the level of accuracy required to trigger this belief, is it still correct to refer to the phenomenon as a "bogus" pipeline?

Thus, although discussions about PCSOT often get bogged down in arguments about accuracy levels and the basis of disclosures, both issues are more complex than they appear at face value.

What the Polygraph Records

That there is an association between deception and physiological activity has been known for centuries. One of the earliest and clearest expressions of this was by Daniel Defoe, who when writing about the prevention of street robberies in the eighteenth century observed that:

> Guilt carries fear always about with it; there is a tremor in the blood of the thief that, if attended to, would effectually discover him … take hold of his wrist and feel his pulse, there you shall find his guilt; a fluttering heart, an unequal pulse, a sudden palpitation shall evidently confess he is the man, in spite of a bold countenance or a false tongue. (Defoe, 1730/ quoted in Matte, 1996)

Fairly, though, Defoe also noted, "The experiment perhaps has not been try'd."

While the phrase "a tremor in the blood" is so often quoted by those who write about the history of the polygraph that it is in danger of becoming a cliché, it nonetheless lays the groundwork for both the basis of polygraph testing and some of the misconceptions associated with it.

The involuntary physiological responses associated with guilt and deception recognized by Defoe are now known to be caused by activity in the autonomic nervous system. These responses, however, are not unique to deception—lots of things can make the blood tremor besides guilt and lying, and no physiological variable has yet been discovered that is specific to deception. Because of this, it is sometimes concluded that polygraphy, or any other techniques that rely on recording and interpreting physiological activity, cannot possibly work. But there need not be a unique physiological lie response for polygraph testing to be effective; instead, what matters is whether physiological reactivity recorded *in the context of a polygraph examination* discriminates truth telling from deception at levels sufficiently above the chance to make the technique meaningful and worthwhile. False-positive and false-negative findings occur with every test and investigation; more relevant is being able to quantify their frequency and ensure that whatever actions follow a test result take this error rate into account.

A second misconception that can be seen in Defoe's observations is that physiological responses associated with deception are the result of emotion, especially the emotions of fear and anxiety. This mistake leads some to argue that anxious individuals, either inherently or because they are made anxious by the circumstances of the test, are likely to wrongly "fail" for this reason. Other critics are concerned that in order for the test to work, polygraph examiners must induce anxiety or fear in examinees, which is ethically dubious (BPS, 1986; Vess, 2011). There is also a belief that psychopathic individuals, because of their low levels of anxiety and emotional responsiveness, are more likely to "beat" the test. But though there is uncertainty regarding the mode of action of polygraphy and the neuropsychological basis of the physiological reactions it records, it is clear that emotional reactivity is only part of the story and that a number of cognitive processes associated with deception contribute to what the polygraph observes. Anxiety and fear, except insofar as they indicate that the examinee takes the examination seriously, are likely to be minor components at best. More will be said about this later.

Cardiovascular, respiratory, and electrodermal activities measured by recording devices as opposed to being observed indirectly began to be used as a means of detecting deception in the late nineteenth and first part of the twentieth centuries, mainly on their own but in some cases together, both in Europe and the United States (Alder, 2007; Krapohl & Shaw, 2015). Criminologists, psychologists, and physicians such as Cesare Lombroso, Hugo Munsterberg, Georg Sticker, Vittorio Benussi, Walter Summers, William Marston, John Larson, and Leonarde Keeler researched and applied their various techniques, sometimes with phenomenal claims of success. In the 1930s this work coalesced into instruments that could simultaneously record data from the three physiological systems, giving rise to what became known as the polygraph. Although the hardware has improved since then, and the process has become digitalized so that ink pens writing on moving paper are no longer required, little has changed in terms of the basic physiology that is recorded.

In what way is activity in these physiological systems associated with deception? Traditionally polygraph examiners are taught that what they are observing is a "fight, flight, or freeze" response caused by the fear of being caught out in a lie and the consequences that follow, implicitly accepting an emotional basis to the test's mode of action. There are a number of major problems with this explanation; however, response characteristics that are associated with deception on the polygraph test are not identical to what is seen in a "fight, flight, or freeze" scenario, deceptive responses are recorded even where there is little anxiety and no consequence attached to being caught out (e.g., in tests where examinees are simply told to pick a number and then to lie when asked if they have done so), and not all polygraph formats require lying at all but instead relate to the "recognition" of relevant items.

The reality is that we are well short of understanding the mode of action of the polygraph, indicated by the number of theories proposed to explain it (National Research Council, 2003; Nelson, 2015), although it is now accepted that a range of mental processes are involved in addition to emotion. Important are concepts and factors such as the "differential salience" (i.e., differing degrees of importance or threat represented by the questions asked on the test), cognitive work involved in lying and in inhibiting truth telling (truth telling being the default position), autobiographical memory, orienting to "threat," and attention (Nelson, 2015; Senter, Weatherman, Krapohl, & Horvath, 2010), which interact to produce arousal in the autonomic nervous system that can be seen in a number of peripheral physiological processes.

While a lengthy discussion regarding the physiological and psychological mechanisms underlying polygraphy cannot be pursued here, the fundamental point is that conducting a successful polygraph test is about more than simply attaching the recording hardware and then asking questions. Instead, the examiner must work at ensuring that whatever reactions are recorded are produced because the examinee is deceptive to the questions being asked, rather than by other possible causes of autonomic arousal. This is achieved in a lengthy pretest interview and requires examiner training and skill, in other words, a competent examiner. Given that the process is so heavily dependent on the examiner's capabilities, it has been argued that polygraphy should not be seen as a "scientific test" (BPS, 2004), but this is perhaps more of a semantic than a practical issue—operator skill is important in all forms of scientific testing. But whether "scientific" or not, what matters is whether, in the hands of a competent examiner, polygraph testing can be shown to be a reliable means of distinguishing truth telling from deception.

In terms of PCSOT, there is no need to induce anxiety in examinees, anxious individuals are no more or less likely to "fail" the test, and, because the generation of fear or anxiety is irrelevant, psychopaths are no more or less likely to wrongly "pass" the test (Patrick & Iacono, 1989; Raskin & Hare, 1978). Furthermore, as will be discussed later, the examinee does not need to be deceived about the accuracy of polygraphy nor manipulated in other ways for the test to be successful.

Polygraph Accuracy

While the physiological targets of polygraph testing have not changed much since the 1930s, numerous testing techniques, question formats, scoring systems, and specialized applications have emerged since then, often introduced with little empirical support. The plethora of approaches and the associated lack of standardization have made it difficult to provide clear estimates of polygraph accuracy.

A number of initiatives have meant that the situation has improved (Krapohl & Shaw, 2015). Chart scoring, as opposed to decisions based on a global overview of the polygraph chart, was introduced in the 1960s, a hardening of testing protocols took place between the 1960s and 1990s, increased acceptance of blind scoring of charts as a means of quality control to overcome the risk of examiner bias became more commonplace in the 1990s, research in the early 2000s better clarified response patterns that are indicative of deception (and just as importantly, response patterns that aren't) and the amount of variance explained by the different physiological channels, and in the late 2000s, the American Polygraph Association undertook an exercise to validate testing techniques (American Polygraph Association, 2011). All of this has provided a better scientific basis on which to evaluate the efficacy of polygraph testing.

The most definitive review of polygraph accuracy to date has been carried out by the National Academies of Science in the United States. It concluded that "polygraph tests can discriminate lying from truth telling at rates well above chance, though well below perfection" (National Research Council, 2003, p. 4). Accuracy for the most commonly used test format, the comparison question test (a version of which is employed in PCSOT), was estimated to be between 81 and 91 %, which is highly supportive of a meaningful association between what the polygraph records, truth telling, and deception.

The National Academies Review was carried out on behalf of the US Department of Energy, triggered by allegations of espionage at the Los Alamos nuclear weapons facility, and was designed to advise on the use of polygraph testing for personnel security vetting. Its overall conclusion was that an error rate of 10–20 % was too high for this type of application given the low levels of deception likely to be found in the population to be tested (one hopes that there are not many spies working in federal agencies) and the disproportionate number of false-positive findings such an error rate would imply. Although polygraph proponents disagree with this conclusion, arguing that it is based on a misconception of the way in which security vetting is undertaken because in this setting it acts as an initial screen rather than providing a definitive outcome, more important in terms of PCSOT is the review's observation that polygraphy becomes viable when the underlying rate of deception is over 10 % — a rate which most observers, even those critical of polygraphy, would accept is probably exceeded in sex offender populations.

For a number of reasons, however, the National Academies Review is not the end of the story, at least in terms of PCSOT. Its estimate of accuracy is based on single-issue, "diagnostic" tests, that is, tests in which a single known issue is being investigated, for example, whether an individual was involved in a bank robbery. Although this is sometimes the case in PCSOT, as when the focus is on specific behaviors reported to have occurred during an offense or where the matter of concern is whether the offender is responsible for a new crime, the majority of tests carried out in PCSOT are screening in nature. In screening tests, a number of behaviors are explored, but there is not a known event that underpins the thrust of the exam.

Screening tests are generally considered to be less accurate then single-issue tests, although there are insufficient trials from which to determine their precise level of accuracy. Screening tests however tend to have higher false-positive rates (tests which wrongly label an examinee as deceptive). Two studies used anonymous surveys with sex offenders in the United States to ask about their experiences of being wrongly accused of deception and also of instances where deception had been missed (Grubin & Madsen, 2006; Kokish, Levenson, & Blasingame, 2005). The findings were very similar, with responses from offenders in both studies suggesting an accuracy rate for PCSOT between 80 and 90 %, reassuringly similar to the National Academies estimate.

Because of its likely error rate, the utility of PCSOT tends to be emphasized rather than its accuracy, with disclosures seen as more important than test outcome. In addition, it is recommended that outcome in screening tests is reported as "significant response" or "no significant response" rather than "deception indicated" or "no deception indicated" as it is in single-issue tests. However, a more recent initiative has expressed polygraph test outcome as a probability statement with confidence intervals derived from data normed on large sets of confirmed tests.

Referred to as the "Empirical Scoring System" (ESS), this allows a better judgment to be made about the degree of confidence one can have in a given test result (Nelson et al., 2011). Although the database on which ESS is built could be larger, and while it still requires independent validation, this type of approach provides greater clarity on polygraph test accuracy in environments such as PCSOT.

The error rate associated with polygraphy, and its screening function in most PCSOT settings, means that it is probably a mistake to talk about an individual 'passing' or 'failing' the test. One doesn't pass or fail a screening exam of any sort. The aim of screening is to identify those who require further investigation. In the case of PCSOT, significant responses to some questions are observed, which might be thought of as 'screening positive', but this is different from failing a test. It is therefore probably more sensible to think in terms of positive and negative predictive values: the former referring to the likelihood of a true positive (that is, deception) when an individual shows a significant response, and the latter to the likelihood of truthfulness when no significant responses are recorded. It is usually the case that one is higher than the other, providing an indication of whether one should be more confident in deceptive or truthful calls (the first where it the positive predictive value is higher, the second when the negative predictive value is).

There remains the problem of examiner competence and its impact on test accuracy. However, if properly trained examiners use correct techniques that are administered properly, then their accuracy rate should be similar to that reported in the research literature. Ensuring that this is the case requires a well-constructed quality assurance and quality control program, which unfortunately many PCSOT programs lack. But this is a reason to improve programs rather than to dismiss polygraphy. Provided it is in place, the important question becomes not whether polygraph is "accurate" but whether accuracy in the range of 80–90 % is accurate enough.

The answer to this question will depend on how test outcome is used. An error rate of 10–20 % is clearly too high to warrant sending someone to prison or taking away their livelihood but not too high to inform decisions about treatment engagement, changes in monitoring conditions, or the need for further investigation into possible transgressions. This is particularly the case when one remembers that typically we make these types of decision based on our own determination of whether or not someone is deceptive, even though in experimental settings the ability of the average person to do so accurately is rarely above 60 % (Bond & DePaulo, 2006; Vrij, 2000).

Utility and Disclosure

Polygraphy is known to increase the likelihood that an examinee will disclose previously unknown information. There are many anecdotal accounts of this phenomenon in both investigative and screening settings, but the best evidence for this effect is found in sex offender testing where numerous studies describe significant increases in self-report of previous offense types and victims, deviant sexuality, and risky behaviors (e.g., Ahlmeyer, Heil, McKee, & English, 2000; Grubin, Madsen,

Parsons, Sosnowski, & Warberg, 2004; Heil, Ahlmeyer, & Simons, 2003; Hindman & Peters, 2001; Madsen, Parsons, & Grubin, 2004). This work, however, lacks robustness in that comparisons are usually made in terms of what was known about an offender before and after polygraph testing rather than with contemporaneous comparison groups in which polygraph testing is not used. As critics readily point out, this makes it difficult to disentangle the effects of polygraphy from other factors such as treatment impact or changes in supervision.

The lack of a comparison group with which to determine polygraph efficacy in facilitating disclosures has been addressed in two large UK studies, both of which confirmed the findings of earlier work that showed increases in disclosure when polygraphy is used. In one of these studies, polygraph testing was voluntary (Grubin, 2010), while in the other it was a mandatory condition of a parole license (Gannon et al., 2014; Gannon, Wood, Vasquez, & Fraser, 2012).

In the trial of voluntary testing (Grubin, 2010), the supervision of nearly 350 polygraphed offenders was compared with 180 sex offenders from probation areas where polygraphy was not used. Just over 40 % of eligible offenders agreed to be tested, of whom 47 % were tested more than once. The majority were taking part in treatment programs. Probation officers reported that new disclosures relevant to treatment or supervision were made in 70 % of the first tests, compared with 14 % of the non-polygraphed offenders making similar types of disclosure in the previous 6 months. A similar difference was found in respect of retests (only in this case the comparison was with 3 months before). The disclosures made by polygraphed offenders were rated as "medium" or "high" severity (the former relating to behaviors indicative of increased risk, the latter to actual breaches or offenses) in over 40 % of cases. The odds of a polygraphed offender making a disclosure relevant to his treatment or supervision were 14 times greater than they were for non-polygraphed offenders.

Although the test and comparison groups reported in Grubin (2010) did not differ on demographic or criminological variables, the fact that those tested were volunteers could have introduced bias. Because of this the mandatory trial described by Gannon et al. (Gannon et al., 2012, 2014) was considered necessary before a decision could be reached about implementing mandatory testing nationwide (it was a requirement set by the UK Parliament). Like the earlier study, a comparison group was used. Unlike it, the mandatory trial was limited to high-risk offenders (defined as those released on parole following a prison sentence of a year or more), and though many had undertaken sex offender treatment in prison, relatively few were involved in community treatment programs. The focus of the mandatory trial, therefore, was on the impact of polygraph testing on supervision only.

There were over 300 offenders in each group, which again did not differ on demographic variables. Although the mandatory trial involved an overall higher risk group and many fewer were in treatment than in the voluntary trial, its findings were similar. Significant increases were found in the number of individuals who made what were referred to as "clinically relevant disclosures" and in the number of disclosures these individuals made in the polygraph group. This was particularly noticeable in respect of sexual- and risk-related behaviors. However, the odds ratio of a disclosure being made was lower at 3.1.

In both studies significantly more actions were taken by probation officers who managed offenders subject to polygraphy than by probation officers supervising comparison offenders. One interesting finding reported in Gannon et al. (2012) was that while 73 % of interviewed probation officers believed the offenders they supervised were "open and honest" with them, this was the case for only 25 % of the probation officers who supervised polygraphed offenders. This is perhaps an explanation for the finding in Grubin (2010) that whereas probation officers of polygraphed offenders were more likely to increase risk ratings, risk ratings were more likely to be decreased in the comparison group.

Although the impact of polygraph testing on disclosures is clear, the question still remains whether it is simply a "bogus pipeline" effect. As described earlier, this refers to the increase in disclosures being the product of a belief that the polygraph "works," the implication being that disclosures would dry up in the absence of such a belief. As one critic commented in a newspaper article, it relies on offenders "not knowing how to use Google" (London Daily Telegraph, 2012).

A number of social psychology studies have demonstrated that subjects who believe they are attached to a "lie detector" appear to be more honest in their answers to questions regarding attitudes and behaviors, which has been interpreted as a reflection of social desirability or acquiescence biases (Jones & Sigall, 1971; Roese & Jamieson, 1993). But the effect is not in fact that great—a meta-analysis of 31 published reports found a mean effect size of $d=0.41$, which is in the small-to-moderate range (Roese & Jamieson, 1993).

Another factor to take into account when considering the "bogus pipeline" hypothesis is that all of the bogus pipeline studies are based on the use of a near 100 % lie detector. It is not clear from them what would happen if, rather than being sold as being 100 % accurate, the "lie detector" was instead said to have an accuracy rate "well above chance, though well below perfection" as described by the National Academies in respect of polygraph testing (National Research Council, 2003). In a yet unpublished research, our group found that a "lie detector" claiming to have a 75 % accuracy rate (i.e., a level below that attributed to polygraphy) appears to elicit disclosures with a frequency similar to that of a near 100 % accurate lie detector. This would seem to suggest that if part of the increase in disclosures brought about by polygraph testing is due to a belief in its lie detecting properties, then whatever else it may be the pipeline is not a bogus one.

Regardless of the merits and impact of the "bogus pipeline effect," the much more psychologically interesting question is what makes individuals disclose in this setting anyway, bogus pipeline or not. It may be that offenders disclose because they believe they will be, or have been, "caught out" by the polygraph, which would be consistent with research showing that one of the best predictors of whether a suspect will confess to a crime is the belief that there is good evidence against them (Gudjonsson, Sigurdsson, Bragason, Einarsson, & Valdimarsdottir, 2004). As indicated above, however, the "bogus pipeline effect" itself is unlikely to be the entire reason for increased disclosures, explaining only a small part of the variance. It could be that a polygraph test allows the offender an opportunity to change his account in a face-saving manner (after all, he was found out by a "lie detector") or it may simply be that the dynamics of the interview itself are different from what takes place in normal supervision. Whatever the reason, the effect deserves increased research attention the words, and consideration given as to how to enhance it.

One further issue to address in respect of disclosures is whether the circumstances of a polygraph test result in offenders making false admissions in order to please polygraph examiners or to explain a "failed" test. Because many of the disclosures made in PCSOT are in any case difficult if not impossible to verify (e.g., how can one determine whether or not an offender has been masturbating to deviant fantasies?), it can be a challenge to confirm their veracity. What little research there is in relation to this suggests that false admissions occur but not often. Two studies have addressed this question using anonymous surveys with sex offenders in the United States who were asked whether they had ever made false disclosures in a polygraph test (Grubin & Madsen, 2006; Kokish et al., 2005). In both studies fewer than 10 % of offenders indicated that they had done so; in the Grubin and Madsen (2006) study, those who reported making false admissions had higher scores on the NEO neuroticism scale and lower scores on the conscientiousness scale, suggesting that those who make false admissions during a polygraph test may share characteristics with those who make false confessions in police interviews (Gudjonnson & Pearse, 2011; Gudjonsson et al., 2004). In any case, while the issue is not trivial, it does not seem to be a major problem.

Proponents of PCSOT argue that whatever the reason for increased disclosure by offenders who undergo polygraph tests, the effect is genuine and valuable. They ask whether critics are really suggesting that this information should not be sought or used because of concerns regarding the evidence base for the mechanisms that generate it. But resolution of this issue perhaps depends more on how PCSOT is implemented than on the academic arguments regarding polygraph itself.

The Implementation of PCSOT

The initial use of polygraph testing with sex offenders was as a clinical assessment to assist treatment providers in gaining fuller histories with which to inform treatment plans. The term "postconviction sex offender test" started to be used in the 1990s in reference to tests administered to individuals under court order, court supervision, or court-ordered treatment, with the intention of enhancing treatment or improving supervision (Holden, 2000). Its aim was to generate more complete information about an offender's history, sexual interests and functioning, and offending behavior based on disclosures and test outcome. This has been referred to as adding "incremental validity to treatment planning and risk management decisions" with which to improve decision-making (Colorado, 2011) and can perhaps be thought of more simply as "information gain."

In the late 1990s, the "Containment Model" was developed by practitioners in Colorado (English, 1998). It has since become the basis of many PCSOT programs in the United States, although it has not taken root in the United Kingdom. The Containment Model refers to a triangle formed by a supervision officer, treatment provider, and polygraph examiner, although others may also be involved, in which the offender is "contained." It depends on good communication between agencies, with information obtained by one informing the actions of others.

While the Containment Model has clear attractions from a public protection perspective, it implies that all sex offenders require high levels of external control to keep them from reoffending. Compliance in the immediate term may be obtained, but whether it leads to longer-term change is uncertain. And though some offenders may require "containment," others genuinely seek to improve their internal controls and engage with treatment and supervision. In other words, there are some offenders who work with treatment providers and supervisors, and there are others who work against them. For the latter group, containment may be necessary, with the polygraph serving primarily as a lie detector to indicate when risk is increasing (related to this is a finding of Cook, Barkley, and Anderson (2014) that recidivism rates were higher in offenders who avoided or delayed their polygraph), but for the former group of offenders, polygraphy can act as a truth facilitator, encouraging them to discuss problematic thoughts and behaviors and providing reassurance that their risk is stable. It should be remembered that polygraphy not only detects lies, it also catches offenders telling the truth.

Whether or not following a strict containment approach, PCSOT has moved away from being an accessory of treatment to assume a more central role in offender supervision. It remains, however, the servant of those working directly with the offender, functioning to provide information about whatever is most relevant at the time. In this respect, different test types are relevant depending on the offender's circumstances.

Test Structure

Before describing the types of test used in PCSOT, the basic structure of a polygraph session needs to be described. The typical format employed in PCSOT is the "comparison question technique." It consists of three phases: a pretest interview, the examination itself, and a posttest interview:

The *pretest* is the longest part of the examination and can take from 1 to 2 h. Among other matters, information is collected about the examinee's background and current behavior, and the test questions are established and reviewed in detail. Many disclosures take place during this part of the process.

The *polygraph examination* consists of 10–12 questions, of which just 3 or 4 target the areas of concern and are referred to as the "relevant questions." Responses to the relevant questions are compared with so-called comparison questions to determine whether or not they are indicative of deception. More will be said about this shortly. Polygraph questions need to be simple, answerable with a yes or no, and relate to specific behavior rather than mental state, intention, or motivation.

In the *posttest* interview, the outcome of the exam is fed back, with the examinee given an opportunity to explain deceptive responses. In the UK study of voluntary testing, one third of disclosures were made during the posttest (Grubin, 2010).

As referred to above, in the comparison question technique, relevant questions are evaluated against comparison ones. If physiological responses to the former are greater than the latter, the examinee is judged to be deceptive; vice versa, the examinee is considered truthful. The comparison questions often take the form of a "*probable lie*," that is, questions that the examinee is unlikely to be able to answer truthfully. Examples of probable lies are "have you ever lied to a loved one?" and "have you ever stolen from a family member?" The theory is that truthful subjects will find these questions more concerning than the relevant ones because of their implications and thus show greater responses to them, while the deceptive examinee will be more responsive to the relevant questions because they represent more of a threat. The strength with which relevant questions exert a greater pull on the examinee than the comparison ones has been called "relevant issue gravity" (Ginton, 2009), which is a tidy way of packaging the various cognitive processes that determine autonomic arousal in response to polygraph questions.

The probable lie approach has been criticized on a number of grounds. First, the underlying theory that the differential response to the two question types relates to truthful individuals being more worried about what are in effect less serious comparison questions is frankly implausible (Ben-Shakhar, 2008; National Research Council, 2003). But given that the technique has been shown to be able to identify deception, this suggests that we need a new theory, not that the technique itself is faulty. Others are concerned that the probable lie approach means the test is based on deceiving the examinee and requires the examinee to be forced into a position of having to lie (Cross & Saxe, 2001; Meijer et al., 2008; Vess, 2011). This ethical objection, however, is based on a misconception—the cognitive work of the probable lie doesn't arise from the lie but from the uncertainty associated with the question. Indeed, comparison questions can take the form of a "*directed lie*" in which the examinee is instructed to lie to a question such as "have you ever made a mistake?," which involves neither manipulation nor dishonesty. More will be said about directed lies later in this chapter.

Test Types

There are four basic types of polygraph test used in PCSOT, some of which have variants to them (American Polygraph Association, 2009).

Sex History Exams

The purpose of this test is to obtain a fuller and more accurate account of an offender's sexual history, including the type and range of deviant behaviors in which he has engaged, the age at which they commenced, and his history of involvement in unknown or unreported offenses. There are two forms of this exam, one that focuses on unreported victims of contact offenses and the other on sexually deviant behavior more generally and offenses that don't involve forces such as voyeurism or Internet-related offending. The rationale for the separation is that the more severe potential consequences associated with the former behaviors may contaminate responses to the latter. Prior to the polygraph exam, the offender completes a sex history questionnaire, usually as part of sex offender treatment. The questionnaire is the focus of the examination, but only selected questions are asked during the test itself.

The intention of the Sex History Exams is to develop a better understanding of risk and of treatment need. There can be a tendency, however, for examiners to dig for much more detail than is needed to achieve these aims, making the procedure an unrealistic exercise in recall for the offender as well as a potentially humiliating one; more information is not necessarily better information. In addition, because it is based on a lengthy questionnaire which covers behaviors that have taken place over many years, the risk of false-positive outcomes (i.e., wrongly "failing" the test) is increased. This is an important consideration given that about half of the American community and a third of residential sex offender treatment programs for adult males require the Sex History Exam to be passed in order for the treatment to be completed successfully.

A further problematic issue associated with Sex History Exams is what to do about self-incriminating disclosures. Programs typically try to get around this ensuring that only general information about past offenses is obtained, but in some states even this minimal level of disclosure needs to be passed to the authorities. In reality, however, this is not a difficulty unique to polygraph testing and applies to treatment programs generally. Whatever solution works for the program should be sufficient for PCSOT.

The following are two examples of how Sex History Exams can be helpful to treatment (these and subsequent examples are taken from the UK polygraph trials):

An offender on parole following a conviction for the indecent assault of his stepdaughter disclosed during a Sex History Examination a large amount of previously unknown pornography use and cross-dressing. Subsequent to the test, he began to discuss this and his sexual fantasies more generally in treatment for the first time.

An offender in his 50s with no sex-offending history was convicted of Internet-related offenses. In a Sex History Examination, he admitted to stealing underwear from his sister's house, to sexual fantasies regarding schoolgirls, and to sitting in cinema car parks to watch young girls. Based on this and other fantasy-related informations he disclosed during the test, new treatment targets regarding fantasy and fantasy modification were identified and delivered.

Critics argue that information from Sex History Exams tell us nothing new in that it would be a surprise if offenders hadn't engaged in deviant behaviors besides their offenses and that there is little evidence to show that the additional information adds meaningfully to risk assessment or treatment provision (Rosky, 2013). This criticism seems odd, however, given that sex history questions are asked routinely in sex offender assessment and are considered an important part of the evaluation;

the only difference being that there is more likelihood of getting an honest account during a polygraph examination.

Instant Offense Exam

This exam type explores behavior that took place during the instant offense where there is inconsistency between victim and offender accounts or where the offender denies important aspects of what took place. A variant of this test relates to prior allegations where there hasn't been a conviction. Like the Sex History Exam, this test is directly relevant to treatment. Also like the Sex History Exam, there is a risk that the examiner will go on a fishing exercise seeking detail that doesn't take treatment any further. Used properly, however, it can overcome denial that is blocking treatment progress.

Below is an example of how an Instant Offense Exam assisted treatment in a perhaps unexpected way:

An offender was on license having committed an indecent assault on a child in a supermarket when intoxicated. He admitted the offense but denied any memory of having pushed his groin into the girl's back as reported by her mother even though he accepted this could have happened. Much time was spent in the treatment group trying to overcome his "denial." On an Instant Offense Exam, he was questioned about his lack of recall, and he was found truthful. The consistency of his self-report taken together with the test result led to his account of partial amnesia being accepting, allowing treatment to move beyond this issue.

Some critics believe this sort of information would be obtained anyway in the course of treatment, but whether or not this is the case, supporters of PCSOT argue that the disclosures come much earlier when polygraphy is used. There is little evidence with which to determine either of these claims.

Offenders may see the Instant Offense Exam as an opportunity to prove their "innocence" in the face of a wrongful conviction. Although there may be a time and place for this issue to be explored, PCSOT is not it. The Instant Offense Exam, therefore, must be used with caution.

Maintenance Exam

The Maintenance Exam is the workhorse of PCSOT. It addresses an offender's compliance with the terms and conditions of probation, parole, or treatment. It is a screening test that typically covers a wide range of issues in the pretest, following which 3 or 4 specific questions are asked on the test itself. Maintenance Exams can address sexual thoughts and fantasies so long as they are linked to masturbatory behavior. The aims of the test are to identify behaviors indicative of increased risk so that interventions can take place, confirm when offenders are not engaging in problematic behavior, and deter offenders from engaging in risky behaviors in the first place. Its primary purpose is to prevent reoffending rather than to detect reoffenses after they have occurred.

Two examples of Maintenance Exams illustrate their potential value:

An offender on parole license disclosed he had recently started a relationship with a young woman (one of his license conditions being that he informed his probation officer of any new relationships). Although that was the extent of his disclosure, his offender manager met with the new girlfriend and found not only that she was a single mother but also that the offender was grooming her child in a manner similar to his instant offense. He was recalled to prison.

An offender with a history of involvement with sex offender networks had a license condition not to associate with known sex offenders. Following a deceptive test, he admitted to breaching this condition. When his probation officer later explored this with him, he admitted to marked feelings of loneliness and isolation following a move from a probation hostel. Steps were taken to address his isolation, and on his next Maintenance Exam, he said he was no longer reliant on his former sex offender contacts and much more settled in himself; he showed no significant responses to questions relating to associating with other sex offenders.

In neither of these cases can it be demonstrated that offenses were prevented, but it would be hard to argue that the outcomes were not worthwhile.

A difficulty faced by Maintenance Exams is how to respond to a deceptive result in the absence of disclosures. Given the 10–20 % error rate of polygraph testing, it is hard to justify sanctions such as prison recall based on a failed test alone (although this does occur in some US states, it is prohibited in the United Kingdom), but a deceptive test does provide a warning sign that all may not be well. Depending on the risk represented by the offender, the response could range from the probation officer addressing the issue in supervision with him to not relaxing restrictions such as curfews or exclusion zones to, in especially high-risk cases, putting the offender under surveillance.

Maintenance Exams are carried out regularly, to set protocols—for example, in the United Kingdom, they take place at 6 monthly intervals, but sooner if the offender fails, tests or concerns emerge between exams. This gives rise to a risk of habituation or sensitization, resulting in fewer disclosures and false-negative test results (Branaman & Gallagher, 2005). To counter this PCSOT, policies usually recommend that a different examiner is introduced after a set number of tests have been undertaken. Again, however, research relating to this issue is sparse, and it is not clear the extent to which habituation occurs or whether the suggested remedy is effective.

Monitoring Exams

Monitoring Exams are specific issue tests that take place where there is concern that an offender may have committed a new offense or breached a license condition. As in Maintenance Exams, no sanction follows a failed test in the absence of disclosure, but a failed test may indicate the need for further investigation. On the other hand, a passed test can offer reassurance to supervisors.

The following is an example of how a Monitoring Exam can contribute to management:

A 24-year-old man was on parole having been convicted of unlawful sexual intercourse with a 14-year-old girl. His probation officer believed he was still in a sexual relationship with his victim, but this was persistently denied by the offender, who was compliant with a night-time curfew and a tag. He denied any wrongdoing during the pretest interview, but he was deceptive on the test. In the posttest interview, he admitted to regular contact with the girl as well as a low level of sexual activity with her. The probation officer passed this information to the police and the offender was arrested. When interviewed by the police, the girl reported regularly spending a night a week in the offender's home (a place his tag confirmed him to be), where in addition to the sexual activity he had described she said they also engaged in sexual intercourse.

Beating the Test

Somewhat incongruously, the same critics who argue that polygraphy does not reliably differentiate truth telling from deception nonetheless also invariably raise the issue of countermeasures, that is, physical or psychological techniques, used to manipulate responses on the test to enable examinees to appear truthful when they are being deceptive (Ben-Shakhar, 2008; London Daily Telegraph, 2012). They argue that false-negative findings, whether the result of error or countermeasures, mean that "dangerous" offenders can "beat" the test and remain free in the community.

It is almost certainly the case that some offenders "beat" the test, but the reality is that without polygraphy, many more "beat" their supervisors and treatment providers. For example, as referred to earlier, in the absence of polygraphy, probation officers are more likely to reduce their risk assessments than they are when polygraphy is used (Grubin, 2010). Decisions, however, should not be based on polygraphy alone—PCSOT is just one part of the information package.

It is also the case that countermeasure techniques exist and can be taught, and there are a number of websites that offer to do so. But in order to be successful, practice is required—theory is not sufficient—and the examinee needs feedback when attached to the polygraph (Honts, Hodes, & Raskin, 1985). Most sex offenders do not have access to this type of coaching, and without it their charts usually show tell-tale signs of their attempts to manipulate the test. It should also be remembered that polygraph examiners read the same websites as their examinees.

Treatment Benefit and Risk Reduction

Probation officers like PCSOT. In the English probation trials (Gannon et al., 2014; Grubin, 2010), over 90 % rated polygraphy as being "somewhat" or "very" helpful, with very few tests considered by officers to have had either no or a negative impact.

But while subjectively probation officers may believe polygraphy makes their jobs easier, this is not the same as being able to demonstrate objectively that PCSOT results in improved treatment outcome or a genuine reduction in risk (Rosky, 2013).

Evidence regarding reduction in recidivism is extremely thin, although the absence of evidence should not be confused with evidence of absence. It is difficult to carry out randomized control trials of PCSOT for a range of reasons, not the least of which is a reluctance by criminal justice agencies to "experiment" with dangerous sex offenders. Furthermore, the low levels of recidivism that make treatment programs difficult to evaluate create similar problems for PCSOT, although significant increases in prison recall for breaches have been demonstrated (Gannon et al., 2014; Grubin, 2010).

Two early studies, although not of PCSOT per se, point in the right direction. Abrams and Ogard (1986) compared recidivism rates of 35 probationers (few of whom were sex offenders) from two counties in Oregon required to take periodic polygraph tests, with 243 offenders from a county where supervision did not involve polygraphy. Over 2 years, 31 % of the polygraphed men committed an offense or infringement compared with 74 % of those who were not polygraphed. But the number of polygraphed offenders was small; the samples were not matched nor is it clear whether there was selection bias in choosing those who underwent polygraphy. Also in Oregon, Edson (1991) reported that 95 % of 173 sex offenders on parole or probation who were required to undertake periodic polygraph testing did not reoffend over 9 years, but there was no comparison group in this study at all.

McGrath, Cumming, Hoke, and Bonn-Miller (2007) carried out the one randomized trial of PCSOT in the literature, comparing 104 sex offenders in Vermont who received treatment in programs that included PCSOT with 104 matched offenders in programs where polygraphy was not used. At 5-year follow-up, they found no difference in sex offense recidivism rates, but they did find a significantly lower rate of reconviction for nonsexual violent offenses. But though the study was well designed, its results are difficult to interpret because while the research was sound, the way in which PCSOT was delivered was not. Offenders undertook polygraph examinations on average just once every 22 months, dissipating the likelihood that polygraphy would have much of an impact on behavior. Even so, the reduction in violent offending is notable.

In trying to determine the impact of PCSOT, there is another issue to consider. It is well established in relation to sex offender interventions generally that to be effective, they should adhere to the "risk-need-responsivity" principle—that is, they should target high-risk individuals, reflect treatment need, and be responsive to cognitive and cultural differences between offenders (Andrews, Bonta, & Wormith, 2011). PCSOT does not tend to be delivered in this way because it is an assessment procedure rather than an intervention as such. After all, a screening technique for a medical condition is not judged on the basis of whether it improves survival rates for that condition—that is, the role of what follows—but on its success in identifying at-risk individuals. Expecting PCSOT to reduce recidivism may be an unreal expectation.

So how then is PCSOT to be judged? Rather than focus on recidivism perhaps, attention should be focused instead on the value of the information gained as one would in an evaluation of screening instruments generally. The frequency and content of disclosures, the impact of test outcome on decision-making, and actions taken after a polygraph test could all form part of a cost-value analysis to determine the value added by PCSOT compared with the cost of administering it. In other words, to what extent does PCSOT better enable probation officers to monitor risk and initiate timely interventions, and are treatment targets better identified, when polygraph is used? The question then becomes, "is PCSOT worth it?"

Internet Offenders

Men who download indecent images of children from the Internet present a particular challenge for those carrying out risk assessments. Typically, little is known about relevant risk factors and they often have no criminal history. It is estimated, however, that around 50 % of men convicted of Internet offenses have committed undetected sexual assaults on children, and the majority show pedophilic sexual arousal patterns (Seto, 2013). It has been suggested that applying PCSOT techniques in a preconviction setting to men arrested for downloading offenses could assist in differentiating low- from high-risk offenders (where risk relates to contact offending against children), enabling police resources to be better focused and criminal justice interventions to be more accurately targeted in terms of custody and treatment. That this can be done was demonstrated in a small study in which 31 apparently low-risk Internet offenders underwent sex history-type polygraph examinations preconviction, where it was found that only 8 (26 %) could be confirmed as genuinely low risk (Grubin, Joyce, & Holden, 2014). A number of police forces in England are now exploring this application of polygraphy further.

Legal Considerations

The legal situation in the United Kingdom is more straightforward than it is in the United States. In the United Kingdom, the Offender Management Act 2007 sets out the statutory position regarding the mandatory testing of sex offenders on parole (Offender Management Act, 2007). Offenders must have been sentenced to a year or more in prison in order to ensure that the polygraph condition is proportionate. The legislation prohibits the use of evidence from polygraph tests in criminal proceedings, although this information can form the basis of criminal investigation, and it can also be used in civil proceedings. The act is supported by a statutory instrument containing polygraph "rules" which govern the conduct of polygraph sessions and set out the requirements that must be met by examiners. The 2007 legislation mandated a time-limited period to allow mandatory polygraph testing to be evaluated on a pilot basis in a small number of probation regions, after which the Secretary of State for Justice was required to return to Parliament for approval to extend mandatory testing nationwide. Following the successful evaluation of the pilot (Gannon et al., 2012), Parliamentary approval was granted in 2013, and mandatory testing throughout England and Wales became effective in January 2014.

Although the Offender Management Act 2007 prohibits the use of the results of mandatory testing in criminal proceedings, there is no legislation that prevents polygraph testing in general from being used as evidence in the British courts. It is sometimes claimed that the law prevents the use of polygraph evidence, but this is not true (Stockdale & Grubin, 2012). Whether polygraphy evidence should be allowed in criminal proceedings is a too complicated issue to be explored here, apart from observing that while polygraphy can be a valuable investigative tool, it is not clear that it can add much to the decision-making process in court.

The position regarding PCSOT in North America is more haphazard. The main issue for the courts has been whether PCSOT breaches the Fifth Amendment rights against self-incrimination. In considering this question, the Supreme Court ruled in McKune v. Lile that it does not, albeit in a tight 5-to-4 decision. It observed that the treatment program of which it was part served "a vital penological purpose." On the other hand, in the United States v. Antelope (2005), the Federal 9th Circuit Appeal Court ruled that a paroled offender could not be compelled to waive his Fifth Amendment rights and take a polygraph exam with the threat of prison recall if he did not. This has made it even more necessary for programs to ensure that they properly address the self-incrimination issue, both in terms of PCSOT and more generally.

PCSOT is hardly used in Canada (McGrath et al., 2010), and it therefore does not appear to have been an issue for the Canadian courts, apart from one case where a prisoner applied for judicial review of a Parole Board decision not to release him partly on the basis that the decision was made before he had undertaken a polygraph examination—in this case the Court decided that the polygraph test results would not have changed anything in the Parole Board's decision (Aney v. Canada, 2005). In general, however, the Canadian Courts allow polygraph disclosures to be used in criminal proceedings so long as the jury is not told that they came from a polygraph test.

Ethics

Commentators rightly distinguish between practice standards and ethical principles, observing that the two do not necessarily overlap (Chaffin, 2011). Even where the delivery of PCSOT is well managed and delivered, potential ethical objections don't go away. When discussing PCSOT, a number of ethical issues are frequently raised. These tend to relate to a lack of respect for autonomy, intrusiveness, and compulsion, as well as special considerations that arise when testing special groups such as adolescents, the intellectually disabled, and individuals with mental disorder.

Some of these objections relate to a misconception of what happens in PCSOT, others to its questionable implementation. For example, Cross and Saxe (2001) refer to PCSOT as "psychological manipulation" on the basis that examiners deceive offenders by telling them that the polygraph is error-free. While this may occur, it is certainly not good practice nor is there any reason for examiners to make out that the test is any more accurate than it actually is. Indeed, the British Psychological Society (2004) observes that participants should be informed of known error rates, a sentiment with which it is hard to disagree. There is no reason to believe that PCSOT would cease to be effective in these circumstances.

Cross and Saxe (2001), Meijer et al. (2008), and Vess (2011) all argue that the test itself is based on deception when the probable lie technique is used given the hypocrisy involved in demanding the offender to be honest. Vess (2011) and McGrath et al. (2010) wonder in addition what damage this might do to the therapeutic relationship. But as indicated earlier, the probable lie technique is not in fact dependent on the examinee lying even though this is what tends to be taught (indeed, as referred to above, other critics refer to this theory being deficient), but on uncertainty. Regardless, the use of "directed lies" overcomes this objection and also avoids the risk of the examinee admitting to transgressions that have nothing to do with his sexual risk.

Chaffin (2011), although concerned mainly with the testing of adolescents, focuses on PCSOT "extracting confessions" from examinees, stating "The polygraph is fundamentally a coercive interrogation tool for extracting involuntary confessions" (p. 320). PCSOT, however, need not, and should not, involve interrogation. It is instead an interview process in which lying is explicitly discouraged. The questions asked during PCSOT are asked by assessors and treatment providers anyway—the fact that PCSOT encourages disclosure of information relevant to treatment and risk management is in itself not an ethical issue.

Mandatory PCSOT is of course coercive in that there are penalties for noncooperation. But PCSOT examinees are convicted offenders, who by virtue of their criminal convictions are required to accept a range of restrictive and coercive measures such as conditions on where they live, limitations on employment, curfews, and treatment requirements. Indeed, the European Court of Human Rights has ruled that penile plethysmography (a technique in which penile arousal in response to sexual stimuli is measured and recorded) can be made a compulsory part of sex offender treatment on the grounds of public safety (Gazan, 2002); one might think this is considerably more "invasive" than polygraphy. Provided that the questions asked during the polygraph test are directly relevant to treatment or supervision, the process does not seem any more coercive then these other measures or any more morally problematic.

Another objection to PCSOT is that it carries with it the implication that sex offenders are not to be trusted and that this itself damages the relationship between supervisors and offenders. There is no evidence, however, that this is the case, while what evidence there is suggests it does not (Grubin, 2010). Indeed, this implication is often implicit in any case. One should not underestimate the benefits of an offender being able to demonstrate that he is being truthful in his dealings with those supervising him and the positive impact this can have on the therapeutic relationship.

There remains the question, however, of special groups. About half of adolescent treatment programs in the United States, for example, incorporate PCSOT (McGrath et al., 2010), and the American Polygraph Association PCSOT model policy allows for testing juveniles down to the age of 12. As Chaffin (2011) points out, given the increased vulnerability of juveniles and adolescents to coercion and suggestion, and differences in the way that risk, treatment, and rehabilitation are conceptualized in this group, one can't assume that PCSOT approaches are appropriate for them. He could have added that it is not even clear that polygraphy itself works in the same way as it does in adults given differences in brain maturity and psychological development and that the American Polygraph Association age threshold appears arbitrary. Because of these and similar issues, mandatory polygraph testing in the United Kingdom does not apply to offenders who are under the age of 18.

Does this mean that polygraph testing of those under 18 is unethical? Testing offenders younger than 18 has its advocates (Jensen, Shafer, Roby, & Roby, 2015). Even Chaffin (2011), who considers the ethical concerns to be "substantial," doesn't go that far, although his view is contingent on the ability of those supporting its use in this group to prove that it provides more benefit than harm. Unless and until this evidence is produced, however, it probably makes sense to use PCSOT with great caution with those under 18, with decisions made on a consideration of individual cases rather than based on a blanket policy of PCSOT for all.

In terms of other special groups, such as those with intellectual disability and mental disorder, the position is similar. PCSOT has the potential to be of benefit, but caution needs to be used, by examiners who are aware of the pitfalls.

Finally, one might ask whether it is unethical *not* to use PCSOT in the treatment and supervision of sex offenders. If the information obtained during polygraph examination adds significantly to what is otherwise known about treatment need and risk, is it right to deny the potential benefits of PCSOT to an offender? When asked, many offenders themselves reported that they find polygraph testing to be helpful (Grubin & Madsen, 2006; Kokish et al., 2005). If PCSOT does reduce risk, how can one explain to a future victim why it did not form part of the offender's treatment and supervision package?

Conclusion

Does PCSOT increase community safety? Does it enhance sex offender treatment? Although the evidence is supportive, the benefits of PCSOT have yet to be conclusively demonstrated. Objections made by many of its critics, however, are based on opinion rather than fact. But what would count as definitive evidence? For ideological reasons, some will never be convinced.

Given the complexity of sex offender management, simply collecting data on numbers of disclosures, reconvictions, and the like will tell us little more than we already know. More thought needs to be directed to which offenders are most likely to benefit, the needs that PCSOT should target in those offenders, and whether modifications are necessary depending on the characteristics of the individual taking part. In other words, consideration should be given to how the "risk-need-responsivity" principle can be made to apply to PCSOT.

In the meantime, those who deliver PCSOT need to ensure that examiners are properly trained and supervised, protocols for the process are sound, and good quality control procedures are in place. In turn, those who make use of it must know the right questions to ask of it, how much weight to give its results, and how to integrate it with everything else they do with an offender. It should not be forgotten, however, that PCSOT remains just one tool in the box, and like any tool if it is not used with care it can cause harm.

References

Abrams, S., & Ogard, E. (1986). Polygraph surveillance of probationers. *Polygraph, 15*, 174–182.

Ahlmeyer, S., Heil, P., McKee, B., & English, K. (2000). The impact of polygraphy on admissions of victims and offenses in adult sexual offenders. *Sexual Abuse: A Journal of Research and Treatment, 12*, 123–139.

Alder, K. (2007). *The lie detectors: The history of an American obsession*. New York, NY: Free Press.

American Polygraph Association. (2009). Model policy for post-conviction sex offender testing. Retrieved from http://www.polygraph.org/files/model_policy_for_post-conviction_sex_offender_testing_final.pdf.

American Polygraph Association. (2011). Committee report on validated techniques. *Polygraph, 40*, 194–305.

Andrews, D. A., Bonta, J., & Wormith, J. S. (2011). The risk-need-responsivity (RNR) model: Does adding the good lives model contribute to effective crime prevention? *Criminal Justice and Behavior, 38*, 735–755.

Aney v. Canada. (2005). 2005 FC 182.

Ben-Shakhar, G. (2008). The case against the use of polygraph examinations to monitor post-conviction sex offenders. *Legal and Criminological Psychology, 13*, 191–207.

Bond, C. F., & DePaulo, B. M. (2006). Accuracy of deception judgments. *Personality and Social Psychology Review, 10*, 213–234.

Branaman, T. F., & Gallagher, S. N. (2005). Polygraph testing in sex offender treatment: A review of limitations. *American Journal of Forensic Psychology, 23*, 45–64.

British Psychological Society. (1986). Report of the working group on the use of the polygraph in criminal investigation and personnel screening. *Bulletin of the British Psychological Society, 39*, 81–94.

British Psychological Society. (2004). A review of the current scientific status and fields of application of polygraphic deception detection. Report (26/05/04) from the BPS Working Party. Retrieved from http://www.bps.org.uk/sites/default/files/documents/polygraphic_deception_detection_-_a_review_of_the_current_scientific_status_and_fields_of_application.pdf.

Chaffin, M. (2011). The case of Juvenile polygraphy as a clinical ethics dilemma. *Sexual Abuse: A Journal of Research and Treatment, 23*, 314–328.

Colorado. (2011). *Colorado Sex Offender Management Board: Standards and guidelines for the assessment, evaluation, treatment and behavioral monitoring of adult sex offenders*. Retrieved from https://cdpsdocs.state.co.us/somb/ADULT/FINAL_2012_Adult_Standards_120712.pdf.

Cook, R., Barkley, W., & Anderson, P. B. (2014). The sexual history polygraph examination and its influences on recidivism. *Journal of Social Change, 6*, 1–10.

Cross, T., & Saxe, L. (2001). Polygraph testing and sexual abuse: The lure of the magic lasso. *Child Maltreatment, 6*, 195–206.

Edson, C. F. (1991). *Sex offender treatment*. Jackson County, OR: Department of Corrections.

English, K. (1998). The containment approach: An aggressive strategy for the community management of adult sex offenders. *Psychology, Public Policy, & Law. Special Issues: Sex Offenders: Scientific, Legal, and Public Policy Perspectives, 4*, 218–235.

Gannon, T. A., Wood, J. L., Pina, A., Tyler, N., Barnoux, M. F., & Vasquez, E. A. (2014). An evaluation of mandatory polygraph testing for sexual offenders in the United Kingdom. *Sexual Abuse: A Journal of Research and Treatment, 26*, 178–203.

Gannon, T. A., Wood, J. L., Vasquez, E. A., Fraser, I. (2012). *The evaluation of the mandatory polygraph pilot (Ministry of Justice Research Series 14/12)*. Retrieved from https://www.gov.uk/government/uploads/system/uploads/attachment_data/file/217436/evaluation-of-mandatory-polygraph-pilot.pdf.

Gazan, F. (2002). Penile plethysmography before the European Court of Human Rights. *Sexual Abuse: A Journal of Research and Treatment, 14*, 89–93.

Ginton, A. (2009). Relevant issue gravity (RIG) strength – A new concept in PDD that reframes the notion of psychological set and the role of attention in CQT polygraph examinations. *Polygraph, 38*, 204–217.

Grubin, D. (2008). The case for polygraph testing of sex offenders. *Legal and Criminological Psychology, 13*, 177–189.

Grubin, D. (2010). A trial of voluntary polygraphy testing in 10 English probation areas. *Sexual Abuse, 22*, 266–278.

Grubin, D., Joyce, A., & Holden, E. J. (2014). Polygraph testing of 'low risk' offenders arrested for downloading indecent images of children. *Sexual Offender Treatment, 9*, 1–10.

Grubin, D., & Madsen, L. (2006). The accuracy and utility of post conviction polygraph testing with sex offenders. *British Journal of Psychiatry, 188*, 479–483.

Grubin, D., Madsen, L., Parsons, S., Sosnowski, D., & Warberg, B. (2004). A prospective study of the impact of polygraphy on high-risk behaviors in adult sex offenders. *Sexual Abuse: A Journal of Research and Treatment, 16*, 209–222.

Gudjonnson, G. H., & Pearse, J. (2011). Suspect interviews and false confessions. *Current Directions in Psychological Sciences, 20*, 33–37.

Gudjonsson, G. H., Sigurdsson, J. F., Bragason, O. O., Einarsson, E., & Valdimarsdottir, E. V. (2004). Confessions and denials and the relationship with personality. *Legal and Criminological Psychology, 9*, 121–133.

Heil, P., Ahlmeyer, S., & Simons, D. (2003). Crossover sexual offenses. *Sexual Abuse: A Journal of Research and Treatment, 15*, 221–236.

Hindman, J., & Peters, J. (2001). Polygraph testing leads to better understanding adult and juvenile sex offenders. *Federal Probation, 65*, 8–15.

Holden, E. J. (2000). Pre and post-conviction polygraph: Building blocks for the future – Procedures, principles, and practices. *Polygraph, 29*, 69–92.

Honts, C. R., Hodes, R. L., & Raskin, D. C. (1985). Effects of physical countermeasures on the physiological detection of deception. *Journal of Applied Psychology, 70*, 177–187.

Iacono, W. G. (2008). Effective policing understanding how polygraph tests work and are used. *Criminal Justice and Behavior, 35*, 1295–1308.

Jensen, T. M., Shafer, K., Roby, C., & Roby, J. L. (2015). Sexual history disclosure polygraph outcomes: Do juvenile and adult sex offenders differ? *Journal of Interpersonal Violence, 30*, 928–944.

Jones, E. E., & Sigall, H. (1971). The bogus pipeline: A new paradigm for measuring affect and attitude. *Psychological Bulletin, 76*, 349–364.

Kokish, R., Levenson, J., & Blasingame, G. (2005). Post-conviction sex offender polygraph examination: Client-reported perceptions of utility and accuracy. *Sexual Abuse: A Journal of Research and Treatment, 17*, 211–221.

Krapohl, D. J., & Shaw, P. K. (2015). *Fundamentals of polygraph practice*. San Diego, CA: Elsevier.

Levenson, J. S. (2009). Sex offender polygraph examination: An evidence-based case management tool for social workers. *Journal of Evidence-Based Social Work, 6*, 361–375.

London Daily Telegraph. (2012). *The Awkward Truth About Lie Detectors.* Retrieved from http://blogs.telegraph.co.uk/news/tomchiversscience/100173508/the-awkward-truth-about-lie-detectors.

Madsen, L., Parsons, S., & Grubin, D. (2004). A preliminary study of the contribution of periodic polygraph testing to the treatment and supervision of sex offenders. *British Journal of Forensic Psychiatry and Psychology, 15,* 682–695.

Matte, J. A. (1996). *Forensic psychophysiology using the polygraph: Scientific truth verification, lie detection.* New York, NY: J.A.M. Publications.

McGrath, R. J., Cumming, G. F., Burchard, B. L., Zeoli, S., & Ellerby, L. (2010). *Current practices and emerging trends in sexual abuser management: The Safer Society 2009 North American Survey.* Brandon, VT: Safer Society Press.

McGrath, R. J., Cumming, G. F., Hoke, S. E., & Bonn-Miller, M. O. (2007). Outcomes in a community sex offender treatment program: A comparison between polygraphed and matched non-polygraphed offenders. *Sexual Abuse: A Journal of Research and Treatment, 19,* 381–393.

McKune v. Lile. (2002). 536 U.S. 24.

Meijer, E. H., Verschuere, B., Merckelbach, H., & Crombez, G. (2008). Sex offender management using the polygraph: A critical review. *International Journal of Law and Psychiatry, 31,* 423–429.

National Research Council. (2003). *The polygraph and lie detection. Committee to Review the Scientific Evidence on the Polygraph.* Washington, DC: The National Academic Press.

Nelson, R. (2015). Scientific basis of polygraph testing. *Polygraph, 44,* 28–61.

Nelson, R., Handler, M., Shaw, P., Gougler, M., Blalock, B., Russell, C., … Oelrich, M. (2011). Using the empirical scoring system. *Polygraph,* 40:67–78.

Offender Management Act. (2007). Retrieved from http://www.legislation.gov.uk/ukpga/2007/21/pdfs/ukpga_20070021_en.pdf.

Patrick, C. J., & Iacono, W. G. (1989). Psychopathy, threat and polygraph test accuracy. *Journal of Applied Psychology, 74,* 347–355.

Raskin, D. C., & Hare, R. D. (1978). Psychopathy and detection of deception in a prison population. *Psychophysiology, 15,* 126–136.

Raskin, D. C., Honts, C. R., & Kircher, J. C. (Eds.). (2014). *Credibility assessment: Scientific research and applications.* San Diego, CA: Elsevier.

Roese, N. J., & Jamieson, D. W. (1993). Twenty years of bogus pipeline research: A critical review and meta-analysis. *Psychological Bulletin, 114,* 363–381.

Rosky, J. W. (2013). The (F)utility of post-conviction polygraph testing. *Sexual Abuse: A Journal of Research and Treatment, 25,* 259–281.

Senter, S., Weatherman, D., Krapohl, D., & Horvath, F. (2010). Psychological set and differential salience: A proposal for reconciling theory and terminology in polygraph testing. *Polygraph, 39,* 109–117.

Seto, M. (2013). *Internet sex offenders.* Washington, DC: American Psychological Association.

Stockdale, M., & Grubin, D. (2012). The admissibility of polygraph evidence in English criminal proceedings. *Journal of Criminal Law, 76,* 232–253.

United States v. Antelope (2005). 395 F.3d 1128.

Vess, J. (2011). Ethical practice in sex offender assessment: Consideration of actuarial and polygraph methods. *Sexual Abuse: A Journal of Research and Treatment, 23,* 381–396.

Vrij, A. (2000). *Detecting lies and deceit.* Chichester: Wiley.

Chapter 7
The Strengths of Treatment for Sexual Offending

Adam J. Carter and Ruth E. Mann

Introduction

The term "sex offender treatment" is generally used to describe psychological programmes delivered to groups of people convicted of sexual offences, in either custody and community settings, for the tertiary prevention of sexual recidivism. Somewhat less commonly, the term is used to describe other approaches such as medication to reduce an individual's level of sexual arousal (e.g. Beech & Harkins, 2012: Lösel & Schmucker, 2005).

The term treatment, used in the context of rehabilitative efforts with people convicted of sexual offences, arguably misrepresents what rehabilitation is both able to achieve and aims to do. To a lay person, the term *treatment* could imply that we know how to reduce sexual recidivism with perpetrators of sexual crimes, suggesting that we can as a matter of course identify and address the s*ymptoms* of sexual offending and take action to ameliorate these symptoms in the same way it can be possible to administer medical care for an illness. This term also suggests that if people haven't received any treatment then they are *untreated* and will continue to offend. However, the extremely low recidivism rates (e.g. 2.2 % sexual recidivism over 2 years; Barnett, Wakeling, & Howard, 2010) for this type of offence suggests otherwise: it seems that, even taking into account the problem of detecting all incidences of sexual offending, most people with sex offence convictions are likely to desist from further offending whether or not they are treated. Another issue with using the term "treatment" is that it risks failing to acknowledge the active role of the treatment participant in the process of change. As the field of desistance research

A.J. Carter, Ph.D. (✉) • R.E. Mann, Ph.D.
National Offender Management Service, Clive House, 70 Petty France,
London SW1H 9EX, UK
e-mail: adam.carter@noms.gsi.gov.uk

© Springer International Publishing Switzerland 2016
D.R. Laws, W. O'Donohue (eds.), *Treatment of Sex Offenders*,
DOI 10.1007/978-3-319-25868-3_7

157

has shown us, treatment programmes do not "make people into non offenders". They offer opportunities for people to learn new cognitive and behavioural skills, but they do not in themselves change people. The individual himself or herself is the person who achieves change through, for example, using the opportunities provided by the programme to examine and alter their attitudes that support sexually abusive behaviour. If there is no intent to change, a treatment programme will be unlikely to make any difference to offending (Webster, 2005; Webster, Bowers, Mann, & Marshall, 2005). This is not to say it is always the client's fault if a treatment programme is ineffective—programmes may also be unengaging or may involve ineffective treatment procedures. The attribution of effectiveness, therefore, is a complex endeavour which must go beyond reflexive finger pointing at either the individual or the programme.

The notion of "treatment" can also distract attention from the wider context that can and is necessary to support desistance from offending outside of the treatment room. Pharmaceutical treatment or surgery could arguably often be expected to work regardless of the context in which it is received by the patient, although even with these types of treatment, the social context also assists with success and recovery. Psychological "treatment", particularly when it is mandated or otherwise not entirely voluntary (as is usually the case with sex offenders), needs to be situated in a context of wider social and professional support. It is important that stigma is actively minimised, and that the sex offender does not fear for his personal safety, which is often the case particularly in prison (Blagden, Winder, & Hames, 2014; Mann, 2016; Mann, Webster, Wakeling, & Keylock, 2013).

For all these reasons, it is widely accepted that the effectiveness of sex offender treatment is difficult to determine. Therefore, we begin this chapter by acknowledging the mixed evaluation findings in this field and the consequent need for most treatment programmes to re-evaluate their curricula and methods. However, our main purpose for this chapter is to look at the evidence for what parts we have got "right". What features of our current treatment approach should remain in rehabilitative programmes aimed at reducing recidivism with people convicted of a sexual offence? Although our brief for this chapter was to focus on the strengths of treatment, it is important to stress that we are highly cognisant of the typical problems in most current treatment approaches. By focussing on the strengths, however, we hope to clarify the most effective and promising parts of treatment that should successfully reduce sexual recidivism.

Sexual Offending Treatment Could Be More Effective

Evaluating sexual offending programmes is complicated in part by the very thing that makes engaging in rehabilitation with this group so challenging: people who have sexually offended represent an extremely heterogeneous group. This heterogeneity is evident in the type and detail of the sexual offence committed, an individual's aetiology, what motivated their offending, co-morbidity issues and their level of risk. Not all risk factors that have been identified for sexual offending perpetrators as a group will apply to each individual convicted of a sexual offence, and the motivation for offending and what drives or maintains it can vary significantly. Therefore, evaluations of programmes may need to consider multicomponent programmes with flexible delivery schedules. From an evaluation point of view, this kind of programme is hard to evaluate, and it will be even harder to draw conclusions about "why" it worked or didn't work.

There are other practical problems in terms of matching treatment and control groups as issues of heterogeneity discussed above would indicate. Those who undertake treatment may differ considerably from comparisons in terms of denial of the offence (maintaining innocence for offending can be a bar to entering treatment) as well as the role that deviance played in offending. Matching is also difficult because international data suggests that offenders selected to undertake treatment are at greater risk of sexual recidivism than routine samples that have not been identified for a programme even after taking static risk into account (Helmus, Hanson, Thornton, Babchishin, & Harris, 2012).

Lastly, although there have been several systematic reviews and meta-analyses of sex offender treatment effectiveness, these reviews mask considerable heterogeneity of treatment approaches. While some differences between programmes can be accounted for in meta-analysis (e.g. theoretical orientation such as psychodynamic or cognitive behavioural), there are many more subtle differences that may not be available to meta-analysts, such as therapist variability, programme context and degree of felt coercion. So, while contemporary treatment programmes across and within jurisdictions share similarities, they can also differ considerably in significant ways that include the methods they use and what they target and the extent by which they constitute evidence-informed practice (McGrath, Cumming, Burchard, Zeoli, & Ellerby, 2010). The variance found across treatment programmes both complicates our ability to reach conclusions about the overall strengths of treatment while paradoxically advancing our understanding. Different practices potentially allow comparisons to be made on what are the more beneficial aspects of treatment against the desired goals, although unfortunately, this kind of research has rarely been undertaken.

Bearing these caveats in mind, the current evidence base for treatment effectiveness is by no means strong. Although evidence from meta-analysis indicates that sex offender treatment programmes *can* bring about reductions in recidivism (e.g. Hanson, Bourgon, Helmus, & Hodgson, 2009), this is by no means routinely the case. The efficacy of sex offender treatment continues to be debated robustly in the rehabilitative literature (e.g. Crighton & Towl, 2007; Ho & Ross, 2012; Mann, Carter, & Wakeling, 2012; Marshall & Marshall, 2007). Sex offender treatment cannot be regarded as an "evidence based treatment" according to Kazdin's (2008) definition of "interventions or techniques that have produced therapeutic change in controlled trials" (p. 147). There have been only a few controlled trials of sex offender treatment, and the largest scale of these studies (Marques, Wiederanders, Day, Nelson, & von Ommeren, 2005) found no effect for the treatment group.

Taking an Evidence-Based Approach to Sex Offender Treatment

There is no approach to sex offender treatment that can be regarded as an "evidence-based treatment" (EBT) according to customary definitions (e.g. Kazdin, 2008). Given this situation, our best efforts can only be described as "evidence-informed practice" or "evidence-based practice", defined by the APA as "the integration of the best available research with clinical expertise in the context of patient characteristics, culture and preferences" (APA Presidential Task Force on Evidence-Based Practice, 2006, p. 273). Taking an evidence-based approach requires that those who deliver treatment are cognisant of the best available research and also that the best available research is at least adequate in its scope and design.

In the sex offender treatment field, arguably more than with other criminal behaviours, there is a strong community of practitioners who take research seriously. Three international organisations—the Association for the Treatment of Sexual Abusers (ATSA), the International Association for the Treatment of Sexual Offenders (IATSO) and the National Organisation for the Treatment of Abusers (NOTA)—exist to support practitioners; each publishes its own research journal and holds regular conferences and training events that repeatedly make the link between research and practice. Although conference programmes can still sometimes reveal a split between research and practitioner interests (e.g. with workshops being labelled as intended for one or the other audience), in our view there is ample opportunity for practitioners working with sex offenders to be exposed to the best available research, and we have experienced little hostility to the notion of evidence-based practice among the many practitioners with whom we have interacted.

In the remainder of this chapter, we will summarise what we consider to be the messages from the "best available research" and the aspects of typical practice to which they refer. As many programmes contain significant components that could be described as evidence based, it is possible that the lack of robust findings of effectiveness are due to one of three reasons. First, it may be that there is simply a lack of robust controlled evaluation designs, as has been argued by many researchers, and that large-scale high-quality studies would reveal effective approaches to sex offender treatment. Second, it is possible that our best available knowledge is still incomplete, and there are treatment targets or techniques still to be evidenced that would improve overall outcomes. Third, it is possible that current treatment approaches do contain evidence-informed components, but the success of these components is offset by poor quality delivery (e.g. inadequately collaborative or supportive) or by a hostile treatment context (e.g. programmes that take place in the unsafe environment of prisons) or wider societal rejection of those convicted of sex offences.

Bearing these issues in mind, we will proceed to discuss what the best available evidence tells us about effective approaches to sex offender treatment. Our assessment of the evidence for effective treatment below relies heavily on four recent comprehensive reviews of treatment outcome studies (Dennis et al., 2012; Hanson et al., 2009; Långström et al., 2013; Schmucker & Lösel, 2009).

We have categorised this discussion according to the three principles of the risk-need-responsivity (RNR) model of correctional rehabilitation (Andrews & Bonta, 2006): who does sex offender treatment seem to work best for, what targets should be addressed by treatment programmes and how should treatment programmes respond to the particular needs of the client group? The RNR model, if followed, has been shown to improve assessment and rehabilitative efforts with those convicted of criminal behaviour. Importantly, it has been demonstrated that RNR is applicable to the assessment and treatment of sexual offenders (Hanson et al., 2009); Hanson et al. were able to demonstrate through reviewing 23 treatment programmes that greater adherence to these principles was met with better reductions in recidivism. Hanson et al. found that those programmes that followed only one or none of the principles had little effect on recidivism while those that followed two or three had the largest impact.

There are other suggestions in the meta-analyses that treatment works better for some individuals than others in terms of other variables than those covered by the RNR principles, but we are not yet at a position where we can say definitively that some people will or will not benefit. For instance, Schmucker and Lösel (2009) found no difference in treatment effect for those who entered treatment voluntarily compared to those who were mandated to treatment. They also found that younger participants fared better, but this finding was confounded with treatment type; younger participants were more likely to have received multisystemic therapy which focuses efforts on improving the offender's family and social systems; older participants were more likely to have received cognitive behavioural treatment, focusing on changing attitudes and behaviour. One as yet unanswered question is whether treatment is more effective with men who have sexually offended against adults or those who have offended against children. The most recent meta-analysis (Schmucker & Lösel, 2009) found it impossible to perform "a sensible analysis" (p. 23) on this question.

For Whom Does Treatment Work?

The RNR model's first core principle, the risk principle, directs that sexual offenders will require different levels of intervention depending upon the risk of recidivism that they present. A number of studies have shown that with low-risk non-sex offenders, treatment has either very little impact on recidivism reduction (Andrews & Bonta, 2006; Andrews & Dowden, 2006) or, in some cases where treatment is intensive, recidivism rates can in fact increase (Andrews, Bonta, & Hoge, 1990; Andrews & Dowden, 2006; Bonta, Wallace-Capretta, & Rooney, 2000; Lowenkamp & Latessa, 2002; Lowenkamp, Latessa, & Holsinger, 2006), and it has been argued that this is likely to be true for sex offenders as well (Wakeling, Mann, & Carter, 2012).

Hanson et al. (2009) examined the applicability of the RNR principles to sex offender treatment but found that the odds ratio for those programmes that targeted only higher-risk offenders (defined as "higher risk than average" (p. 871) but not linked to scores on any particular risk tool) was not significantly better than the odds ratio for programmes that targeted all risk groups. They noted that the risk principle was the weakest of the three RNR principles and concluded that "the magnitude of these differences is sufficiently small as to be of little practical value in most settings" (p. 884) but that "noticeable reductions in recidivism are not to be expected among the lowest risk offenders" (p. 886).

A stronger effect by risk was reported by Schmucker and Lösel (2009) who stated that: "… the results revealed a clear picture. The higher the risk for reoffending, the higher the resulting treatment effect. Treatment for low risk participants showed no effect at all" (p. 24). Although there may need to be exceptions, e.g. those low-risk but high-criminogenic need offenders (Carter, 2014), the best available evidence seems to suggest that treatment programmes are best targeted at higher-risk offenders.

Treatment Targets

The RNR principles provide an important framework to help consider the strengths of sex offender treatment. The need principle requires that criminogenic needs (dynamic risk factors that are amenable to change) are assessed then targeted in treatment. The four most recent comprehensive reviews (Dennis et al., 2012; Hanson et al., 2009; Långström et al., 2013; Schmucker & Lösel, 2009) of sex offender treatment programmes all concluded that as a consequence of mixed findings of effectiveness, treatment providers should ensure that their programmes are focused on issues that have been shown to have strong links with recidivism. For example:

> Attention to the need principle would motivate the largest changes in the interventions given to sexual offenders…Consequently it would be beneficial for treatment providers to carefully review their programs to ensure that the treatment targets emphasised are those empirically linked to sexual recidivism. (Hanson et al., 2009, p. 886)

It is fortunate that, perhaps more so than with any other type of criminal behaviour, the factors associated with sexual recidivism have been extensively researched, mainly by Karl Hanson and his associates. There have been several high-quality large-scale studies and meta-analyses of the predictors of sexual recidivism (e.g. Hanson & Bussière, 1998; Hanson & Harris, 2000; Hanson & Morton-Bourgon, 2005; Helmus, Hanson, Babchishin, & Mann, 2013; Mann, Hanson, & Thornton, 2010; see Table 7.1 below).

The importance of focusing on these factors as priority targets for treatment is well understood by the practitioner community, and in the last 5 years particularly, considerable effort has been made to bring treatment programmes in line with the outcomes of this research. The key elements of programmes from the 1980s through

Table 7.1 Psychological risk factors for sexual recidivism (from Mann et al., 2010)

Empirically supported risk factors	Promising risk factors	Not risk factors
Sexual preoccupation	Hostility towards women	Depression
Any deviant sexual interest	Machiavellianism	Poor social skills
Offence supportive attitudes	Callousness	Poor victim empathy
Emotional congruence with children	Dysfunctional coping	Lack of motivation for treatment at intake
Lack of emotionally intimate relationships with adults		
Lifestyle instability		
General self-regulation problems		
Poor cognitive problem solving		
Resistance to rules and supervision		
Grievance/hostility		
Negative social influences		

to the 2000s (Mann & Marshall, 2009) comprised (1) encouraging treatment participants to "take responsibility for their offending", (2) developing victim empathy and (3) relapse prevention, where treatment participants are trained to anticipate high-risk situations and develop plans to avoid or control them (Laws, 1989).

McGrath et al.'s survey of treatment providers in 2010, and several essays critiquing these treatment goals (e.g. Mann & Barnett, 2013; Maruna & Mann, 2006; Ware & Mann, 2012), encourages those providing treatment programmes to place less emphasis on these areas. We do not yet have sufficient research to justify removing these components from treatment programmes altogether, however. Participant feedback studies typically find that treatment participants value these components of treatment more than any other (Levenson, Macgowan, Morin, & Cotter, 2009; Levenson, Prescott, & D'Amora, 2010; Wakeling, Webster, & Mann, 2005) and on this basis, it may be premature to disregard them altogether.

We can conclude that the best available evidence provides clear direction on the treatment targets for an evidence-informed treatment programme. Table 7.1 summarises a review of the risk factor literature by Mann et al. (2010) and presents a list of the best-evidenced risk factors as well as those variables which have been explored in fewer studies but show promise as factors which predict recidivism and those variables which have been shown not to predict recidivism.

Treatment Approaches

High-Level Approach

The responsivity principle consists of what Andrews and Bonta (2010) term *general* and *specific* responsivity. General specificity refers to the adoption of cognitive social learning methods as being most effective in bringing about a change in behaviour. Consequently, the responsivity principle states that offenders generally benefit most from programmes that take a cognitive behavioural approach. Cognitive behavioural programmes are by no means homogeneous activities but should be based on a model of teaching both attitudes and new behavioural skills. General responsivity principles for programmes addressing criminal behaviour also stress the importance of the therapeutic relationship between the facilitator and offender as well as the use of prosocial modelling, reinforcement and other appropriate methods to modify change are highlighted. Specific responsivity requires that programmes recognise the individual needs of participants, such as their intellectual ability, cultural background and personal strengths.

With people convicted of sexual offences, three high-level approaches can be described as evidence informed on the basis of the best available evidence: cognitive behavioural programmes, pharmacological therapies such as anti-androgen treatment, and multisystemic therapy for juvenile offenders, which involves expanding the focus of treatment beyond the individual to his family, peers, school and community systems (Borduin, Henggeler, Blaske, & Stein, 1990). These approaches have not been found to consistently reduce recidivism through controlled studies (see earlier discussion), but across the meta-analyses, their outcomes are consistently superior to counselling, psychotherapy and nonbehavioural methods. For example:

> Cognitive-behavioral and multisystemic treatment had larger effects than other approaches. (Schmucker & Lösel, 2009, p. 2)
>
> In practice, it is likely that both pharmacological and psychological therapies will need to be used in unison in order to obtain the greatest benefit. (Dennis et al., 2012, p. 28)

Another popular approach to treatment is the Good Lives Model (e.g. Ward, 2002; Ward & Mann, 2004; Ward, Mann, & Gannon, 2007), which could be described as a version of cognitive behavioural treatment but with a focus on building strengths rather than addressing risk factors, which is the more traditional approach to sexual offending treatment. Good Lives programmes have a strong intuitive appeal for many therapists who prefer to take a positive and future-oriented approach to working with clients, but as yet, there has been insufficient empirically robust outcome research to demonstrate a treatment effect for this approach.

As noted above, however, sexual offending programmes that describe themselves as cognitive behavioural are by no means homogeneous approaches (Hanson et al., 2009). A broad variety of treatment techniques can be described as cognitive behavioural, and so it is necessary to consider the evidence for not just the overall model but also the specific techniques used within a programme. There is research to support methods used for some of the treatment targets listed in Table 7.1 but not all, and there has also been considerable research into treatment style. Further, there is considerable complexity in getting the context right for sex offender treatment, which is an important issue in ensuring treatment is responsive. We will consider these issues separately in more depth below.

Specific Treatment Techniques

Following the groupings of risk factors used by Mann et al. (2010) as set in Table 7.1, we will consider effective methods for (a) sexual deviance risk factors, (b) attitudinal risk factors such as pro-sexual offending attitudes and (c) self-management risk factors including the management of emotions and impulsive urges. The quality of research varies across these different issues, and in addition, it is likely that some of these risk factors are harder to change than others. For instance, it is unlikely to be possible to change a deviant sexual preference such as paedophilic preference. However, there is greater cause for optimism in relation to risk factors such as offence supportive attitudes and self-management.

Sexually Deviant Interests

Conditioning theory, which purports that behaviour experienced as pleasurable will be repeated while behaviour that is unpleasant will not, has given rise to a number of methods to address sexually deviant interests (Laws and Marshall 1990). In accordance with conditioning theory, techniques have been employed to modify deviant interests through *aversive therapies* that aim to negate the enjoyment of fantasies, e.g. olfactory aversion and *masturbatory reconditioning techniques*, e.g. directed masturbation aimed at raising sexual arousal to suitable stimuli that are nondeviant. There is no large-scale or controlled research into the efficacy of these technique but only case study reports, few of which are recent. While aversion techniques, such as covert and modified covert sensitisation, are unlikely to eradicate deviant sexual interests, some case study reports have described using these methods to help an individual manage sexual arousal related to offending, and in some cases it has been reported that benefits made can be sustained over time, e.g. Earls and Castonguay (1989). The evidence for directed masturbation, a reconditioning technique, was considered as hopeful in 1991 (Laws & Marshall, 1991), but unfortunately, no further evidence has been forthcoming since this time. The position is similar for thematic shift methods, used in conjunction with aversion techniques (Marshall, 1979) and verbal satiation (Laws & Marshall, 1991).

Therefore, although behavioural techniques have been used to attempt to modify sexual interests since the 1960s, there remains an absence of evidence to support the effectiveness of these approaches. The existing studies are characterised by being of poor quality (e.g. Marshall, Anderson, & Fernandez, 1999; Quinsey & Earls, 1990) or involve small samples sizes or single case studies (e.g. Maletzky, 1985). Existing research has also failed to isolate the role of behaviour modification techniques from the range of different treatment approaches an individual can undertake. Therefore, the effectiveness of behavioural conditioning techniques in changing sexual arousal is unclear.

While the focus of this chapter is on psychological treatments, we note that medication, particularly as an adjunct to psychological approaches, is also used to both change the nature and intensity of sexual arousal. These techniques have been shown to have the best results if used alongside psychological therapies such as cognitive behavioural programmes (Beech & Harkins, 2012; Lösel & Schmucker, 2005).

Cognitive Risk Factors

In terms of cognitive risk factors, we have examined the evidence for various treatment methods that have been employed to target cognitive factors such as cognitions about the world (e.g. the world is dangerous and uncontrollable), cognitions about others (e.g. suspiciousness, hostile attributional bias), cognitions about the self (e.g. seeing the self as damaged or disadvantaged), cognitions about sexual offending in general (e.g. sex with children is not harmful) and cognitions about one's own offending (e.g. my victim was not harmed by the offence). From the review by Beech, Bartels, and Dixon (2013), it can be concluded that several treatment techniques could be considered to have a reasonable evidence base. First, *cognitive restructuring* has been shown in at least three studies to be associated with a decrease in offence supportive cognitions for child molesters (Bickley & Beech, 2003; Bumby, 1996; Williams, Wakeling, & Webster, 2007), although this technique should not be used to push treatment participants towards "taking responsibility" for their offending, because taking responsibility is not an established risk factor for sexual offending (Ware & Mann, 2012).

Second, *schema therapy* (e.g. Mann & Shingler, 2005) has been shown to have some success with people convicted of sexual offences in terms of leading to attitude change (e.g. Thornton & Shingler, 2001; Barnett, 2011) although both these studies emanated from HM Prison Service England and Wales and did not examine reoffending as an outcome. Studies in other settings have not yielded positive effects on measures of cognitive change (Tarrier et al., 2010; see also Eccleston & Owen, 2007)—again, reoffending has not been studied as an outcome from schema therapy.

Third, *experiential techniques* such as role-play of interpersonal situations where the treatment client takes on different roles within the situation can improve perspective taking, which may be effective in future potential offending situations. These techniques have typically been used in sexual offending programmes to develop victim empathy (e.g. Mann, Daniels, & Marshall, 2002; Webster et al., 2005), but Mann and Barnett argued that this use was based on insufficient evidence and carried dangers, and there is no evidence that these techniques have led to a reduction in reoffending.

Techniques to improve self-management, including emotional management and urge management, are well established in criminal justice settings. Cognitive skills training programmes are widely used for people who have been convicted but not for a sexual offence to considerable effect, especially given that they are relatively short and cheap to run. While the tradition for sexual offence perpetrators has been to eschew this type of programme in favour of offence-focused programmes, two studies have shown that cognitive skills programmes alone are associated with reduced recidivism for people convicted of sexual offences. Robinson (1995) studied 4072 prisoners referred to the Reasoning and Rehabilitation programme while

Table 7.2 Techniques to address risk factors associated with sexual offences

Treatment target	Documented techniques
Sexually deviant interests	Behaviour modification
Offence supportive attitudes and cognitions/schemas associated with sexual offending	Cognitive restructuring
	Schema therapy
	Experiential techniques, e.g. role-play
Self-management	Cognitive skills training[a]

[a]Supported by recidivism outcome studies

in custody and found that the people convicted of sexual offences within this sample who completed the programme showed a 57.8 % drop in recidivism compared to a control group, Similarly, Travers, Mann, and Hollin (2014) studied the effect of another cognitive skills programme, the Enhanced Thinking Skills (ETS) course, on over 21,000 prisoners in England and Wales, examining impact by risk and offence type. Their sample contained about 1800 men convicted of sex offences (589 rapists and 1235 men convicted of sex offences against children), for whom ETS had been the only intervention they received (i.e. they did not participate in any specialised sexual offending treatment).

On average (although there were some differences according to risk level), the rapists who participated in ETS had a reconviction rate about 20 percentage points less than predicted, and the child molesters had a reconviction rate about 10 percentage points less than predicted. In both these studies, only general reconviction was reported, so it cannot be concluded that cognitive skills training reduced *sexual* recidivism. However, it appears clear from these studies that cognitive skills training is beneficial for people convicted of sexual offences.

Table 7.2 below summarises what the best-documented techniques for the various risk factors shown in Table 7.1. Of these techniques, only cognitive skills training has been shown to have an impact on recidivism. The other techniques in Table 7.2 lack sufficient evidence and can still only be described as experimental, but they do have supportive theoretical models, and they have been reasonably well described in the literature. A programme combining these various techniques, if individualised to participants, could be considered an evidence-informed approach to reducing sexual recidivism, but not an evidence-based approach. It is clear that sexual offending treatment components need to be evaluated more robustly for their impact on reoffending.

Treatment Style

Alongside the programme theory, our understanding of the nature of the therapy style and the therapist-client relationship needed to encourage change has advanced and changed over the decades. The confrontational approach, originally advocated for sexual offending treatment (Salter, 1988), is now recognised to be detrimental to group cohesion and individual change. Research has shown that the anxiety raised from a confrontational style could impact upon understanding (Beech & Fordham, 1997). Instead, Mann et al. (2002) found that facilitators who showed a warm, honest and direct approach with expressions of empathy and verbal reward were associated with those groups that achieved their aims.

The treatment style that Marshall et al. identified was consistent with the principles of motivational interviewing (MI; Miller & Rollnick, 2002) techniques that were similarly revolutionising substance misuse treatment, another field where confrontational approaches had previously dominated. MI research had already challenged practitioners that confrontation when tackling addiction problems impeded change by causing defensiveness.

Building on practitioner enthusiasm for delivering treatment in a more motivational way, the Good Lives Model (GLM; Ward, 2002) proposed a theoretical framework by which sexual offending treatment can become part of a positive psychology, helping motivate treatment participants to reach the primary goods that all humans want as part of a fulfilling life. The GLM encourages primary goods to be achieved in prosocial ways, e.g. intimacy with age appropriate adults as part of seeking relatedness, rather than simply identifying the things that an offender must avoid, e.g. seeking intimacy with a child. The GLM has been adopted as a unifying framework by many sexual offending programmes. We regard the GLM as a theoretically sound model for treatment programmes which has the potential to radically change the way in which treatment programmes conceptualise their targets and relate to their clients. However, we must add the caution that despite claims of effectiveness, there have as yet been insufficient robust evaluation designs to enable the GLM to be considered an evidence-based treatment approach.

More recently, treatment providers have begun to explore more biologically informed approaches to treatment delivery. A biopsychosocial approach recognises the role that biological and social factors play in making an individual vulnerable to offending (Carter & Mann, in press). In this model, treatment engagement can be enhanced by making treatment accessible to individuals, regardless of their biological vulnerabilities. For example, developing positive and trusting relationships with facilitators and other group members may be extremely challenging for individuals who have deficits in their neurocognitive functioning. Keeping track and understanding verbal arguments, particularly if they require extended periods of concentration, can also be problematic for these individuals. Incorporating visual, auditory and kinaesthetic methods into programmes to allow a more active and less verbally dependent method of engagement in contrast to the more common talking and introspective methods of therapy could help improve responsivity and engagement.

Treatment Context

The culture in which a treatment programme is set, from the narrow culture of the immediate setting, through the wider culture of the system within which treatment is located, to the broadest level of societal culture, can affect the impact of sexual offending treatment. People with convictions for sex offences know that they are universally reviled. It is perhaps unsurprising that in this context, they are wary of treatment professionals, especially when these same professionals also often have the power to dictate or withhold their release from custody or their freedoms in the community. Furthermore, even if someone attends the best treatment programme and is agreed by all to have made excellent progress, these gains can potentially be quickly undone by experiences of public hostility, disgrace and rejection in the community.

There is evidence that treatment programmes are more effective when delivered in the community rather than in prison. Schmucker and Lösel (2009) reported from their meta-analysis that treatment in prisons failed to show a significant effect overall and noted that this finding accorded with earlier studies (Aos, Miller, & Drake, 2006; Hall, 1995; Lösel & Schmucker, 2005) as well as with the general "what works" literature. They suggested that effectiveness of treatment in prisons may be negated by contamination effects (where participants are mixing socially with more deviant peers), difficulty with the delay in transferring learning to the real world or difficulties during resettlement. Also, there can be differences in clients, offence history and therapists in prison programmes compared to community settings. However, Schmucker and Lösel also noted that inpatient hospital treatment was effective, suggesting that the iatrogenic effects may be particular to a prison environment rather than any inpatient setting. This finding might suggest that being treated away from the "real world" is not necessarily ineffective, so perhaps the key issue is that the wider setting is therapeutically rather than punitively oriented.

In the UK, there has been a long-running debate over the desirability of keeping people convicted of sexual offences in prison in separate units from people serving sentences for offences that are not sexual. The available evidence seems to suggest that this kind of separation aids participation in programmes because it removes, to a large extent, fears for physical and psychological safety (Blagden et al., 2014), freeing up "headspace" to focus on rehabilitation. In contrast, when sex offenders are integrated with non-sex offenders, they have to focus their cognitive resources on survival (Schwaebe, 2005). This is not to say that separate units for people convicted of sexual offences are entirely desirable (Mann, 2016), but on balance they may be able to provide more therapeutic environments akin to that of a hospital, as long as the staff are carefully trained.

Other features of a positive organisational context for treatment include having highly trained and well-supervised nontreatment staff who can listen to offenders, understand their perspectives and build constructive relationships; a strategy to identify and counter myths; treatment aims that are strengths-based; sensitive referral-making; clear and transparent information about treatment; use of intrinsic rather than extrinsic motivators; involvement of family members; provision of choice about the nature of treatment; and involvement of men who have completed treatment in the support of those considering it or participating in it (see Mann, 2009 for a more detailed discussion).

Conclusions

Given the significant and lasting harm sexual offending can cause, it is understandable that victims, policymakers and members of the public may expect perpetrators of these crimes to undergo *treatment* to stop them from offending again. Reasonable as this expectation may be, it fails to address the paradox that treatment to reduce sexual reoffending presents: that is, for many people who have committed a sexual offence, it is probably not necessary; for others it will be insufficient on its own to achieve this goal. That is not to say that effective rehabilitative programmes should be removed from a range of different measures to help with addressing the risk of sexual recidivism. However, recognition of the limitations of sexual offending treatment is important if we are to realise its strengths.

Hanson et al. (2009) concluded that "not all interventions [for sex offenders] reduce recidivism" (p. 881), but their meta-analysis and those by others all indicate that some interventions do reduce recidivism. The important challenge, therefore, is to isolate the effective components of treatment programmes and to differentiate them from the components of programmes that hinder effectiveness. In this chapter, we have set out to propose which parts of treatment that we have got right. In doing so, we have identified treatment components that could be considered as weaknesses to be removed from programmes or require further research to determine if we should continue with them.

The evidence indicates that programmes are most effective when closely bound to the principles of risk, need and responsivity. It seems reasonable to conclude that programmes addressing sexual offending risk should not be provided to those offenders who are at low risk of recidivism. There is clear guidance on what we should target in terms of need, and we have also highlighted those techniques to employ in programmes that have evidence to support their use in relation to these targets.

We have also highlighted the importance of the context that programmes are delivered in and the wider supporting environment. A stronger public acknowledgement that not all people convicted of sexual offences are high risk, and that many will desist from further offending in the absence of any psychological therapy, could help create environments and a society that better support successful reintegration back into the community or do not alienate those convicted of an offence from living in them. By not automatically viewing perpetrators of sexual offences as persistent offenders and highly risky, we may help people to see past the crime and reduce stigma and negative labelling that people who have committed a sexual offence experience. These attitudes can hinder an ex-offender's ability to play a constructive role in society. We recognise that some perpetrators of sexual offences raise significant concerns about their risk of further offending and will need to be managed very carefully to rightly meet public protection responsibilities. Nevertheless, more accepting and supporting environments will still be of benefit to poeple who have committed offences with the most complex or difficult needs to address who present the greatest challenges to correctional staff.

In this chapter, we have argued that some aspects of current sexual offending programmes could be described as evidence informed, although few can be termed "evidence based". The mixed findings for treatment effectiveness likely reflect a combination of poor quality studies, programme aims or techniques that lack internal coherence or consistency (e.g. a mixture of rehabilitative and punitive aims), weak adherence to the RNR model and the iatrogenic effect of hostile cultures outside the treatment environment. These issues vary in the extent to which they are in the control of treatment providers. The content of treatment programmes is obviously important but is not the only thing that determines whether a person convicted of a sexual offence is likely to desist from further offending.

Our aim in this chapter was to consider what aspects of current or typical sexual offending programmes can be considered evidence based or, at a minimum, evidence informed. Our summary shows that it is possible to select appropriate targets for a treatment programme based on robust research. However, effective treatment methods and techniques have been less robustly established or, in some cases, not established at all. It is not possible to conclude that treatment programmes for people convicted of sexual offences constitute evidence-based practice, yet, but the jigsaw is being assembled. To ensure that sexual offending treatment is as strong as it can be, we must continue to research our practice, evaluate our efforts and be prepared to adjust our approach when evidence indicates this is necessary.

References

Andrews, D. A., & Bonta, J. (2006). *The psychology of criminal conduct* (4th ed.). Cincinnati, OH: Anderson.

Andrews, D. A., & Bonta, J. (2010). *The psychology of criminal conduct* (5th ed.). New Jersey: Matthew Bender.

Andrews, D. A., Bonta, J., & Hoge, R. D. (1990). Classification for effective rehabilitation: Rediscovering psychology. *Criminal Justice and Behavior, 17*, 19–52.

Andrews, D. A., & Dowden, C. (2006). Risk principles of case classification in correctional treatment: A meta-analytic investigation. *International Journal of Offender Therapy and Comparative Criminology, 50*, 88–100.

Aos, S., Miller, M., & Drake, E. (2006). *Evidence-based adult corrections programs: What works and what does not.* Olympia, WA: Washington State Institute for Public Policy.

APA Presidential Task Force on Evidence-Based Practice. (2006). Evidence-based practice in psychology. *American Psychologist, 61*, 271–285.

Barnett, G. D. (2011). What is grievance thinking and how can we measure this in sexual offenders? *Legal and Criminological Psychology, 16*(1), 37–61.

Barnett, G., Wakeling, H., & Howard, P. (2010). An examination of the predictive validity of the Risk Matrix 2000 in England and Wales. *Sexual Abuse: A Journal of Research and Treatment, 22*, 443–470.

Beech, A. R., Bartels, R. M., & Dixon, L. (2013). Assessment and treatment of distorted schemas in sexual offenders. *Trauma, Violence & Abuse, 14*(1), 54–66.

Beech, A., & Fordham, A. S. (1997). *Sexual Abuse: A Journal of Research and Treatment, 9*, 219–237.

Beech, A., & Harkins, L. (2012). DSM-IV paraphilia: Descriptions, demographics and treatment interventions. *Aggression and Violent Behaviour, 17*, 527–539.

Bickley, J. A., & Beech, A. R. (2003). Implications for treatment of sexual offenders of the Ward and Hudson model of relapse. *Sexual Abuse: A Journal of Research and Treatment, 15*(2), 121–134.

Blagden, N., Winder, B., & Hames, C. (2014). "They treat us like human beings"—Experiencing a therapeutic sex offenders prison impact on prisoners and staff and implications for treatment. *International Journal of Offender Therapy and Comparative Criminology*, 0306624X14553227.

Bonta, J., Wallace-Capretta, S., & Rooney, R. (2000). A quasi-experimental evaluation of an intensive rehabilitation supervision program. *Criminal Justice and Behavior, 27*, 312–329.

Borduin, C. M., Henggeler, S. W., Blaske, D. M., & Stein, R. J. (1990). Multisystemic treatment of adolescent sexual offenders. *International Journal, 996*(3), 1.

Bumby, K. M. (1996). Assessing the cognitive distortions of child molesters and rapists: Development and validation of the MOLEST and RAPE scales. *Sexual Abuse: A Journal of Research and Treatment, 8*(1), 37–54.

Carter, A. J. (2014). Sexual offending treatment programs: The importance of evidence-informed practice. In K. McCartan (Ed.), *Responding to sexual offending: Perceptions, risk management and public protection* (pp. 111–127). Hampshire: Palgrave Macmillan.

Carter, A. J., & Mann, R. E. (in press). Organising principles for an integrated model of change for the treatment of sexual offending. In Beech, A. R., & Ward, T. (Eds.). *The Wiley Blackwell Handbook on assessment, treatment and theories of sexual offending* (Vol. 1). Chichester: Wiley.

Crighton, D., & Towl, G. (2007). Experimental interventions with sex offenders: A brief review of their efficacy. *Evidence-Based Mental Health, 10*, 35–37.

Dennis, J. A., Khan, O., Ferriter, M., Huband, N., Powney, M. J., & Duggan, C. (2012). Psychological interventions for adults who have sexually offended or are at risk of offending. *Cochrane Database of Systematic Reviews, 12*, CD007507

Earls, C. M., & Castonguay, L. G. (1989). The evaluation of olfactory aversion for a bisexual pedophile with a single case study multiple baseline design. *Behaviour Therapy, 20*, 137–146.

Eccleston, L., & Owen, K. (2007). Cognitive treatment "Just for Rapists": Recent developments. In T. A. Gannon, T. Ward, A. R. Beech, & D. Fisher (Eds.), *Aggressive offenders' cognition: Theory, research, and practice* (p. 135). Oxford: John Wiley & Sons Ltd.

Hall, G. C. (1995). Sexual offender recidivism revisited: A meta-analysis of recent treatment studies. *Journal of Consulting and Clinical Psychology, 63*(5), 805–809.

Hanson, R. K., Bourgon, G., Helmus, L., & Hodgson, S. (2009). The principles of effective correctional treatment also apply to sexual offenders; A meta-analysis. *Criminal Justice and Behavior, 36*, 865–891.

Hanson, R. K., & Bussière, M. T. (1998). Predicting relapse: A meta-analysis of sex offender recidivism studies. *Journal of Consulting and Clinical Psychology, 66*, 348–362.

Hanson, R. K., & Harris, A. J. R. (2000). Where should we intervene? Dynamic predictors of sexual offense recidivism. *Criminal Justice and Behavior, 27*, 6–35.

Hanson, R. K., & Morton-Bourgon, K. E. (2005). The characteristics of persistent sexual offenders: A meta-analysis of recidivism studies. *Journal of Consulting and Clinical Psychology, 73*, 1154–1163.

Helmus, L., Hanson, R. K., Babchishim, K. M., & Mann, R. E. (2013). Attitudes supportive of sexual offending predict recidivism: A meta-analysis. *Trauma Violence Abuse, 14*, 34–53.

Helmus, L., Hanson, R. K., Thornton, D., Babchishin, K., & Harris, A. (2012). Absolute recidivism rates predicted by Static-99R and Static 2002R sex offender risk assessment tools vary across samples: A meta-analysis. *Criminal Justice and Behavior, 39*, 1148–1171.

Ho, D. K., & Ross, C. C. (2012). Cognitive behaviour therapy for sex offenders: Too good to be true? *Criminal Behaviour and Mental Health, 22*, 1–6.

Kazdin, A. E. (2008). Evidence-based treatment and practice: New opportunities to bridge clinical research and practice, enhance the knowledge base, and improve patient care. *American Psychologist, 63*(3), 146.

Långström, N., Enebrink, P., Laurén, E.-M., Lindblom, J., Werkö, S., & Hanson, R. K. (2013). Preventing sexual violence against children: Systematic review of medical and psychological interventions. *BMJ, 347*, f4630. doi:10.1136/bmj.f4630.

Laws, D. R. (1989). *Relapse prevention with sex offenders*. New York, NY: Guilford Press.

Laws, D. R., & Marshall, W. L. (1990). An integrated theory of the etiology of sexual offending. In W. L. Marshall, D. R. Laws, & H. E. Barbaree (Eds.), *Handbook of sexual assault: Issues, theories and treatment of the offender* (pp. 257–275). New York, NY: Plenum Press.

Laws, D. R., & Marshall, W. L. (1991). Masturbatory reconditioning with sexual deviates: An evaluative review. *Advances in Behaviour Research and Therapy, 13*, 13–25.

Levenson, J. S., Macgowan, M. J., Morin, J. W., & Cotter, L. P. (2009). Perceptions of sex offenders about treatment: Satisfaction and engagement in group therapy. *Sexual Abuse: A Journal of Research and Treatment, 21*(1), 35–56.

Levenson, J. S., Prescott, D. S., & D'Amora, D. A. (2010). Sex offender treatment: Consumer satisfaction and engagement in therapy. *International Journal of Offender Therapy and Comparative Criminology, 54*(3), 307–326.

Lösel, F., & Schmucker, M. (2005). The effectiveness of treatment for sexual offenders: A comprehensive meta-analysis. *Journal of Experimental Criminology, 1*, 117–146.

Lowenkamp, C., & Latessa, E. (2002). Evaluation *of Ohio's community based correctional facilities and halfway house programs.* Unpublished manuscript

Lowenkamp, C., Latessa, E., & Holsinger, A. (2006). The risk principle in action: What have we learned from 13,676 offenders and 97 correctional programs? *Crime and Delinquency, 52*, 77–93.

Maletzky, B. M. (1985). Orgasmic reconditioning. In A. S. Bellack & M. Hersen (Eds.), *Dictionary of behaviour therapy techniques* (pp. 157–158). New York, NY: Pergamon.

Mann, R. E. (2009). Getting the context right for sex offender treatment. In D. Prescott (Ed.), *Building motivation for change in sexual offenders*. Brandon, VT: Safer Society Press.

Mann, R. E. (2016). Sex offenders in prison. In Y. Jewkes, B. Crewe, & J. Bennett (Eds.), *Handbook on Prisons*. Routledge.

Mann, R. E., & Barnett, G. (2013). Victim empathy intervention with sexual offenders: Rehabilitation, punishment or correctional quackery? *Sexual Abuse: A Journal of Research and Treatment, 25*, 282–301.

Mann, R. E., Carter, A. J., & Wakeling, H. C. (2012). In defence of NOMS' view about sex offending treatment effectiveness: A reply to Ho and Ross. *Criminal Behaviour and Mental Health, 22*, 7–10.

Mann, R. E., Daniels, M., & Marshall, W. L. (2002). The use of role plays in developing empathy. In Y. M. Fernandez (Ed.), *In their shoes: Examining the issue of empathy and its place in the treatment of offenders* (pp. 132–148). Oklahoma City, OK: Wood 'N' Barnes.

Mann, R. E., Hanson, R. K., & Thornton, D. (2010). Assessing risk for sexual recidivism: Some proposals on the nature of psychologically meaningful risk factors. *Sexual Abuse: A Journal of Research and Treatment, 22*, 172–190.

Mann, R. E., & Marshal, W. L. (2009). Advances in the treatment of adult sexual offenders. In A. R. Beech, L. A. Craig, & K. D. Browne (Eds). Assessment and treatemnt of sexual offenders: A Handbook. Chichster: Wiley & Sons.

Mann, R. E., & Shingler, J. (2005). Schema-driven cognition in sexual offenders: Theory, assessment and treatment. In W. L. Marshall, Y. M. Fernandez, L. E. Marshall, & G. Serran (Eds.), *Sexual offender treatment: Controversial issues* (pp. 173–185). New York, NY: Wiley.

Mann, R. E., Webster, S. D., Wakeling, H. C., & Keylock, H. (2013). Why do sex offenders refuse treatment? *Journal of Sexual Aggression, 19*(2), 191–206.

Marques, J. K., Wiederanders, M., Day, D. M., Nelson, C., & von Ommeren, A. (2005). Effects of a relapse prevention program on sexual recidivism: Final results from California's Sex Offender Treatment and Evaluation Project (SOTEP). *Sexual Abuse: A Journal of Research and Treatment, 17*, 79–107.

Marshall, W. L. (1979). Satiation therapy: A procedure for reducing deviant sexual arousal. *Journal of Aplied Behavior Analysis, 12*, 377–389.

Marshall, W. L., Anderson, D., & Fernandez, Y. M. (1999). *Cognitive behavioral treatment of sexual offenders*. Chichester: John Wiley & Sons.

Marshall, W. L., & Marshall, L. E. (2007). The utility of the random controlled trial for evaluating sexual offender treatment: The gold standard or an inappropriate strategy? *Sexual Abuse, 19*, 175–191.

Maruna, S., & Mann, R. E. (2006). A fundamental attribution error? Rethinking cognitive distortions. *Legal and Criminological Psychology, 11*, 155–177.

McGrath, R. J., Cumming, G. F., Burchard, B. L., Zeoli, S., & Ellerby, L. (2010). *Current practices and trends in sexual abuser management: The Safer Society 2009 North American Survey.* Brandon, VT: Safer Society Press.

Miller, W., & Rollnick, S. (2002). *Motivational interviewing: Preparing people for change* (2nd ed.). New York, NY: Guilford.

Quinsey, V. L., & Earls, C. M. (1990). The modification of sexual preferences. In W. L. Marshall, D. R. Laws, & H. E. Barbaree (Eds.), *Handbook of sexual assault: Issues, theories and treatment of the offender* (pp. 279–295). New York, NY: Plenum.

Robinson, D. (1995). *The impact of cognitive skills training on post-release recidivism among Canadian federal offenders* ((Report No. R-41)). Ottawa, ON: Public Safety Canada.

Salter, A. (1988). *Treating child sex offenders and victims: A practical guide.* Newbury Park, CA: Sage Publications.

Schmucker, M., & Lösel, F. (2009). A systematic review of high quality evaluations of sex offender treatment. In *Annual Conference of the European Society of Criminology, Ljubljana, Slovenia.*

Schwaebe, C. (2005). Learning to pass: Sex offenders' strategies for establishing a viable identity in the prison general population. *International Journal of Offender Therapy and Comparative Criminology, 49*(6), 614–625.

Tarrier, N., Dolan, M., Doyle, M., Dunn, G., Shaw, J., & Blackburn, R. (2010). Exploratory randomised control trial of schema modal therapy in the personality disorder service at Ashworth Hospital. *Ministry of Justice Research Series, 5/10.*

Thornton, D., & Shingler, J. (2001). Impact of schema level work on sexual offenders' cognitive distortions. Paper presented at the 20th Annual Research and Treatment Conference for the Treatment of Sexual Abusers, San Antonio, TX.

Travers, R., Mann, R. E., & Hollin, C. R. (2014). Who benefits from cognitive skills programs? Differential impact by risk and offense type. *Criminal Justice and Behavior, 41*(9), 1103–1129.

Wakeling, H., Mann, R. E., & Carter, A. J. (2012). Are there any benefits in treating low risk sexual offenders? *The Howard Journal of Criminal Justice, 51*, 286–299.

Wakeling, H., Webster, S. D., & Mann, R. E. (2005). Sexual offenders' treatment experiences: A qualitative and quantitative investigation. *Journal of Sexual Aggression, 11*, 171–186.

Ward, T. (2002). The management of risk and the design of good lives. *Australian Psychologist, 37*, 172–179.

Ward, T., & Mann, R. E. (2004). Good lives and the rehabilitation of sex offenders: A positive approach to treatment. In A. L. Linley & S. Joseph (Eds.), *Positive psychology in practice* (pp. 598–616). Hoboken, NJ: Wiley.

Ward, T., Mann, R. E., & Gannon, T. A. (2007). The good lives model of offender rehabilitation: Clinical implications. *Aggression and Violent Behavior, 12*, 87–107.

Ware, J., & Mann, R. E. (2012). How should "acceptance of responsibility" be addressed in sexual offending treatment programs? *Aggression and Violent Behavior, 17*, 279–288.

Webster, S. D. (2005). Pathways to sexual offense recidivism following treatment. An examination of the Ward and Hudson self-regulation model of relapse. *Journal of Interpersonal Violence, 20*(10), 1175–1196.

Webster, S. D., Bowers, L. E., Mann, R. E., & Marshall, W. L. (2005). Developing empathy in sexual offenders: The value of offence re-enactments. *Sexual Abuse: A Journal of Research and Treatment, 17*(1), 63–77.

Williams, F., Wakeling, H., & Webster, S. (2007). A psychometric study of six self-report measures for use with sexual offenders with cognitive and social functioning deficits. *Psychology, Crime & Law, 13*(5), 505–522.

Chapter 8
Responsivity Dynamic Risk Factors and Offender Rehabilitation: A Comparison of the Good Lives Model and the Risk-Need Model

Tony Ward and Gwenda M. Willis

Introduction

There has been a lot of ink spilt over the last 12 years or so concerning the comparative merits of the Risk-Need-Responsivity (RNR) and the Good Lives Models (GLM) of offender rehabilitation (e.g., Andrews, Bonta, & Wormith, 2011; Ward, Yates, & Willis, 2012). The proponents of the RNR) and)GLM have critically engaged each other along a number of theoretical, empirical, ethical, and practice dimensions, (a) typically finding fault with their critics' formulation of their own model and (b) pointing to putative conceptual confusions and logical flaws in the other's model. The trouble is that while much heat has been generated in this debate, there has been little progress in developing an integrated approach to offender rehabilitation that incorporates the best from the GLM and RNR. Relatedly, there has been a notable lack of any real understanding of exactly what are the core differences between the two approaches and if in fact they amount to anything of theoretical or practice significance. In our view, writing yet another paper that compares the core values, assumptions, and practice implications of the two models in a comprehensive way is unlikely to change the repetitive and somewhat acrimonious nature of the debate. It certainly will not move the field further forward, which is a pity as theoretical and practice innovation is sorely needed in the correctional and sexual offending fields (Ward, 2014). Furthermore, there have been comprehensive recent summaries of both the RNR and the GLM in the general correctional and sexual offending

T. Ward, Ph.D., Dip.Clin.Psyc., (Canty) MNZCCP (✉)
School of Psychology, EA 604, Victoria University of Wellington, PO Box 600,
Wellington, New Zealand
e-mail: Tony.Ward@vuw.ac.nz

G.M. Willis, Ph.D., P.G.Dip.Clin.Psyc.
School of Psychology, University of Auckland, Tamaki Innovation Campus,
Private Bag 92019, Auckland, New Zealand

© Springer International Publishing Switzerland 2016
D.R. Laws, W. O'Donohue (eds.), *Treatment of Sex Offenders*,
DOI 10.1007/978-3-319-25868-3_8

literature that can be consulted by interested readers (e.g., Andrews & Bonta, 2010a, 2010b; Laws & Ward, 2011; Thornton, 2013; Willis, Ward, & Levenson, 2014; Yates, Prescott, & Ward, 2010). We do not intend to provide such a summary here.

In our opinion, there are important theoretical differences between the RNR and the GLM that would profit from sustained analysis and which have been somewhat neglected so far. This is a pity as at least one of the neglected issues may be key in understanding what we have got right so far in correctional treatment, why we have become side tracked, and where we need to go. The topic we refer to is the nature of the need principle and its associated concepts of dynamic risk factors, risk prediction and management, and causal explanation. According to Andrews and Bonta (2010a), the *need* principle proposes that potentially changeable variables associated with reductions in recidivism (i.e., dynamic risk factors or *criminogenic needs*) should be targeted in treatment to create safer communities. The need principle in conjunction with the principles of risk and responsivity constitutes the theoretical core of the RNR. In recent years, sex offender researchers and practitioners have increasingly recruited the need principle to explain offending and to structure treatment (Mann, Hanson, & Thornton, 2010; Thornton, 2013). The assumption is that dynamic risk factors referred to by the need principle directly track causal processes and as such should be used to develop sex offender treatment programs. Certainly, preliminary evidence suggests that programs that incorporate the principles of the RNR are likely to be more effective than those that do not (Hanson, Bourgon, Helmus, & Hodgson, 2009; Marshall & Marshall, 2012).

We argue that the assumption that dynamic risk factors track causal process in any straightforward sense is incorrect and therefore the RNR is unable to provide a comprehensive guide for treatment on its own. We are assuming that comprehensive rehabilitation frameworks/theories should be theoretically coherent and not crucially depend on problematic ideas or false assertions. By "coherency," we mean that the concept of dynamic risk factors and its expression in the need principle should not refer to incompatible causal processes or be formulated in logically inconsistent ways. We would also add that important distinctions implicit in the concept of dynamic risk factors should be carefully drawn out rather than run together. On the other hand, the GLM with its basis in agency theory is able to incorporate the concept of dynamic risk in a theoretically coherent manner and apply these insights directly to treatment and offender rehabilitation. The key and pivotal theoretical difference between the RNR and the GLM is that the former is based on shaky conceptual foundations while the latter is not. And given that the need principle is arguably *the* distinctive theoretical idea in the RNR, its lack of coherency means that the rehabilitation framework collapses into a patchwork of guidelines and practices. While the specific principles and intervention suggestions of the RNR are useful, they need to be underpinned by additional theory if it is to provide a theoretically sound practice framework.

In this chapter, we critically examine the need principle and its associated concepts of dynamic risk factors, risk management, and causal explanation. Concluding that the RNR need principle is theoretically incoherent because the concept of dynamic risk factors does not refer to genuine causal processes in any straightforward sense, we turn to the GLM. In our examination of the GLM's ability to conceptualize dynamic risk factors, we present the agency model of risk, a recent theoretical innovation, to explain how this composite construct can be employed to explain sexual offending and, ultimately, to guide sex offender treatment. Finally, we conclude the chapter with some brief comments on the comparative empirical and theoretical status of the RNR and GLM and the implications of this standing for future research and practice.

The RNR Need Principle: Dynamic Risk Factors and Causal Explanation

The RNR Basic Principles

The principal architects of the RNR model of offender rehabilitation are the Canadian researchers James Bonta, Don Andrews, and Paul Gendreau (e.g., Andrews & Bonta, 2010a; Andrews, Bonta, & Wormith, 2006; Gendreau & Andrews, 1990). Exactly what constitutes the RNR rehabilitation model is not entirely clear, but typically researchers and practitioners have understood and implemented it according to its three primary principles of risk, need, and responsivity and their associated assumptions (Ward, Yates, & Melser, 2007). In brief, the *risk* principle suggests offenders at higher risk of reoffending will benefit most from more intensive levels of intervention, including high intensity treatment. The *need* principle proposes that changeable features of the offender reliably associated with reductions in recidivism (i.e., dynamic risk factors or *criminogenic needs*) should be targeted in treatment programs in preference to those that have no demonstrated empirical relationship to crime. The *responsivity principle* states that correctional programs should use empirically supported treatment models (i.e., cognitive behavioral therapy) and be tailored to offender characteristics such as learning style, level of motivation, and the individual's personal and interpersonal circumstances. The first two principles (risk and need) are used to select treatment intensity and targets, and the whole set of principles are employed to guide the way practice is actually implemented.

The need principle is the central theoretical component of the RNR as it defines intervention targets in terms of risk of reoffending and specifies what kind of factors should be considered dynamic risk factors or criminogenic needs. That is, according to the RNR, dynamic risk factors are changeable features of offenders and their life circumstances that are good predictors of reoffending. In terms of the four key concepts associated with causality identified by Illari and Russo (2014), causal inference, explanation, prediction, and control, the concept of dynamic risk factors emerged from the context of risk prediction and has over time extended its conceptual reach to include all four. That is, researchers and practitioners applying the need principle and the concept of dynamic risk factors to the sexual offending field use them to make causal inferences, explain sexual offending, predict reoffending, and control offense-related propensities and situations. The formulation of the need principle in the RNR and its subsequent role as the core intervention guideline has meant that it has increasingly been used to inform correctional policy (Mann et al., 2010; Thornton, 2013; Ward, 2014; Ward & Beech, 2015).

The other two principles rely on the need principle conceptually and practically. They rely on it *conceptually* because risk is partly defined in terms of dynamic factors and/or refers indirectly to dynamic factors by way of static variables. That is, static variables are viewed as indicators or pointers to features of offenders that need to be modified if their chances of reoffending are to be reduced. The risk and responsivity principles are *practically* dependent upon the need principle because their application depends on its acceptance. The risk principle assumes that offender risk bands have been identified, based on a combination of dynamic and static risk variables. Without identified risk factors, the principle is unable to be employed. Relatedly, the responsivity principle concerns the way treatment for moderate- to high-risk offenders is conducted and practically depends on (a) the listing of intervention targets and (b) the development of interventions to alter them in ways that are likely to reduce recidivism rates. The validity and applicability of the need principle with its concept of dynamic risk factors is presupposed by the risk and responsivity principles.

Dynamic Risk Factors and the Sexual Offending Domain

In the sexual offending area, there has been a recent surge of research, clinical, and policy interest in risk assessment, predication, and management (Ward, 2014). Third-generation risk assessment measures and protocols have been developed that incorporate both static and dynamic risk factors, and practitioners are turning to these measures and assessment guidelines for help in formulating cases and planning interventions with sex offenders (Beech & Craig, 2012; Brouillette-Alarie, Babchishin, Hanson, & Helmus, in press; Hanson et al., 2009; Hanson & Morton-Bourgon, 2005; Mann et al., 2010; Thornton, 2013). Ward (2014) recently commented on the increasing reliance on dynamic risk factors and risk management strategies to structure and deliver treatment and raised some concerns:

> The status of theory construction has fallen significantly and there is very little cooperation between researchers working on the conceptualization of risk factors and those seeking to explain the causes of sexual offending. In addition, assessment and case formulation seems to revolve largely around the detection of dynamic risk factors and the classification of offenders and their problems amounts to formulating risk profiles. (p. 30)

The concept of dynamic risk factors and its encapsulation in the need principle is arguably a major reason for this shift in theoretical preferences and associated practice. Research on dynamic risk factors in the sexual offending domain has converged on a list of empirically supported factors which are reasonably good predictors of sexual reoffending (Beech & Craig, 2012; Mann et al., 2010; Russell & Darjee, 2013; Thornton, 2013). The empirically supported dynamic risk factors include sexual preoccupation, any deviant sexual interest, sexual interest in children, sexualized coping, sexualized violence, pro-offending attitudes, pro-child molestation attitudes, pro-rape attitudes, generic sexual offending attitudes, emotional congruence with children, lack of sustained marital-type relationships, conflicts in intimate relationships, general self-regulation problems, grievance thinking, impulsivity/recklessness, noncompliance with supervision, antisocial personality disorder, poor problem solving, employment instability, negative social influences, and violation of conditional release.

A notable feature of the above list is the sheer number of dynamic risk predictors, which raises the grain problem. What level should the predictors be categorized at? Do they cluster together into natural groups (kinds) or should they be lumped together at finer levels of resolution and considered separately? Opting for the larger grain solution, Thornton (2013) recently grouped the above risk factors into the four general dynamic risk domains of sexual interest (deviant), distorted attitudes, relational style (problems), and self-management (difficulties). The question of how best to categorize dynamic risk factors is theoretically important once the issue of their coherency is raised. We will return to this issue later in the chapter.

A final general comment on the concept of dynamic risk factors concerns terminology. While most authors seem to use the terms "dynamic risk factors" and "criminogenic needs" interchangeably, others prefer to flag their potential causal role and refer to them as offense-related propensities, psychological traits, vulnerability factors, or dispositions. For example, in a recent paper, Mann et al. (2010) identify a number of what they call *psychologically meaningful* risk factors which they believe to be prima facie causes of sexual offending and validated predictors of recidivism. They propose that to qualify as psychological meaningful risk factors, (a) there should be plausible reasons for regarding the factor in question as a cause of sexual offending and (b) strong evidence should exist that it actually predicts sexual offending.

Critical Comments

The concept of dynamic risk factors and its utilization in sexual offending research and practice contexts is an important innovation and has lead to significant advances in risk assessment and treatment. What remains to be determined is its degree of theoretical coherency as an explanatory concept as opposed to its utility in risk prediction contexts. The shift from risk prediction to explanatory (etiological) and practice domains is a major one that should be matched by conceptual analysis and if necessary theoretical refinements. The danger in not subjecting such an important concept to theoretical investigation with respect to its ability to function in explanations of sexual offending is that its subsequent use in clinical assessment and case formulation is unjustified. We shall see later on that there are problems with the concept of dynamic risk factors currently relied on in the sexual offending field that render its unmodified incorporation into clinical explanation and research contexts unwarranted (Ward, 2015). A critical question is then: do dynamic risk factors refer to, or pick out, the processes and their associated component structures that cause sexual offending/reoffending in an acceptably transparent and coherent way?

Or is the general concept, and the specific examples of dynamic risk factors (e.g., deviant sexual interests), characterized by confusion, incompatible causal elements, and vagueness? In the following discussion, we will be referring to the *concept* of dynamic risk factors and make the assumption that the concept and its theory and practice utilizations are intended to refer to real processes. That is, we adopt a realist view of scientific theory and accept that our scientific theories and their constituent concepts (which refer to entities, properties, processes, etc.) represent objective, offense-related phenomena and their causes; they exist independently of our individual viewpoints and perspectives (Haig, 2014).

A first general point is that once you start to talk about dynamic risk factors in causal terms, you are obligated to provide a theoretical account of them at some point. While theoretical entities are initially formulated in relatively vague terms such as psychological meaningful causes or offense-related propensities, sooner or later it is expected that a more refined theoretical account is produced, that is, an account that (a) spells out the nature of the underlying causes (structure and processes), (b) details the processes by which they create offense-related problems and outcomes, and (c) describes their relationships to each other. While researchers such as Mann et al. (2010), Beech and Ward (2004), and Thornton (2013) understand this requirement, at this stage they have not provided any such analysis. An encouraging sign has been the recent work by Brouillette-Alarie et al. (in press) on the latent constructs underpinning the Staic-99R and Static-2002R actuarial measures of reoffending risk in sex offenders. In this study, they discovered that the three factors of persistence/paraphilia, youthful stranger aggression, and general criminality could be viewed as potential psychological meaningful constructs, or cutting to the chase, as possible causes of sexual offending. However, Brouillette-Alarie et al. did not unpack the constructs in a theoretically coherent way, and the level of categorization was so broad it is difficult to know whether they are best conceptualized as summaries of predictive factors or references to putative causes (see below).

A second problem with the concept of dynamic risk factors concerns their degree of coherency. At the most general level of dynamic risk factor formulation, some of the conceptual subcomponents appear to be inconsistent with one another. In his recent summary of risk and protective factors in adult male sexual offenders, Thornton (2013) listed sexual violence and sexual interest in children as subdomains of the general dynamic risk factor of sexual interests. The problem is that the "umbrella," so to speak, of deviant sexual interests consists of qualitatively different variables, which arguably refer to distinct causal processes and their associated problems. This issue highlights the challenges when shifting the zone of application of concepts from one domain to another without making the appropriate conceptual adjustments. In the case of dynamic risk factors, the shift has occurred from the arena of risk prediction to those of explanation and treatment planning.

The problem of construct coherency remains even if you shift from the broad categorization to the specific list of dynamic risk factors identified by researchers such as Mann et al. (2010). To recall, this list includes specific dynamic risk factors such as deviant sexual interests, sexual interest in children, sexualized coping, pro-offending attitudes, emotional congruence with children, lack of sustained marital-type relationships, conflicts in intimate relationships, general self-regulation problems, grievance thinking, and impulsivity/recklessness (to take one example, that of emotional congruence with children). Mann et al. (2010) state that emotional congruence

> refers to feeling that relationships with children are more emotionally satisfying than relationships with adults. The offender who is emotionally congruent with children may find children easier to relate to than adults, may feel he is still like a child himself, and may believe that children understand him better than adults do. He often feels himself to be "in love" with his child victims, as if the relationship was reciprocal...... (p. 201)

The above passage comes from the Mann et al. (2010) description of this dynamic risk predictor and is intended to capture the various facets of the emotional congruence construct such as feeling less anxious around children, feeling psychologically like a child, believing children are more understanding or compassionate, and experiencing greater emotional fulfillment with relationships with children. These are all potentially distinct causal processes and may in fact be incompatible as a group. There is no problem with the "composite" nature of the construct in the context of a paper on dynamic prediction; arguably it improves its performance as a predictor to sample diverse aspects of emotional congruence. The difficulty is that when you present the dynamic risk factor of emotional congruence as a possible causal factor and use it to formulate treatment plans and guide treatment, you need to be clear (a) which of the above senses of the concept is applicable, (b) what exactly do you mean by the facet or process in question, and (c) link the causal processes and structures to the outcome variable of interest (offending, relationships etc.). So far, no researcher or theorist has done this with dynamic risk factors except in a very rudimentary sense (see Brouillette-Alarie et al., in press; Mann et al., 2010; Thornton, 2013; Ward & Beech, 2015). The other dynamic risk factors share this problem, and therefore, we conclude that there is a degree of indeterminacy and possible incoherence evident in the concept of sexual offending dynamic risk factors which make its routine use in explanatory and treatment planning domains unjustified.

A third problem is related to the issue of vagueness and incoherency described above (Durrant & Ward, 2015; Ward, 2015). The specific dynamic risk factors are composite constructs in an additional sense as well; they include both trait-like (enduring) and state (temporary) aspects. The stable dynamic factor of general self-regulation includes negative emotionality (a mental state) and poor problem solving (a trait or enduring psychological feature). Another example is the dynamic risk factor of poor cognitive problem solving. Deficient problem solving may involve (a) trait-like features such as lack of relevant knowledge, dysfunctional core beliefs, difficulty integrating information, and problems anticipating future possibilities and/or (b) current states such as feeling anxious, having trouble focusing on relevant features, or experiencing conflicting motivation. The only way to clarify what type of factor is involved, the degree to which it is a cause or an effect, or whether it is an internal or contextual feature is to present a detailed theoretical account of the dynamic risk factor in question and its underlying causal properties and their impact on the person and situation. To date this has not been provided by sexual offending researchers.

A final difficulty with the concept of dynamic risk factors and its incorporation into sexual offending research and treatment is a lack of theoretical attention to their interaction with one another. When researchers and theorists attempt to dig beneath the surface and explain why—and how—an offender sexually abused a child or raped an adult, they are engaged in the causal problem of *explanation*. The task is to provide an account of how a cause actually produces a specific effect rather than resting content with the demonstration that there is a statistical relationship between two (or more) factors. In an attempt to describe the relevant causal processes in detail, researchers often construct mechanistic explanations that depict how certain entities interact to produce an outcome. According to contemporary theories, the causes of a phenomenon of interest typically consist of a number of interacting processes, none of which are necessary or sufficient for the outcome to occur. In other words, it is more accurate to conceptualize the causes of something like sexual offending as plural in nature, consisting of background conditions, triggers, and interacting mechanisms, that it makes sense to think about causal fields rather than specific causes. In applying causal thinking to case formulation and treatment planning, practitioners need to think in terms of an array of causes and their interaction (Hart, Sturmey, Logan, & McMurran, 2011). The integration of information on risk variables, psychological problems, and situational factors is likely to require the availability of theories that explain how dynamic risk factors exert causal influence and how they combine to create a propensity to offend.

Conclusions

In the above analysis, we identified a number of conceptual problems in the concept of dynamic risk factors. These problems apply to all uses of the concept within the correctional domain and in the sexual offending field. In brief, we argue that the concept of dynamic risk factors is a composite construct and, as such, is valuable within risk assessment contexts. However, once extended beyond this area, it fails to deliver on its explanatory promises. More specifically, the concept is vague, refers to incompatible and/or distinct causal processes, and does not distinguish between trait and state factors. Given that the concept of dynamic risk factors is theoretically problematic, any theory or theoretical framework that depends on this concept is substantially weakened. The RNR presupposes the validity and theoretical cogency of the concept of dynamic risk factors and is therefore markedly weakened by these conceptual flaws. We conclude that the RNR rehabilitation framework, or theory, is not a coherent rehabilitation framework and collapses into a loose patchwork of practices, guidelines, and norms.

The GLM, Dynamic Risk Factors, and the Agency Model of Risk

The theoretical dependence of the RNR on the concept of dynamic risk factors has undermined its coherency as rehabilitation theory. One of the points of contrast between the RNR and the GLM is the latter's emphasis on personal agency and goal-directed behavior. In our view, this view of human functioning and motivation provides a way of conceptualizing dynamic risk factors that enable it to accommodate their composite or hybrid nature. We will now briefly outline the GLM and then describe the agency model of risk recently developed in a number of publications (Durrant & Ward, 2015; Ward, 2015; Ward & Beech, 2015). We conclude that because the GLM is able to satisfactorily integrate the important concept of dynamic risk factors into its structure by way of the agency view of risk, it is in this respect a more coherent rehabilitation theory than the RNR.

The Good Lives Model of Offender Rehabilitation

The Good Lives Model (GLM) is a strength-based approach to offender rehabilitation because it is responsive to offenders' particular interests, abilities, and aspirations (Ward & Maruna, 2007; Ward & Stewart, 2003; Willis et al., 2014). It also asks practitioners to explicitly construct intervention—good lives plans—plans that help offenders acquire the capabilities to achieve personally meaningful goals. From the perspective of the GLM, sexual offending results when individuals lack the internal and external resources necessary to realize their values in their everyday lives using pro-social means. In other words, criminal behavior represents a maladaptive attempt to secure valued outcomes (Purvis, Ward, & Shaw, 2013; Ward & Stewart, 2003; Yates et al., 2010). Rehabilitation plans should therefore aim to equip offenders with the knowledge, skills, opportunities, and resources necessary to satisfy their life values in ways that do not harm others. Related to its strong focus on offenders' core commitments and lifestyles that reflect these, there is a corresponding stress on agency. That is, because of the assumption that offenders like the rest of us actively seek to satisfy their life values through whatever means available to them, any rehabilitation plan should be pitched at the level of agency, goals, planning, and facilitative environments. In this sense, it is an ecological model and always keeps in mind the relationship between the environments in which persons live and the capabilities and resources they need to live meaningful and crime-free lives (Ward & Stewart, 2003).

Criminogenic needs or dynamic risk factors are conceptualized within the GLM as internal or external obstacles (i.e., flaws within a good life plan) that make it difficult for individuals to secure primary goods in personally meaningful and *socially acceptable* ways. These flaws take the form of insufficient attention to the range of goods required for individuals to have a chance at fulfilling lives, lack of internal and external capabilities, the use of inappropriate and counterproductive means to achieve personal goals, and conflict within a person's good life plan (Ward & Maruna, 2007; Yates et al., 2010). There is no assumption that dynamic risk factors are anything other than individual, social, and environmental problems that are causally related to sexual offending. It is understood they are composite constructs developed in the domain of risk prediction that are expected to break apart when recruited to perform explanatory roles.

According to the GLM, there are two ways rehabilitation programs can reduce dynamic risk factors. First, the establishment of the internal and external capacities needed to achieve a primary good (or more broadly, implement a good life plan) in socially acceptable and personally fulfilling ways can directly modify dynamic risk factors. For example, learning the skills necessary to become a mechanic might make it easier for an offender to develop the skills for concentration and emotional regulation, thereby reducing impulsivity, a criminogenic need. Second, the reduction of risk can occur indirectly when an offender is strongly motivated to work hard in treatment because of his involvement in projects that personally engage him.

The Agency Model of Risk

Dynamic risk factors in the correctional domain are intended to predict harm related to reoffending, typically to victims and the community. Protective factors are features that lessen the chances of risk factors having this effect, or more generally, if present they reduce the likelihood of offending occurring. As argued above, dynamic risk factors have no reality apart from prediction contexts and do not refer uniquely to causal processes that result in sexual offending. They are composite variables best conceptualized as predictive devices rather than explanatory constructs. In this sense, we agree with Borsboom (2005, p. 158) that

> If term is treated as referential but has no referent, then one is reifying terms that have no other function than that of providing a descriptive summary of a distinct set of processes and attributes. For instance, one then comes to treat a name for a group of test items as if it were a common cause of the item responses. That of course is a mistake.

In our opinion, one useful way of thinking about dynamic risk factors in sex offenders is by conceptualizing them in terms of the components of agency, that is, viewing dynamic risk factors as composite constructs that are useful predictors because they cover important aspects of goal-directed actions, within an offending context. The capacity for agency is inherent in all living things; however, in human beings, the level of sophistication is ratcheted up several notches because of their ability to intentionally structure learning and physical environments (i.e., niche construction). The key components of agency are (1) goals, plans, and strategies; (2) implementation of plans and their evaluation; and (3) the subsequent revision of goals and plans in light of outcomes. Furthermore, in our recent Agency Model of Risk, there are three levels of agency, each associated with its own distinct set of goals, plans, and strategies and each capable of influencing the other types of agency. The levels of agency in the AMR are the system level (goals related to physical integrity and functioning), social role (goals concerned with specific social roles such as being teacher), and personal (concerns individuals overall sense of identity and core normative commitments). The type of goals offenders possess and the plans they construct to achieve their goals and to evaluate their effectiveness are partly a function of the contexts in which they live and the resources available to them. Goals are activated or selected in response to external contexts and their cues such as the presence of threats and by internal cues such as hunger, fear, sexual desire, or anger. Dynamic risk factors can be viewed as flaws in individual functional capacities, social supports, and opportunities. Thus, dynamic risk factors once broken down into their causal elements are seen as psychological and social processes (i.e., those associated with goals, plans, strategies, and action implementation) that impair normal functioning and hence disrupt persons' internal and external relationships to their social, cultural, and physical environments. This disruption can occur at multiple levels or can be confined to incorrect actions within a single practice (e.g., relationship repair task). Protective factors, once stripped down into their core elements, work in multiple ways across the various levels of agency to inhibit and/or disrupt dysfunctional systems and to restore normal functioning. Sometimes, the constraints exerted by protective factors are external, such as the construction of supportive social networks around high-risk offenders.

The implications of this depiction of dynamic risk factors and their division into criminogenic needs and lifestyle destabilizers are far reaching. For example, the dynamic risk factor (criminogenic need) of intimacy deficits in sex offenders can be understood as (1) maladaptive beliefs and norms concerning relationships (e.g., adults are untrustworthy); (2) interpersonal and emotional regulation strategies that damage relationships with adults (e.g., do not talk about feelings and avoid social contact with adults) and that isolate individuals from social support; and (3) the active search for, and construction of, social environments in which such individuals feel comfortable and where their needs seem to be met (e.g., pedophilic networks and spending a lot of time with vulnerable children). The idea is to break down dynamic risk factors into several causal elements that in certain environments create, and maintain, antisocial values or behavior. Furthermore, it then becomes much easier to dig beneath the surface to redirect research and practice to relevant targets.

The GLM—and arguably other strength-based treatment approaches (see Marshall, Marshall, Serran, & O'Brien, 2011)—is able to theoretically ground a conceptualization of dynamic risk factors in the AMR because of its strong emphasis on offender agency and the central role that values, goals, strategies, and environmental variables play in non-offending and offending spheres. The point of creating the AMR was to provide detail on possible ways dynamic risk factors could be causally related to offending. The conceptual link between the GLM and an agency view of dynamic risk factors is its assumption that individuals translate important values into concrete goals and actively strive to realize them in their everyday lives. Therapeutically, the construction of good lives plans around offenders' most heavily weighted primary goods (and their associated personal goals) encourages practitioners to build desistance elements into rehabilitation initiatives (Laws & Ward, 2011; Scoones, Willis, & Grace, 2012). After all, a good life plan is a plan for living a different kind of lifestyle, and this means understanding the dependence of human beings on their relationships with others and the environment if significant change is to be maintained once they leave prison. Relevant desistance factors include access to social models that promote a non-offending lifestyle, employment, a stable emotional relationship, good social support, cognitive competencies, development of an adequate self-concept, and the acquisition of a sense of meaning in life.

GLM and RNR Empirical Research

Our major aim in this chapter has been to examine the way the RNR and GLM conceptualize dynamic risk factors. Of course, we understand that empirical considerations are also critical in evaluating rehabilitation theories and their associated treatment programs: are the constructs valid and treatment based on them effective in reducing reoffending rates? Understanding the causes of offending and reoffending should help practitioners to predict, explain, and control aspects of crime. We will now briefly describe recent work on the RNR and GLM and identify areas where empirical research is required to assist theorists and practitioners to determine the strengths and weaknesses of the RNR and GLM.

Risk-Need-Responsivity Model

There is considerable meta-analytic support indicating that adherence to the three major RNR principles is associated with reductions in sexual reoffending and also that adhering to more principles is associated with greater reductions in reoffending (Hanson et al., 2009). According to the RNR model, changes in dynamic risk factors should be associated with reductions in reoffense risk (Andrews & Bonta, 2010a, 2010b). Some research supports this assumption. The Violence Risk Scale: Sex Offender version (VRS:SO; Olver, Wong, Nicholaichuk, & Gordon, 2007; based on the Violence Risk Scale, VRS; Wong & Gordon, 2006) incorporates within-treatment change into sex offender risk assessment. Included are clinician-rated static and stable dynamic risk scales, and change in each of the dynamic domains is measured using a modified application of the transtheoretical model of change (Prochaska, DiClemente, & Norcross, 1992). Olver et al. (2007) found that post-treatment pro-social change was significantly related to reductions in sexual recidivism after controlling for static risk, pretreatment dynamic scores, and follow-up time (Olver et al., 2007).

Several researchers/clinicians have highlighted the importance of the responsivity principle and its poor adherence among sexual offending treatment providers (e.g., L. E. Marshall & Marshall, 2012). Narrow operationalization of the RNR principles and even narrower assessment of their adherence likely obscure detection of the most effective sexual offending treatment programs. Missing from large-scale meta-analyses are consideration of therapist characteristics, group cohesion, use of approach goals, assessment of agency capacity, etc., which have all been demonstrated to enhance treatment effectiveness (Marshall et al., 2011). Finally, one of the weakest aspects of the RNR is its theoretical looseness and tendency to concentrate on the application of the RNR principles to correctional practice at the expense of establishing its coherency as a rehabilitation framework (Ward & Maruna, 2007).

The Good Lives Model of Offender Rehabilitation

The GLM was first proposed by the lead author in 2002 (Ward, 2002) and since then has undergone several theoretical and practical developments (e.g., Laws & Ward, 2011; Purvis et al., 2013; Ward & Maruna, 2007; Ward & Stewart, 2003; Willis, Yates, Gannon, & Ward, 2013; Yates et al., 2010). Emerging research supports the conceptual underpinnings of the GLM when applied to individuals who have sexually offended (Barnett & Wood, 2008; Willis et al., 2013). Substantial variation has been observed in terms of how the GLM has been operationalized in practice (Willis et al., 2014). It is therefore not surprising that empirical support for the GLM has been somewhat mixed, and studies investigating recidivism outcomes have not yet been conducted. However, studies to date suggest that closer adherence to the model is associated with better outcomes (see below). In addition, research suggests that widening the net of risk assessment practices to include assessment of offenders' strengths might further enhance the predictive validity of sex offender risk assessment (e.g., Scoones et al., 2012).

The three group-based studies to date that have explored the effectiveness of adopting the GLM as an overarching rehabilitation framework in sexual offending treatment programs compared to traditional risk-oriented approaches have provided preliminary, although *mixed*, evidence concerning its superiority (although it was never inferior to traditional approaches—see Barnett, Manderville-Norden, & Rakestrow, 2014; Harkins, Flak, Beech, & Woodhams, 2012; Simons, McCullar, & Tyler, 2006). For example, Simons et al. (2006) found that offenders who received the GLM approach were more likely to complete treatment, remain in treatment longer, and be rated by therapists as more motivated to participate in treatment compared to clients who received traditional relapse prevention treatment. In addition, clients who received the GLM approach demonstrated significantly better coping skills posttreatment, and no such gains were observed for clients who received the RP approach.

Compared to the RNR, there has been a lack of good quality treatment outcome studies using the GLM as a rehabilitation framework with which to construct treatment plans. Part of the problem is that the GLM was always intended to include the RNR principles, and therefore, treatment derived from these theories that simply compares the two is missing the point. The superiority of the GLM was seen to reside in its greater degree of theoretical coherency and ability to incorporate aspects of desistance and treatment that the RNR struggles to find room for (e.g., treatment alliance, agency, approach goals, core values, personal identity, etc.). What is required is further research into the two models that (a) explicitly evaluates them as *rehabilitation frameworks* and (b) provides detailed specification of the differences between strict RNR treatment programs and those augmented or underpinned by GLM principles (see Willis et al., 2014).

Conclusions

The RNR consists of a loose coalition of rehabilitation principles, theoretical assumptions concerning the relationship between psychological variables and offending, and concrete practice guidelines. It is not an integrated theoretical framework because the foundational concept of dynamic risk factors does not travel well away from prediction contexts. It is a composite or hybrid construct and as such a poor candidate for recruitment into etiological theories of sexual offending and reoffending. The problem means practitioners should not rely on dynamic risk factors without recourse to a "translation" model such as the AMR when they set about constructing case formulations and delivering treatment. On the other hand, the GLM is able to incorporate the concept of dynamic risk factors into its theoretical structure, by accepting that they are unable on their own to explain sexual offending and therefore should not be relied on in assessment and treatment planning. Another reason the GLM is friendly to dynamic risk factors is that it does not have a strong commitment to them as explanatory concepts or psychological causes and insists on taking them apart when setting out to understand why offenders sexually abuse others. The stress the GLM places on agency and the associated requirement to construct meaningful good lives plans for sex offenders make it much easier to deconstruct dynamic risk factors into their multiple causal elements. If researchers and practitioners within the sexual offending field want to continue referring to dynamic risk factors in an explanatory sense or, more broadly, structure practice according to the RNR, they will need to supplement their theoretical resources with something like the AMR. Another alternative is to use the core normative, etiological, and practice assumptions of the GLM and the AMR and to embed the RNR principles and allied concepts within this theoretical framework. What they should not do is to carry on as usual. In our view, such a decision is likely to push the field rapidly into theoretical rehabilitation dead ends (Ward & Beech, 2015).

What does all this mean for the RNR as a rehabilitation theory? An obvious question is: why has there been so little discussion about problems with importing dynamic risk factors into etiological, assessment, and treatment domains or more expressed concern about their composite nature? Perhaps, the issue is merely a semantic one and too trivial to bother about. Sooner or later the promissory note issued by the RNR theorists will be made good, and a reworked, more powerful, and coherent account of dynamic risk factors will be presented. We think this is all beside the point and that the arguments outlined in the chapter speak for themselves: the RNR suffers from a fatal case of conceptual incoherence and therefore fails as a rehabilitation theory. The GLM does not suffer from the same problem (although it may be subject to other difficulties—see Andrews et al., 2011) and, in *this respect*, is a stronger rehabilitation model. If researchers and practitioners in the sexual offending and the broader correctional fields are committed to the ideal of *evidence-based practice*, this means becoming theoretically literate as well as being familiar with the empirical evidence for assessment measures and treatment programs (Gannon & Ward, 2014). Theories, models, concepts, and principles are cognitive tools, and if we are to do our jobs as well as we can, they are necessary to sharpen our practice.

References

Andrews, D. A., & Bonta, J. (2010a). *The psychology of criminal conduct* (5th ed.). New Providence, NJ: Matthew Bender.

Andrews, D. A., & Bonta, J. L. (2010b). Rehabilitating criminal justice policy and practice. *Psychology, Public Policy, and Law, 16*, 39–55. doi:10.1037/a0018362.

Andrews, D. A., Bonta, J., & Wormith, J. S. (2006). The recent past and near future of risk and/or need assessment. *Crime & Delinquency, 52*, 7–27.

Andrews, D. A., Bonta, J., & Wormith, J. S. (2011). The risk-need-responsivity (RNR) model: Does adding the good lives model contribute to effective crime prevention? *Criminal Justice and Behavior, 38*, 735–755. doi:10.1177/0093854811406356.

Barnett, G. D., Manderville-Norden, R., & Rakestrow, J. (2014). The Good Lives Model or relapse prevention: What works better in facilitating change? *Sexual Abuse: A Journal of Research and Treatment, 26*(1), 3–33. doi:10.1177/1079063212474473.

Barnett, G., & Wood, J. L. (2008). Agency, relatedness, inner peace, and problemsolving in sexual offending: How sexual offenders prioritize and operationalize their good lives conceptions. *Sexual Abuse: Journal of Research and Treatment, 20*, 444–465.

Beech, A.R., & Craig, L. (2012). The current status of static and dynamic factors in sexual offending risk assessment. *Journal of Aggression and Peace Research, 4*, 169–185.

Beech, A. R., & Ward, T. (2004). The integration of etiology and risk in sexual offenders: A theoretical framework. *Aggression and Violent Behavior, 10*, 31–63.

Borsboom, D. (2005). *Measuring the mind: Conceptual issues in contemporary psychometrics.* Cambridge: Cambridge University Press.

Brouillette-Alarie, S., Babchishin, K. M., Hanson, R. K., & Helmus, L. (in press). Latent constructs of the static-99R and static-2002R: A three-factor solution. *Assessment.*

Durrant, R., & Ward, T. (2015). *Evolutionary criminology: Towards a comprehensive explanation of crime and its management.* New York, NY: Academic.

Gannon, T. A., & Ward, T. (2014). Where has all the psychology gone? A critical review of evidence-based psychological practice in correctional settings. *Aggression and Violent Behavior, 19*, 435–436. doi:10.1016/j.avb.2014.06.006.

Gendreau, P., & Andrews, D. A. (1990). Tertiary prevention: What a meta-analysis of the offender treatment literature tells us about 'what woks'. *Canadian Journal of Criminology, 32*, 173–184.

Haig, B. D. (2014). *Investigating the psychological world: Scientific method in the behavioural sciences.* Cambridge, MA: MIT Press.

Hanson, R. K., Bourgon, G., Helmus, L., & Hodgson, S. (2009). The principles of effective correctional treatment also apply to sexual offenders: A meta-analysis. *Criminal Justice and Behavior, 36*, 865–891. doi:10.1177/0093854809338545.

Hanson, R. K., & Morton-Bourgon, K. E. (2005). The characteristics of persistent sexual offenders: A meta-analysis of recidivism studies. *Journal of Consulting and Clinical Psychology, 73*, 1154–1163. doi:10.1037/0022-006X.73.6.1154.

Harkins, L., Flak, V. E., Beech, A., & Woodhams, J. (2012). Evaluation of a community-based sex offender treatment program using a Good Lives Model approach. *Sexual Abuse: A Journal of Research and Treatment, 24*, 519–543. doi:10.1177/1079063211429469.

Hart, S., Sturmey, P., Logan, C., & McMurran, M. (2011). Forensic case formulation. *International Journal of Forensic Mental Health, 10*, 118–126.

Illari, P., & Russo, F. (2014). *Causality: Philosophical theory meets scientific practice.* New York, NY: Oxford University Press.

Laws, D. R., & Ward, T. (2011). *Desistance and sex offending: Alternatives to throwing away the keys.* New York, NY: Guilford Press.

Mann, R. E., Hanson, R. K., & Thornton, D. (2010). Assessing risk for sexual recidivism: Some proposals on the nature of psychologically meaningful risk factors. *Sexual Abuse: A Journal of Research and Treatment, 22*, 191–217. doi:10.1177/1079063210366039.

Marshall, L. E., & Marshall, W. L. (2012). The risk/needs/responsivity model: The crucial features of general responsivity. In E. Bowen & S. Brown (Eds.), *Perspectives on evaluating criminal justice and corrections* (Advances in program evaluation, Vol. 13, pp. 29–45). Bingley: Emerald Group Publishing Limited.

Marshall, W. L., Marshall, L. E., Serran, G. A., & O'Brien, M. D. (2011). *Rehabilitating sexual offenders: A strength-based approach*. Washington, DC: American Psychological Association.

Olver, M. E., Wong, S. C. P., Nicholaichuk, T., & Gordon, A. (2007). The validity and reliability of the Violence Risk Scale-Sexual Offender version: Assessing sex offender risk and evaluating therapeutic change. *Psychological Assessment, 19*, 318–329. doi:10.1037/1040-3590.19.3.318.

Prochaska, J. O., DiClemente, C. C., & Norcross, J. C. (1992). In search of how people change: Applications to addictive behaviors. *American Psychologist, 47*(9), 1102–1114.

Purvis, M., Ward, T., & Shaw, S. (2013). *Applying the Good Lives Model to the case management of sexual offenders*. Brandon, VT: Safer Society Press.

Russell, K., & Darjee, R. (2013). Managing the risk posed by personality-disordered sexual offenders in the community. In C. Logan & L. Johnstone (Eds.), *Managing clinical risk: A guide to effective practice* (pp. 88–114). Abingdon: Routledge.

Scoones, C., Willis, G. M., & Grace, R. C. (2012). Beyond static and dynamic risk factors: The incremental predictive validity of release planning in sex offender risk assessment. *Journal of Interpersonal Violence, 27*, 222–238. doi:10.1177/0886260511416472.

Simons, D. A., McCullar, B., & Tyler, C. (2006). *Evaluation of the Good Lives Model approach to treatment planning*. Paper presented at the 25th Annual Association for the treatment of sexual abusers research and treatment and research, Chicago, IL

Thornton, D. (2013). Implications of our developing understanding of risk and protective factors in the treatment of adult male sexual offenders. *International Journal of Behavioral Consultation and Therapy, 8*, 62–65.

Ward, T. (2002). Good lives and the rehabilitation of sexual offenders: Promises and problems. *Aggression and Violent Behavior, 7*, 513–528.

Ward, T. (2014). The Explanation of sexual offending: From single factor theories to integrative pluralism. *Journal of Sexual Aggression, 20*, 130–141.

Ward, T. (2015). The detection of dynamic risk factors and correctional factors. *Criminology & Public Policy, 14*, 105–111.

Ward, T., & Beech, A. (2015). Dynamic risk factors: A theoretical dead-end? *Psychology, Crime & Law, 21*, 100–113.

Ward, T., & Maruna, S. (2007). *Rehabilitation: Beyond the risk assessment paradigm*. London: Routledge.

Ward, T., Melser, J., & Yates, P. M. (2007). Reconstructing the Risk Need Responsivity Model: A Theoretical Elaboration and Evaluation. *Aggression and Violent Behavior, 12*, 208–228.

Ward, T., & Stewart, C. A. (2003). The treatment of sex offenders: Risk management and good lives. *Professional Psychology: Research and Practice, 34*, 353–360. doi:10.1037/0735-7028.34.4.353.

Ward, T., Yates, P., & Willis, G. (2012). The good lives model and the risk need responsivity model: A critical response. *Criminal Justice and Behavior, 39*, 94–110.

Willis, G. M., Ward, T., & Levenson, J. S. (2014). The Good Lives Model (GLM): An evaluation of GLM operationalization in North American treatment programs. *Sexual Abuse: A Journal of Research and Treatment, 26*, 58–81. doi:10.1177/1079063213478202.

Willis, G. M., Yates, P. M., Gannon, T. A., & Ward, T. (2013). How to integrate the Good Lives Model into treatment programs for sexual offending: An introduction and overview. *Sexual Abuse: A Journal of Research and Treatment, 25*, 123–142. doi:10.1177/1079063212452618.

Wong, S. C. P., & Gordon, A. (2006). The validity and reliability of the violence risk scale: A treatment-friendly violence risk assessment tool. *Psychology, Public Policy, and Law, 12*, 279–309. doi:10.1037/1076-8971.12.3.279.

Yates, P. M., Prescott, D. S., & Ward, T. (2010). *Applying the Good Lives and Self Regulation Models to sex offender treatment: A practical guide for clinicians*. Brandon, VT: Safer Society Press.

Chapter 9
Early Detection and Intervention for Adolescents at Risk for Engaging in Abusive Sexual Behavior: A Case for Prevention

Daniel Rothman

Adolescents Who Have Engaged in Abusive Sexual Behavior

Sexually abusive behavior by adolescent youth is a serious problem, accounting for more than one third of all sexual offenses against minors (Finkelhor, Ormrod, & Chaffin, 2009). However, it is also known that most of these youth do not continue to sexually offend and most do not develop into sexually abusive adults (Caldwell, 2010; Taylor, 2003). In fact, most adolescents will desist from engaging in sexually abusive behavior after contact with the criminal justice system (van Wijk, Mali, & Bullens, 2007). Decades of studies indicate that between 80 and 95 % of adolescents who have engaged in abusive sexual behavior will not reoffend—even without formal therapeutic intervention—with the higher end of this range more often typifying those who complete some sort of treatment program, and the lower end more often describing those who do not (Alexander, 1999; Caldwell, 2002; Rasmussen, 1999; Reitzel & Carbonell, 2006; Worling, Litteljohn, & Bookalam, 2010). Although the vast majority of sexually abusive adolescents are boys, at least 7 % are girls, a population about which much less is known (Snyder, 2002).

Targeted interventions are effective for children and adolescents who have engaged in sexually abusive behavior (Fanniff & Becker, 2006; Reitzel & Carbonell, 2006; St. Amand, Bard, & Silovsky, 2008). Sexually abusive adolescents who have participated in specialized treatment to address their sexual offending are approximately 12 % less likely to reoffend sexually than youth who have not participated in such treatment (Reitzel & Carbonell, 2006; Worling et al., 2010). Interventions are particularly successful when they are caregiver inclusive, strengths-based, develop-

D. Rothman, Ph.D. (✉)
Forensic Psychological Services — Ellerby, Kolton, Rothman & Associates,
500 - 287 Broadway, Winnipeg, MB, Canada R3C 0R9
e-mail: daniel@fps-ea.com

© Springer International Publishing Switzerland 2016
D.R. Laws, W. O'Donohue (eds.), *Treatment of Sex Offenders*,
DOI 10.1007/978-3-319-25868-3_9

mentally appropriate, matched to the youth's dynamic risk and needs, and attentive to factors that can impact the youth's responsiveness to intervention such as early childhood neglect and trauma, neurodevelopmental disorders, cognitive ability, learning style, and culture (Association for the Treatment of Sexual Abusers, 2012). Although this description does not yet characterize the majority of North American treatment programs for sexually abusive youth, recent surveys indicate that an increasing number of clinicians are becoming attentive to these principles (McGrath, Cumming, Burchard, Zeoli, & Ellerby, 2010).

Despite the fact that most adolescents who have engaged in abusive sexual behavior do not persist with this behavior into adulthood, it is also known that about half of adults who have sexually offended report that their first sexual offenses occurred when they were adolescents (Abel, Mittelman, & Becker, 1985; Groth, Longo, & McFadin, 1982). Furthermore, in consideration of the low sexual reoffense rates for youth, it follows that the high proportion of sexual offending perpetrated by adolescents must be largely representative of first-time offenses. Therefore, if one were interested in having a maximal impact on reducing sexual offending against young children, an especially promising approach would involve early detection and intervention with adolescents at risk for engaging in abusive sexual behavior. This requires a public health perspective and the methods of prevention.

Prevention

The field of sexual abuse prevention has a lengthy history, and there have been considerable gains over the last 30 years in terms of public education and awareness, legal protections for victims, funding, community mobilization, and research on the prevalence, etiology, and prevention of sexual violence (DeGue et al., 2014). Sexual violence has been recognized as a significant public health problem impacting millions of people on a global scale (Krug, Dahlberg, Mercy, Zwi, & Lozano, 2002). Public health is a population-based approach that is ultimately concerned with strategies that address the health of a population—as opposed to an individual—and a public health prevention strategy aims to benefit the largest group of people possible, recognizing that the problem is pervasive and typically affects the entire population, either directly or indirectly (Centers for Disease Control and Prevention, 2004). A public health intervention is also a community-oriented approach that depends upon collective action of an entire community to prevent the problem at hand (Krug et al., 2002). A clear advantage of a population-based intervention is that, if a strategy is widely enough implemented, even a small effect on perpetration behavior may have a large overall impact. Furthermore, large-scale public health initiatives targeting sexual violence promise significant cost savings over reactive measures to sexual abuse, when one considers the extraordinary costs of child sexual abuse in terms of health care, social services, and criminal justice (Freyd et al., 2005; Letourneau, Eaton, Bass, Berlin, & Moore, 2014). Public health interventions for sexual violence are often grouped into three prevention categories based on when the intervention occurs:

1. *Primary prevention* strategies are aimed at preventing sexual violence before it has happened (Centers for Disease Control and Prevention, 2004). These approaches include universal interventions directed at the general population as well as selected interventions aimed at those who may be at increased risk for sexual violence perpetration. They can focus either on preventing perpetration of sexual harm (e.g., implementing a media campaign to educate the public about the negative effects of child pornography) or preventing victimization (e.g., a school-based curriculum teaching children how to recognize abuse and avoid and report it). Historically, sexual violence prevention efforts have focused on education, safety promotion, and risk reduction for potential victims (Cook-Craig, 2012). While these strategies can be effective at changing the attitudes of potential victims, research has so far failed to demonstrate their effectiveness in actually changing key behaviors or preventing sexual violence (Morrison, Hardison, Mathew, & O'Neil, 2004). A truly high-impact public health approach to sexual violence prevention would primarily aim to prevent violence perpetration, rather than victimization or risk reduction, as it has been recognized that a decrease in the number of actual and potential perpetrators in the population is necessary to achieve measurable reductions in the prevalence of sexual violence (DeGue et al., 2012). As such, primary prevention strategies aimed at perpetrators of sexual violence have been increasingly recognized as being critical to prevention and necessary to complement approaches aimed at preventing victimization or recidivism and addressing the adverse impact of sexual violence on victims (DeGue et al., 2014).

2. *Secondary prevention* strategies represent an immediate response after sexual violence has been perpetrated and deal with the short-term consequences of violence (Centers for Disease Control and Prevention, 2004). Examples include attempts to reduce the harm to the victims in the immediate aftermath of the violence (e.g., separating the victim and the perpetrator; providing immediate crisis counseling for the victim) and address the perpetrators. Both secondary and tertiary prevention (defined below) can be directed toward affected populations including individuals who have perpetrated sexual violence or those who have been victimized (Association for the Treatment of Sexual Abusers, 2014).

3. *Tertiary prevention* strategies characterize long-term responses after sexual violence has been perpetrated (Centers for Disease Control and Prevention, 2004). Tertiary prevention approaches address the longer-term consequences of sexual victimization (e.g., by providing ongoing counseling for victims) and the provision of specialized intervention and risk management for the perpetrators of sexual violence to minimize the possibility of reoffending (Association for the Treatment of Sexual Abusers, 2014).

Most sexual abuse perpetration prevention initiatives to date have been aimed at the tertiary level of prevention—preventing further sexually abusive behavior—which, overall, are the least likely to be effective in promoting healthy communities, principally because of their limited scope (Laws, 2000, 2008). Efforts at early detection and intervention for adolescents at risk for perpetration of sexual violence could and should include prevention strategies at all three of these levels. However, because secondary and tertiary prevention strategies (particularly intervention approaches for adolescents who are known to have engaged in abusive sexual behavior) have frequently been discussed elsewhere (see Fanniff & Becker, 2006; Letourneau & Borduin, 2008; Reitzel & Carbonell, 2006), the current chapter will focus on primary prevention strategies for this population.

Primary Prevention Strategies for Sexual Violence

One of the first critical steps in designing an effective primary prevention program is to ensure that its implementation is well timed, so that the intervention happens prior to the development of the problem (Nation et al., 2003; Nation, M, Keener, Wandersman, & DuBois, 2005). From a public health perspective, the target group for primary prevention of adolescent sexually abusive behavior is reasonably well defined: research indicates that the average age of onset for sexually abusive conduct is in early adolescence, between 12 and 15 years of age (Caldwell, 2002; Finkelhor et al., 2009). Therefore, primary prevention strategies should focus on preadolescent children and should target risk and protective factors identified for that population.

Risk Factors for Adolescents at Risk for Sexual Offending

Risk factors for the perpetration of sexual violence describe individual, relational, community, and societal characteristics that increase the probability of an individual engaging in sexually abusive behavior (Centers for Disease Control and Prevention, 2004). A large amount of research has been conducted in this field over the past 20 years, resulting in a number of important findings. One of the more important discoveries has been that most of the factors that predict adolescent sexually abusive behavior are not specific to sexual offending but also predict general delinquency (Caldwell, 2002). In fact, it has become well understood that youth who have engaged in sexually abusive behavior are far more likely to engage in future *nonsexual* offending (e.g., nonsexual violence and general delinquency) than sexual offending, indicating that there is substantial overlap between sexually and non-sexually delinquent youth (Caldwell, 2007, 2010; Seto & Lalumiere, 2010).

At the same time, there are some specific differences between these populations. Although research has identified some of the risk factors for general delinquency among adolescents who have offended sexually—including prior nonsexual delinquency, age at first commission of a nonsexual offense (youth who were younger at the time of their first nonsexual offense being at greater risk for future nonsexual delinquency), and peer delinquency (Spice, Viljoen, Latzman, Scalora, & Ullman, 2012) and school functioning (Worling & Langton, 2015)—there has been less clarity in identifying risk factors unique to sexual offending among adolescent populations. Risk assessment instruments designed to predict adolescent sexual recidivism—although certainly better than unstructured clinical judgment—remain works in progress, in need of further research and development (Viljoen, Elkovitch, Scalora, & Ullman, 2009). Differences in the methodologies and sample populations between studies, as well as the overall low base rate of sexual recidivism among youth, have made it difficult to form strong conclusions from these studies.

Nevertheless, research has thus far identified a number of potential risk factors for the perpetration of sexual violence among adolescents. Listed here are the ones that have received empirical support in multiple investigations: opportunities to sexually offend/inadequate adult supervision, atypical/deviant sexual interests or arousal (i.e., sexual arousal to prepubescent children and/or violence), childhood sexual victimization, witnessing and experiencing intrafamilial violence, parental neglect, having ever resided in a family with poor sexual boundaries, sexual preoccupation, poor self-regulation, social isolation, precocious sexual behavior/prepubescent nonnormative sexual behavior, having engaged in multiple types of sexual behaviors, antisocial personality characteristics, and attitudes supportive of sexual offending (Carpentier, Leclerc, & Proulx, 2011; Curwen, Jenkins, & Worling, 2014; Hanson & Morton-Bourgon, 2005; McCann & Lussier, 2008; Nunes, Hermann, Malcom, & Lavoie, 2013; Salter et al., 2003; Seto & Lalumiere, 2010; Spice et al., 2012; Tharp et al., 2012; Wanklyn, Ward, Cormier, Day, & Newman, 2012; Worling & Langstrom, 2006). It is important to note, however, that these risk factors are only known (or suspected) to be relevant to sexual *recidivism* among adolescent populations. Risk factors for the *initiation* of sexual offending behavior among adolescents remain yet unknown. It is certainly possible that there exist differences between those factors that place a teenager at risk for initially engaging in sexually abusive behavior and those factors that predict subsequent sexual offending, but this remains an empirical question.

Another problem that impacts on the implementation of primary prevention efforts for this population is the tremendous diversity among adolescents known to have offended sexually. Individual youth who have engaged in sexually abusive behavior can and often do differ from other youth within this population in terms of family history, intellectual functioning, learning style, mental health, motivation, personality, and specific offending behaviors, among so many other characteristics (Caldwell, 2002; Chaffin, 2008; Chaffin, Letourneau, & Silovsky, 2002; Hunter, Figueredo, Malamuth, & Becker, 2003; Knight & Prentky, 1993; Oxnam & Vess, 2008). While some of these youth have offended against prepubescent children, others (though far fewer) have offended against peers or adults (Finkelhor et al., 2009). And even among those adolescents who have sexually abused younger children, it is likely that the majority does not exhibit sexual arousal to prepubescent children (Seto, Lalumiere, & Blanchard, 2000; Worling, 2012; Worling, Bookalam, & Litteljohn, 2012).

Atypical Sexual Interests

The early development of atypical sexual interests (i.e., sexual arousal to prepubescent children, violence, or other nonnormative stimuli) and their role in offending is not well understood. Recent advances in neuroscience have implicated a number of possible biological mechanisms in the development of pedophilia, such as alterations in brain structure and function (Mohnke et al., 2014). Psychosocial factors have also long been theorized to contribute to the development of atypical sexual preferences, and conditioning theories (see Laws & Marshall, 1990) continue to hold strong explanatory power (Santtila et al., 2010). Among adult offenders, the presence of a child victim suggests pedophilic interests, and a pedophilic arousal pattern has been found to be one of the most reliable predictors of risk for persistent sexual offending for adults (Hanson & Morton-Bourgon, 2005).

However, the meaning of adolescent-perpetrated sexual offenses against young children is far less clear. While atypical sexual interests in adolescents have been associated with a higher probability for future sexual offending (Carpentier et al., 2011; Hanson & Morton-Bourgon, 2005; McCann & Lussier, 2008; Seto & Lalumiere, 2010), the fact remains that most adolescents who have engaged in abusive sexual behavior do not exhibit sexual arousal to prepubescent children (Seto et al., 2000; Worling, 2012; Worling et al., 2012). Current research indicates that, depending on the sample studied, approximately 60–75 % of adolescent males who have offended sexually are, in fact, primarily sexually interested in consensual activities with age-appropriate partners (Worling, 2013). Although atypical sexual arousal likely plays a role in the development and/or maintenance of adolescent sexual offending for some adolescents, there are many other factors that clearly play roles as well. Indeed, one of the most resilient findings in the research on adolescents who have sexually offended is that they comprise an extremely heterogeneous group (Caldwell, 2002).

The meaning and motivations of an adolescent's abusive sexual behavior will vary between individual youths and situations. Adolescents who sexually abuse younger children include but are not limited to teenagers reacting to their own sexual victimization; persistently delinquent or aggressive teens who commit both sexual and nonsexual crimes; otherwise normal adolescent boys who are curious about sex and act experimentally but irresponsibly; immature, impulsive, and poorly self-regulated youth acting without thinking; callous youth who are indifferent to others and selfishly take what they want; youth misinterpreting what they believed was consent or mutual interest; children imitating actions they have seen in movies or television or online; youth ignorant of the law or the potential consequences of their actions; youth attracted to the thrill of rule violation; those imitating what is normal in their own family; depressed or socially isolated teens who turn to younger children as substitutes for peers; youth with serious mental illness; teens responding primarily to peer pressure; youth preoccupied with sex; youth under the influence of drugs and alcohol; or youth with emerging sexual deviancy problems (Chaffin, 2008). And as observed by Caldwell (2002):

> The difficulty with identifying sexual deviance in teen offenders is that teen sexual behaviors are so varied, and juvenile sexual offenders are so heterogeneous, that offenses against young children committed by younger teens serves as a poor proxy for pedophilic deviance.

Even though some teens that commit this type of offense will probably develop into lifelong pedophilic offenders…for the majority of these offenders, there is a strong trend toward desisting pedophilic offending as the offender age increases just a few years. Concluding then, that sexual assault of a young child by an offender in their early teens indicates developing high-risk sexual deviancy or pedophilia does not appear warranted. (p. 296)

Protective Factors for Adolescents at Risk for Sexual Offending

As difficult as it has been to identify risk factors for adolescent-perpetrated sexually abusive behavior, the search for protective factors—those individual, relational, community, and societal characteristics that would reduce the likelihood of sexual offending—has yet to provide clarity. First, there is some debate about whether protective factors should be conceptualized as mirror images of risk factors (i.e., whether an absence of a particular risk factor should be considered a protective factor) or as entities that are entirely distinct (Spice et al., 2012). Secondly, although some studies have identified protective factors for general delinquency among adolescents who have offended sexually—such as strong attachments or bonds (Klein, Rettenberger, Yoon, Köhler, & Briken, 2015; Spice et al., 2012; Worling & Langton, 2015)—research has so far failed to distinguish factors that specifically promote desistance from adolescent sexual offending.

The difficulty in identifying risk and protective factors for this population highlights the population's diversity, as discussed above, as well as the dynamic nature of childhood development. Arguably the defining characteristic of adolescence is change, and it has been observed that a child's level of risk and needs changes quickly as he or she matures (Chaffin, 2008; Prentky & Righthand, 2003; Worling, 2004). Also in support of this notion is that, for both adolescents and adults who have engaged in abusive sexual behavior, risk and protective factors appear to interact and combine in multiple and nuanced ways to increase or decrease the likelihood of sexual violence perpetration, suggesting that these factors are activated in certain situations and may be most relevant during particular developmental periods (Tharp et al., 2012). Nevertheless, the identification of protective factors for adolescents at risk for sexual offending remains an important task, as a greater understanding of risk and protective elements promises to guide the refinement of primary prevention strategies for this population.

What Works in Primary Prevention for Sexual Violence?

Nation and colleagues (2003, 2005) identified nine "principles of prevention" (see Table 9.1) that are strongly associated with positive effects across multiple studies in multiple domains, indicating that effective prevention-oriented interventions have the following characteristics: (a) comprehensive, (b) appropriately timed, (c) utilize varied teaching methods, (d) have sufficient dosage, (e) administered by well-trained staff, (f) provide opportunities for positive relationships, (g) socioculturally relevant,

Table 9.1 Definitions of the principles of effective programs (Nation et al., 2003)

Principle	Definition
Comprehensive	Multicomponent interventions that address critical domains (e.g., family, peers, community) that influence the development and perpetuation of the behaviors to be prevented
Appropriately timed	Programs are initiated early enough to have an impact on the development of the problem behavior and are sensitive to the developmental needs of participants
Varied teaching methods	Programs involve diverse teaching methods that focus on increasing awareness and understanding of the problem behaviors and on acquiring or enhancing skills
Sufficient dosage	Programs provide enough intervention to produce the desired effects and provide follow-up as necessary to maintain effects
Well-trained staff	Program staff support the program and are provided with training regarding the implementation of the intervention
Positive relationships	Programs provide exposure to adults and peers in a way that promotes strong relationships and supports positive outcomes
Socioculturally relevant	Programs are tailored to the community and cultural norms of the participants and make efforts to include the target group in program planning and implementation
Theory driven	Programs have a theoretical justification, are based on accurate information, and are supported by empirical research
Outcome evaluation	Programs have clear goals and objectives and make an effort to systematically document their results relative to the goals

(h) theory driven, and (i) include outcome evaluation. It has also been recognized that effective prevention programs for sexual violence need to focus on actual skill building and not solely knowledge enhancement or attitude change (Nation et al., 2003, 2005).

Contrary to many of these principles, the majority of sexual violence prevention strategies have been brief, psychoeducational programs focused on increasing knowledge or changing attitudes, and, unsurprisingly, none have shown evidence of effectiveness in preventing sexually violent *behavior* (DeGue et al., 2014).

To date, one initiative aimed at child and adolescent populations has clearly demonstrated its effectiveness in reducing the perpetration of sexually abusive behavior in a rigorous evaluation study (DeGue et al., 2014). *Safe Dates* is a universal dating violence prevention program for middle- and high-school students involving a ten-session curriculum teaching about the consequences of dating violence and addressing attitudes (including gender stereotyping, attributions for violence), social norms, and healthy relationship skills (including conflict management skills), a 45-min student theater production about dating violence, and a poster contest aimed at changing school norms by immersing and exposing students to violence prevention messaging. The program also facilitates access to community services for victims of dating violence. Over a 4-year follow-up period (that included a booster session to reinforce the program's impact), students who received the intervention were significantly less likely to be victims or perpetrators of self-reported sexual violence involving a dating partner, relative to students who did not participate in the program (Foshee et al., 2004). Clearly, the Safe Dates program follows a number of the principles of effective prevention. It utilizes a thoroughly evaluated comprehensive, community-based approach aimed at middle adolescents that combines a variety of educational and skill building methods with social norm campaigns over an extended period of time. More recently, the program has evolved to engage and include parents in these efforts, to promising early results (Foshee et al., 2012). And although not specifically intended by the developers, the Safe Dates initiative has also been effective in preventing other kinds of youth violence (Foshee et al., 2014).

In addition to Safe Dates, the literature has identified some other promising sexual violence prevention practices for school-aged children, although sufficient evidence has not yet been collected to form conclusions about their efficacy in terms of actual behavior change. These include *Coaching Boys Into Men* (Miller et al., 2012), a coach-delivered norm-based dating violence prevention program for high-school students, and *Expect Respect–Elementary Version*, a bullying- and sexual harassment-focused program for elementary school-aged children (Meraviglia, Becker, Rosenbluth, Sanchez, & Robertson, 2003). Both programs provide a reasonable dose of intervention (11–12 sessions), and the *Expect Respect* program also involves parent education and engages youth in facilitated peer support groups.

It is also worth noting that some bystander intervention programs (e.g., *Bringing in the Bystander*; Banyard, Moynihan, & Plante, 2007) have shown promise, but none have yet been geared toward school-aged children. These approaches generally involve bystander education and training aimed at engaging potential witnesses to violence and providing them with skills to help when they see behavior that puts others at risk, including speaking out against rape myths and sexist language, supporting victims, and intervening in potentially violent situations (DeGue et al., 2014). There remains a significant gap in the literature, however, when it comes to the primary prevention of adolescent-perpetrated sexual abuse of young children.

The First Wave of a Primary Prevention Initiative: A School-Based Primary Prevention Program for Adolescents at Risk for Engaging in Abusive Sexual Behavior

A comprehensive primary prevention program for adolescents at risk for engaging in sexually abusive behavior would be tailored to the intellectual, cognitive, and social development level of the participants, target known or suspected risk and protective factors, and be guided by the known principles of effective prevention programs (Nation et al., 2003, 2005). Because the most frequently endorsed principles (comprehensive, varied teaching methods, appropriately timed) encourage multicomponent, coordinated preventive interventions (Nation et al., 2003), a primary prevention strategy for adolescent-perpetrated sexual violence should address as many risk factors as possible and involve stakeholders throughout the community, including school personnel, parents, child welfare/child protection agencies, and community mental health service providers.

Ideally, such efforts would also be informed by the input of individuals who currently struggle or who have struggled in the past with sexual behavior problems in adolescence. Certainly, one way to increase the sociocultural relevance of a program (and thereby attend to one of the principles of effective prevention programming) is to include participants in the program's planning and implementation. In fact, participants who are involved in planning are more likely to be invested in good outcomes and may have ideas that can be used to complement or enhance the program design (Nation et al., 2005). It happens surprisingly often that the developers of intervention efforts—perhaps especially those directed at offenders or children—tend to ignore input from the affected individuals, themselves. Indeed, the research literature on adolescent sexually abusive behavior has rarely incorporated feedback from adolescents about their treatment experiences. The following recommendations incorporate data gathered from the above literature review with information provided by individuals who, in their adolescence, struggled with their own sexual interests in prepubescent children (Malone, 2014; Oliver, 2005).

Before implementing a program around a problem as frequently misunderstood and potentially incendiary as adolescent-perpetrated sexual abuse, it will be necessary to first assess the target community's readiness to address the problem. *Community readiness assessments* are tools that can be helpful in matching primary prevention strategies to the specific needs of the communities that will implement them, partnering with the stakeholders in a truly collaborative sense (DeWalt, 2008). These assessments measure the extent to which a community is prepared to take action on an issue by exploring the culture and resources that the community currently has to address the defined problem (see Oetting et al., 2014 for a detailed manual on how to conduct this process). Among other things, the process allows one to assess the level of buy-in from community stakeholders while also allowing the community to evaluate the resources it has (and the ones that will be needed) for strategy implementation, identify potential implementation sites, and assess how available strategies might need to be adapted to address local culture (Cook-Craig, 2012). As is common practice with victimization prevention efforts or sexual health education programs in schools—and out of consideration of different families' beliefs and values—parents of participating schools should be provided with a description of the program and its goals and should be afforded the opportunity to have their children opt out of the program or withdraw from it at a later date if that is what they wish.

According to current and recent research in the fields of child development, public health, and assessment and intervention for youth with sexual and other conduct problems—and subject to any required adaptations to facilitate its implementation within targeted communities—a comprehensive strategy to prevent adolescent sexually abusive behavior might include the components outlined below.

Preadolescent Children

Given that the average age of onset for adolescent sexually abusive behavior is between 12 and 15 years, primary prevention efforts should be geared toward children before the development of the problem behaviors, when they are 10–11 years old or in Grade 5.

Prompt Intervention for Child Victims of Sexual Abuse

Although there remains some disagreement in the literature, there exists enough evidence of a link between childhood sexual victimization and subsequent adolescent sexual offending—whether as a risk factor for the initiation of offending or its persistence over time—to indicate that targeted intervention for sexually abused youth could play a role in the prevention of subsequent sexual abuse perpetration (Grabell & Knight, 2009; Hartinger-Saunders et al., 2011; McGrath, Nilsen, & Kerley, 2011; Nunes et al., 2013). While it is known that (a) an abuse experience is neither a necessary nor a sufficient factor in the development of sexually abusive behaviors (Chaffin, 2008), (b) that most child victims of sexual violence do not go on to sexually abuse others (Salter et al., 2003), and (c) that not all children who have been sexually abused suffer long-term psychological injury or require intervention (Child Welfare Information Gateway, 2013; Dykman et al., 1997), it is also known that victims of childhood sexual abuse are far more likely than their non-abused cohorts to experience a range of negative developmental outcomes through adolescence and adulthood including higher rates of psychosis; posttraumatic stress; other anxiety, mood, personality, substance abuse, and psychotic disorders; sexual risk taking; life dissatisfaction; and contacts with the mental health system (Cutajara et al., 2010; Putnam, 2003; Senn, Carey, & Vanable, 2008; Silverman, Reinherz, & Giaconia, 1996).

Although the mechanisms through which a victim sometimes becomes an offender are not yet well understood, recent research suggests that psychological distress caused by childhood victimization, if left untreated or unidentified, tends to accumulate over time, and this *cumulative* effect may increase the probability of an adolescent offending (Hartinger-Saunders et al., 2011). It is also understood that *early starters*—prepubescent children who engage in antisocial, aggressive, or sexualized behavior—have a higher likelihood of persisting with those behaviors into adolescence and adulthood than peers whose conduct problems begin in adolescence (Carpentier et al., 2011; Moffitt, 1993, 2003). Therefore, in addition to the obvious benefits of alleviating distress and improving developmental outcomes, prompt intervention for sexually abused children—if judged as needed and appropriate through professionally guided screening or assessment—may actually reduce the likelihood of subsequent offending. Trained school staff would ideally conduct this initial screening, and this is discussed further, below.

Screening should also be attentive to those risk factors associated in the literature with the perpetration of sexually abusive behavior (as discussed earlier in this chapter), including but not limited to signs of precocious sexual behavior, indications of sexual interest much younger children or violence, sexual preoccupation, and more general conduct problems or antisocial behavior. Also worthy of attention is another set of behavioral indicators that has been linked to a propensity for involvement in adolescent sexually abusive behavior (see Stop It Now!, 2008). This includes such things as a child preferentially seeking out younger playmates, engaging in secretive play with younger playmates, persisting in unwanted physical touch with other children, viewing sexual images of children, and frequently using age-inappropriate, sexualized language. Although many of these indicators have not yet been subjected to empirical investigation, they are a product of some consensus among child protection and treatment providers in the field. As with all sources of information, appropriate caution is recommended in interpreting and applying this kind of information, since there can be many different reasons and explanations for concerning behavior in children, and most of the time these behaviors will not be indicative of special sexual behavior concerns.

Screening should also look for the most common signs of trauma-related psychological distress in children (see National Child Traumatic Stress, 2005; National Institute of Mental Health, 2013). Indeed, expanding this intervention effort to the provision of prompt screening and intervention services for children who have experienced *any* trauma (including exposure to nonsexual violence) would very likely assist in the prevention of many other forms of adolescent delinquency, as well (Adams, 2010). Multiple problem prevention programs make good sense because at-risk children tend to be at risk for multiple negative outcomes as a result of dysfunctional families, neighborhoods, schools, and peer relationships (Nation et al., 2003).

School-Based Programming

Due to the fact that children spend a considerable portion of their early lives in school, schools have the potential to reach some of the largest populations of children and are ideally positioned to provide a wealth and breadth of universal primary prevention programming for a target group of 10- and 11-year-old children. Delivery in a school setting can and should create an environment, culture, and set of norms in which sexual violence is not accepted. In many cases, it may be possible to integrate sexual abuse perpetration prevention programs with existing sexual education, anti-bullying, or health curricula without significant extra expenditure related to delivery or personnel. Consistent with what is known about successful or promising programs for other populations, curricula should involve diverse and active teaching methods (e.g., teacher-facilitated classroom discussions, role-plays, student presentations, posters, and theatrical productions) that focus on increasing awareness and understanding of sexually abusive behavior and obtaining or enhancing skills. Content might focus on a number of different related areas, including:

- A comprehensive definition of abusive sexual behavior.
- Education about *consent* to sexual contact that anticipates common misinformation and distorted beliefs (e.g., teaching that sexual contact with a younger child is never okay, even if the child doesn't resist, appears to consent, and actively participates in the behavior).
- Education about the negative effects of sexual abuse on children.
- Education about the crimino-legal consequences of sexual abuse.
- Education and skills development in setting healthy sexual boundaries.
- Education to acknowledge sexual feelings and arousal as normal.
- Education about healthy versus unhealthy sexual thoughts, feelings, and behaviors.
- Skills development for healthy management of thoughts and feelings (self-regulation).
- Healthy relationship skills development.
- Engaging students in advocating for and creating a healthy environment at school and at home that does not tolerate abusive sexual behavior.
- Instruction about when and who to ask for help, if a child becomes concerned about him-/herself or the behavior of another person.

Anticipating the negative reactions that parents and community members sometimes have toward curricula focused on sexuality, it is worth noting that some of the specific skills development need not focus solely or specifically on sexual arousal but could involve practice in managing different kinds of emotional arousal—such as anxiety—using commonly used self-regulation procedures (such as relaxation breathing, mindfulness techniques, and visualization). And particularly given that one of the desired outcomes of such a program would be for children to seek and receive help when needed, special efforts should be made to deliver content and facilitate discussion in a manner that—while clearly communicating the wrongness of sexually abusive behavior—withholds negative judgment and shaming of youth who might struggle with unhealthy thoughts or arousal.

Based on other programs that have demonstrated efficacy, the school-based portion of the program should be approximately ten sessions in length. Based upon the content of the program and the developmental level of the participants, sessions of approximately 50 min would likely be sufficient. Nation and colleagues (2003, 2005) also note that, because the effects of most strategies diminish over time, effective interventions often include some type of follow-up or booster sessions to support the continued use of information and skills learned in the original activities. Although the prevention literature does not provide any guidelines regarding optimal timelines for effective booster sessions, given that the known mean age for the onset of sexually abusive behavior is 12–15 years, a booster session to review the program content should probably occur within 1 year of completion of the main set of sessions.

Caregiver Involvement

Consistent with what is known about the risk factors for sexually abusive behaviors in children and adolescents, the ingredients of effective interventions for this population, and the *positive relationships* principle of effective prevention, parent/caregiver involvement is key to any prevention efforts. One of the most frequently found risk factor for this population—in terms of both sexually abusive behavior and other serious conduct problems—involves opportunities to offend, inadequate parental supervision, or parental neglect (Hartinger-Saunders, Rine, Wieczorek, & Nochajski, 2012; Carpentier et al., 2011; Spice et al., 2012). This factor is usually conceptualized as an environment that supports reoffending, as evidenced by such things as unsupervised access to potential victims, poor monitoring of the adolescent's whereabouts, and proximity to adults who are unaware of the adolescent's risk factors, engage in denial, or blame the victim (Worling & Curwen, 2001).

Conversely, parental monitoring and a strong parent–child bond have been identified as protective factors for antisocial conduct in adolescents, though not specifically for sexual conduct problems (Klein et al., 2015; Spice et al., 2012; Worling & Langton, 2015). However, early, healthy parent–child attachments have certainly been postulated as a protective factor that may inhibit the development of sexually abusive behavior (Borowsky, Hogan, & Ireland, 1997; Marshall & Marshall, 2010). It is also known that effective interventions for adolescents who have engaged in sexual offending tend to have strong family involvement (Association for the Treatment of Sexual Abusers, 2012). Whether or not failures in parental supervision might on occasion signal disruptions in the child–parent bond or relationship remains an empirical question. Regardless, embedded in this risk factor are a number of rather concrete intervention targets that could be implemented in a comprehensive prevention strategy.

It has been observed that family-based programs for preventing adolescent behavior problems often present with a number of obstacles to parent involvement that can result in low participation, such as high time demands or the requirement that parents travel to locations outside the home in order to participate in the program (Kumpfer & Alvarado, 2003; Spoth & Redmond, 2000). An effective program will need to address these limitations. In their successful family-focused prevention program for teen dating violence, Foshee and colleagues (2012) mailed parent booklets conveying a combination of information and interactive activities for the parents and their teens to do together, designed to address known risk factors for dating violence. Parents additionally received phone calls every 2 weeks by a health educator to determine whether activities were completed, encourage family participation, answer questions, and assess caregiver satisfaction and other reactions to the materials.

A program for preventing sexual abuse perpetration by adolescents would do well to follow this structure, and the family component could complement the school-based portion of the program. An initial mailing containing information about sexual abuse could be directed at the parents. The mailed materials might include a definition of sexual abuse, the impact and consequences of sexual abuse on children, clarification around facts versus myths about the perpetration of sexual abuse (including the fact that many perpetrators begin in adolescence and most sexual abuse is perpetrated by individuals known to the child), known risk factors and early warning signs for sexually abusive behavior, and the contact information for specific individuals with whom parents can consult if they have questions about the material or become concerned about their child's behavior. Special emphasis should be placed on the importance of parents properly monitoring their children. Subsequent mailings could include activities to reinforce the concepts and skills being taught to the children in school (including healthy self-regulation and relationship skills). The number of mailings should not be overly burdensome. If the school curriculum is ten sessions, mailings might occur every two sessions. Follow-up by phone or email should be initiated every 2 weeks, as well.

Staff Training and Access to Specialized Services

Effective delivery of the program would, of course, require training for the individuals delivering it (presumably teachers and guidance counselors, primarily), the individuals responsible for follow-up phone calls with the caregivers, and the school administrators, who need to be fully informed about the program so they can best support their teachers and respond to concerns. There should also be staff within the school that are specifically trained in screening for signs of trauma and recognizing at-risk behaviors. These staff should also be equipped for making referrals of children for further assessment by a psychologist or child and adolescent behavior specialist, if necessary. Before implementing a prevention program for sexual abuse perpetration, schools will need to ensure that they have identified and established relationships with child and adolescent mental health/behavior service providers in their communities, in the likely event the schools do not have the capacity to manage these referrals internally. Local child welfare agencies should also be made aware of the purpose, content, and process of the program so they are prepared and able to best collaborate in the event of any disclosures or child protection concerns that might become known through the program.

Outcome Evaluation

The final component of a good prevention strategy involves an evaluation of its outcome (Nation et al., 2003). Outcomes such as a reduction in sexual abuse perpetration are often too difficult to assess, given the low base rates for these kinds of behaviors and the long follow-up intervals necessary to detect any desired effects (Worling & Langstrom, 2006). Outcomes should be tracked at at least two points in time: within a year of completion of the program (just before the booster session is delivered) and again at a later time. Foshee and colleagues (2004) evaluated their

Safe Dates program 4 years after its delivery and were able to detect positive outcomes. Given the very low base rates for sexual offending behavior in adolescent populations and the fact that rates of sexual offending among adolescents decline dramatically after age 15 (Finkelhor et al., 2009), one might be interested in obtaining outcome measurements at 1 year following completion and then again 3 years later (4 years after the main components of the program are delivered).

Self-report methodologies have been used successfully to evaluate other sexual violence prevention initiatives with youth (see Foshee et al., 2004, 2012; 2014) and likely could be adapted and validated to suit the purposes of this initiative. Actual behavior change would be of the greatest interest to this initiative, as changes in attitudes or accumulation of knowledge are not necessarily associated with changes in the target behavior, the perpetration of sexual abuse (DeGue et al., 2014). Rates of sexual violence perpetration for the population participating in the intervention would need to be compared with rates in a matched comparison sample, such as students at other schools who are similar in important demographics (such as age, family socioeconomic status, etc.) and who have not taken part in the intervention. In order to ensure that the initiative has the capacity for a thorough outcome evaluation in terms of both funding and expertise, partnerships should be sought with universities, government departments, and private agencies and foundations with an interest in effectively addressing critical public health problems.

It is unknown whether a program aimed at preventing adolescents from sexually abusing younger children would also be effective for preventing other kinds of sexual offending behavior, such as sexually abusive behavior toward peers. However, as demonstrated by the Safe Dates program, it is not unreasonable to expect that a well-designed violence prevention initiative, particularly one that includes components targeting known correlates of general and sexual violence—such as early detection and intervention of childhood abuse and trauma—might have a number of positive, ancillary benefits. An evaluation of this program's outcomes would do well to consider these kinds of questions.

It should also be mentioned that general prevention programs focused on healthy youth development, conducted in place of (or in addition to) programs more specifically focused on sexual violence prevention, could be effective in reducing sexual violence (Morrison et al., 2004). *Positive Youth Development (PYD)* is an alternative approach to prevention that, instead of focusing on risk factors for negative health outcomes (such as sexual violence), concentrates on building youth capacities that have long been associated with positive health outcomes (Mannes, Benson, Scales, Sesma, & Rauhouse, 2010). For example, a set of interventions of a PYD program might support the development of youth resiliency—a known protective factor for a wide range of negative health outcomes—by targeting some of its constituent elements such as family support, caring adults, positive peer groups, a strong sense of self and self-esteem, and engagement in school and community activities (Catalano, Berglund, Ryan, Lonczak, & Hawkins, 1998). Although beyond the scope of this chapter and the proposed program, assessing the effect of such general prevention approaches on adolescent sexual violence—with and without the integration of more specialized components—will no doubt be an additional, important step in understanding and preventing sexual violence (Morrison et al., 2004).

The Second Wave of a Primary Prevention Initiative: Reaching Out to Potential Abusers

Over the past number of years, some interesting, alternative public health approaches have emerged with regard to the prevention of sexual abuse of children. These approaches are grounded in the evidence-based understanding that many individuals with sexual interests in children experience distress due to the problems associated with their sexual preference, and therefore many would be inclined to seek treatment if it were available and safe for them to do so (Beier et al., 2009; Stop It Now!, 2000). These kinds of approaches hold promise for reaching large numbers of individuals struggling with pedophilia before they engage in actual abusive sexual conduct (primary prevention) as well as those who have already engaged in sexually abusive behaviors but have made contact with the program on their own, wishing to stop (secondary prevention). They are conceptualized here as the second wave of a comprehensive primary prevention strategy, reaching out to those who might have been missed or unaffected by the universal school-based program of the first wave.

Stop It Now!

Stop It Now! is a community-based public health organization in the United States that has been successful in educating large numbers of people about sexual abuse and soliciting contact from individuals seeking help regarding their sexual attraction to children and obtaining them professional help (Donovon Rice, Hafner, & Pollard, 2010; Stop It Now!, 2000). Its methods have included a public education/social marketing campaign raising awareness about sexual abuse perpetration (providing definitions, discussing consequences, dispelling myths, educating about early warning signs, and providing tips for prevention), a free and confidential help line and online help center, and a referral database of treatment providers. The program has succeeded in facilitating treatment access for both adults and adolescents, the latter as a result of a parent or guardian soliciting help (Chasan-Taber & Tabachnick, 1999).

Prevention Project Dunkelfeld

The *Prevention Project Dunkelfeld* (Beier et al., 2009; Schaefer et al., 2010) is another prevention effort directed at self-identified individuals with pedophilic sexual preferences, encouraging them to seek professional help through their program. The project, based at the Institute of Sexology and Sexual Medicine at the Charité University Hospital in Berlin, is comprised of a large-scale social marketing campaign communicating empathy, hope, and personal accountability for individuals struggling with pedophilia ("You are not guilty because of your desire, but you are responsible for your sexual behavior. There is help! Don't become an offender!"), as well as confidentiality and anonymity for those who reach out to the program. Individuals who make contact with the program are screened over the telephone and, if appropriate, given the opportunity to participate in a free-of-charge assessment and treatment program designed to support their desistence from sexual offending. The program has reported success in making contact with hundreds of individuals struggling with pedophilic sexual interests who might not otherwise have come into contact with treatment providers. These have included individuals who have never acted on their pedophilic sexual urges as well as individuals who have sexually abused a child in the past but want to prevent future offending. Early results of the treatment program (which reportedly includes cognitive behavior therapy, sexological components, and pharmacological options) are encouraging in terms of self-reported reductions in dynamic risk factors for sexual abuse perpetration (Beier et al., 2015), although data is not yet available regarding the impact on actual offending behavior.

Project Primary Prevention of Sexual Child Abuse by Juveniles (PPJ)

In November 2014, researchers at the Charité in Berlin began piloting a primary prevention program that borrows from the methodology of Prevention Project Dunkelfeld but is specifically directed at adolescents aged 12–18 years. The program, *Project Primary Prevention of Sexual Child Abuse by Juveniles* (*PPJ*; https://www.just-dreaming-of-them.org), involves a social marketing campaign that conveys empathy, a nonjudgmental stance, and confidentiality, as well as a message of personal responsibility for one's own behavior ("You are not responsible for your sexual feelings, but you are responsible for your actions"). And like Prevention Project Dunkelfeld, it offers a specialized, no-cost intervention program for youth who feel sexually aroused by prepubescent children. According to the developers, youth who have contacted the project include those who have never acted on their urges as well as those who have already sexually abused a child or used child abuse images (E. Schlinzig, personal communication, January 23, 2015).

It is worth noting that both of the Charité prevention initiatives are able to guarantee confidentiality to their participants because, unlike the United States, Canada, and Australia, Germany does not have mandatory child abuse reporting laws for mental health professionals. According to German law, it would be a breach of confidentiality to report either a committed or a planned act of child sexual abuse (Beier et al., 2009). The adults and adolescents who contact the program can therefore feel assured that project staff will not report any disclosures of pedophilic interest to child protection or criminal justice authorities.

Help Wanted

Inspired in part by Prevention Project Dunkelfeld, another primary prevention initiative is currently in development in the United States, called *Help Wanted* (Letourneau, 2014). The purpose of Help Wanted is to bring together experts from law enforcement, mental health, victim advocacy, prevention, research, and policy to develop, evaluate, and disseminate a primary prevention intervention for adolescents with sexual interests in prepubescent children. The project is intended to create a safe place for young people to seek early, effective professional intervention, helping them develop the skills and resources needed to prevent them from harming children while at the same time promoting healthy adolescent development. Recognizing how little is known about non-offending youth with child-oriented sexual interests, Help Wanted's initial phase involves conducting qualitative interviews with young adults who have self-identified as attracted to children. Interviews will be focused on aspects of their sexual attraction, their coping strategies, and problems that resulted from their sexual interests or the need to keep it hidden. Additionally, interviewees will be asked about what might have helped them during adolescence. Results from these interviews will help inform development of the subsequent intervention. Based on the results of these interviews, a literature review, and the expertise of the development team, assessment and intervention protocols and outreach strategies and materials will be developed, followed by a pilot testing of the program. The final phase will involve revisions based on the pilot evaluation followed by delivery of the intervention as a large-scale, randomized controlled trial (Letourneau, 2014).

A significant strength of the Help Wanted approach to designing a primary prevention program for this population is that embedded in its development is an investigation into the risk, protective factors, and intervention needs of adolescents with child-oriented sexual interests but who have never acted on them, a population about which very little is actually known. This investigation in itself will help determine the design of the intervention program.

Challenges of a Targeted Primary Prevention Plan for Adolescents

A primary prevention approach directed at a selected population of teens at risk for sexually abusive behavior will certainly have a number of unique challenges. First, it might be difficult to protect the confidentiality of the adolescent participants. The nature of mandatory child abuse reporting laws in a number of jurisdictions in the United States, in particular, compels treatment providers to report not only instances of past child abuse but also concerns about potential, future child abuse (Mathews & Kenny, 2008). Therefore, program participants who disclose not only past sexual offenses but also current child-oriented sexual fantasies or interests might be subject to reporting to child protection or law enforcement authorities, depending upon the wording (and the treatment provider's interpretation) of the reporting statute. Statutes can sometimes be ambiguous, leaving much discretion to the reporter and leading, alternately, to problems with underreporting as well as overzealous reporting (Mathews & Kenny, 2008). This places obvious limitations on a prevention program that attempts to solicit contact from adolescents seeking help in managing their sexual arousal to children, who might be unwilling to contact the program for fear of legal repercussions.

Another challenge relates to the provision of health-related services to minors. Different jurisdictions have different laws when it comes to the age at which a teenager can consent to receiving treatment. Some jurisdictions view decision-making as a developmental process, by which an adolescent's ability to consent to health care depends upon her/his ability to understand and communicate relevant information; think and choose with some degree of independence; assess potential benefit, risk, or harms of multiple options; and consider their consequences (Harrison et al., 2004). Others use strict, age-based guidelines for determining an adolescent's capacity to consent to health-care services (Coleman & Rosoff, 2013). Depending upon the adolescent's age and the jurisdiction in which they reside, the consent of her or his parents or caregivers may need to be obtained before intervention can be provided. It is reasonable to assume that some adolescents would be at least initially reluctant to make their parents aware of their struggles with pedophilic sexual interests and therefore disinclined to seek help if they believe their parents will need to become involved.

These challenges, although not insurmountable, will require careful consideration. Clarification around mandatory reporting laws will need to be obtained in those jurisdictions intending on delivering the program, and it is possible that the laws in some states might preclude the implementation of the program there. Regardless, it will also be necessary to formulate a process for responding to situations in which there are concerns about potential risk. Dialogue and collaboration between the program and child protection and law enforcement authorities will be instrumental in developing a process that balances the need for confidentiality while also responding decisively to child protection concerns.

And while some teenagers may be hesitant to inform their caregivers about their struggles with sexuality, they may become amenable to this if engaged in a supportive therapeutic process through which the risks and benefits of caregiver involvement are discussed and caregivers are assisted in responding therapeutically to their children's disclosures. In some situations, conflict may arise if the values and beliefs of the caregivers differ from those of their child or the treatment providers. It seems likely that, in many of these cases, conflicts will be resolvable through better communication about the risks and benefits of treatment. However, parental decision-making ought to be accepted unless it is obvious to many that the decision is demonstrably not in the best interest of the adolescent (Harrison et al., 2004). If disagreement persists and the treatment providers believe that the caregiver's wishes are clearly inconsistent with the adolescent's best interests, the treatment provider could provide the opportunity for a second opinion (either within his or her own center or from another center) or may, in some cases, even involve local child protection authorities, if deemed necessary (Harrison et al., 2004). Although the latter course of action should, of course, only be used as a last recourse, its ethical basis rests firmly on the treatment provider's duty to ensure that the best interests of the adolescent are being prioritized (Harrison et al., 2004).

It bears mention here that the effectiveness of mandatory child abuse reporting laws—in terms of whether or not they serve to protect children—is unknown. Although these laws are doubtlessly well intentioned, an empirical question remains: "What evidence is there that children are abused and neglected less in jurisdictions where mandatory reporting exists by comparison with jurisdictions where it does not exist?" (Ainsworth, 2002). Although the implementation of mandatory reporting has verifiably increased the number of reports of suspected abuse, there is no evidence that it has actually increased the detection of substantiated cases of abuse or resulted in improved outcomes (Ainsworth, 2002). Additionally, questions have been raised about the cost of mandatory reporting and the extent to which it diverts financial resources away from support services for families in need and at risk as well as the negative consequences on families in which abuse has been misidentified (Ainsworth, 2002; Hutchison, 1993). Although these issues are beyond the scope of the current chapter, they hold relevance to the successful implementation of a primary prevention program for at-risk adolescents and may be worth revisiting with legislative authorities at a future time.

Possible Components of a Targeted Intervention

In some cases, teens will likely contact a prevention program such as Help Wanted on their own initiative. In other cases (as with Stop It Now!, Dunkelfeld, and PPJ), concerned parents will likely be the ones to bring their teenagers to the program's attention. In either case, a comprehensive assessment of the teen's and her/his family's strengths and liabilities will need to be conducted in order to identify appropriate, individualized targets for intervention. Information from the youth, her/his parents, and any other relevant collateral sources (such as the child's school), as appropriate, would be invaluable. In addition to specific sexual behavior concerns, treatment targets might include such things as reducing symptoms of posttraumatic stress, strengthening parent–child relationships, or ensuring the child has a safe and stable place to live, if/as needed.

Although not all teens who present to the program will have histories of sexual abuse perpetration, treatment would likely be guided by the known, effective elements of intervention for adolescents who have engaged in abusive sexual behavior, including caregiver involvement; a developmentally sensitive, strengths-based orientation; and a matching of treatment methods and intensity to the youth's dynamic risk, needs, and factors that impact their responsiveness to intervention. Given that teens will presumably present themselves to the program based, in part, on concerns about their sexual interests or behavior, the initial assessment will need to specifically evaluate their sexual interests and arousal patterns and consider their range of possible implications, as discussed above.

Procedures for Assessing Sexual Interests of Adolescents. Clinicians have historically used a variety of methods for evaluating the sexual interests of individuals with suspected atypical or deviant arousal patterns. Penile plethysmography (PPG) is a physiological measurement procedure that involves attaching an instrument to a person's penis in order to measure changes in penile arousal in response to stimulation such as videos, photos, and/or audio cues. If assessing for pedophilic sexual preferences, individuals being assessed would be exposed to cues involving sexualized depictions of children while measuring the individual's erectile responses to the stimuli (Freund, 1991).

Penile plethysmography is a methodology originally developed for measuring adult sexual arousal. Although it has also been used to assess the sexual interests of adolescents, its use with young populations is problematic for a variety of reasons. First, normative data on adolescents has never been collected. In the absence of data describing what "normal" sexual arousal patterns look like in adolescents, it would be impossible to determine the degree of atypical or deviant sexual arousal in a teen who becomes aroused to sexual stimuli depicting young children. It has been found that adolescents who have engaged in abusive sexual behavior report a wider variety of atypical sexual interests than do comparable adults who have committed sexual offenses (Zolondek, Abel, Northey, & Jordan, 2001), and it is suspected that the "normal" range of sexual interests in teenagers is actually quite broad (Ogas & Gaddam, 2012; Rothman & Letourneau, 2013). Secondly, the reliability and validity of PPG with adolescents are known to be lacking, making the method problematic with this population (Association for the Treatment of Sexual Abusers, 2012; Mackaronis, Byrne, & Strassberg, 2014; Worling, 2012). Thirdly, there exist significant ethical grounds for objecting to PPG use with adolescents, a methodology that has been outlawed in several jurisdictions (Worling, 2012). It has been observed that the procedure is intrusive and potentially degrading, models sexually coercive behavior, and has the potential for inducing harm (particularly if used with adolescents with personal histories of sexual victimization) or even inadvertently contributing to the development of pedophilic arousal (Rothman & Letourneau, 2013; Worling, 2012). Until these concerns have been investigated, the continued use of PPG on adolescents is difficult to justify.

Thankfully, there exist empirically supported and ethically supportable alternatives. Viewing time methodologies have shown some utility with adolescents (Abel et al., 2004; Mackaronis et al., 2014). The principle behind viewing time is that individuals look longer at images of people to whom they are sexually attracted. Individuals are presented with images of models in different age groups and asked to rate the attractiveness of each model while the time that the individual takes to provide the ratings is recorded unobtrusively. In most viewing time software packages, the models are fully clothed and are not presented in sexualized poses. And adolescents undergoing viewing time assessments have reported not finding the experience upsetting (Worling, 2006). These findings address some of the ethical concerns related to PPG methods. Viewing time has been shown to correlate significantly with both adolescent self-report and PPG findings, although the reliability and validity data to date is only moderately supportive of the use of the methodology with adolescents (Worling, 2012).

Service providers who work with adolescent forensic populations have long assumed that their teenaged clients cannot be relied upon to tell the truth about their sexual interests and behaviors (Chaffin, 2011; Worling, 2013). In fact, the use of polygraph ("lie detectors") by treatment providers in the United States for adolescents who have sexually offended has doubled since 1996 (McGrath et al., 2010), despite the fact that polygraphy fails to meet even the most basic scientific standards for validity and reliability; does not contribute to reduced sexual recidivism; is known to elicit false disclosures; may be biased against anxiety prone, immature, and naïve individuals; is rarely used in other countries; and is an ethically questionable, coercive practice that may cause harm (Chaffin, 2011). Nevertheless, there is little empirical evidence to support the belief that adolescents are inclined to be deceptive about their sexuality. A number of studies have demonstrated that teenagers can actually be quite forthcoming about these topics and that adolescents' self-report regarding their sexual interests and arousal tends to be quite consistent with physiologically measured arousal (Daleiden, Kaufman, Hilliker, & O'Neil, 1998; Seto et al., 2000; Worling, 2006).

Mindful of these findings, Worling (2006) developed a structured method for assessing the sexual interests and arousal patterns of teens, in which adolescents—guided by a clinician—are asked to graph their own sexual interests and levels of arousal to males and females in different age groups using a chart prepared for this purpose. The method also allows for ratings of arousal to other subjects of interest to the clinician (such as arousal to specific individuals, animals, inanimate objects, etc.). Self-report information gathered through this methodology has been shown to correlate well with physiologically measured sexual arousal (Worling, 2006). This approach has utility not only as a concrete, easy-to-use assessment strategy for adolescent sexual interests but also as a method for facilitating further exploration of these topics in a client- and child-centered, developmentally sensitive, therapeutic manner.

Interventions for Addressing Atypical Sexual Arousal with Adolescents From the time that the sexual offender treatment field began to evolve in the 1970s, the most common intervention approaches for addressing atypical or deviant sexual interests have been based on behavioral principles and have included aversion therapies (using electrical shocks, noxious odors, or shaming to reduce arousal), covert sensitization, masturbatory satiation, and orgasmic conditioning (Marshall & Laws, 2003). Although these procedures were developed for adults, many practitioners report that they currently use them with adolescent populations (McGrath et al., 2010), despite a number of ethical concerns and the absence of any controlled investigations to examine their effectiveness with youth or their potential to cause iatrogenic harm (Worling, 2012). And more recent and popular cognitive behavioral strategies such as *thought stopping*—where the adolescent is taught procedures to interrupt and remove a deviant sexual thought from conscious awareness and replace it with a thought that is healthier—have actually been shown to cause an unintentional (and ironic) rebound effect where the consciously suppressed thought often recurs even more frequently and with greater intensity than it did prior to using the technique in the first place (Johnston, Ward, & Hudson, 1997; Shingler, 2009; Worling, 2012).

Although a number of treatment programs use medications with adolescents to reduce atypical sexual arousal (McGrath et al., 2010), these pharmacological approaches were developed for adult males, and there is currently almost no empirical basis to support the use of medication with adolescents for this purpose

(Bradford & Federoff, 2006). Some of the medications typically used to control sexual arousal have been shown to cause a range of undesirable side effects in teenagers, and their long-term effects on physical and sexual maturation are unknown (Bradford & Federoff, 2006). It is also important to note that most governmental health regulatory bodies do not recognize the use of medication to treat deviant sexual interests (Bradford & Federoff, 2006).

In the absence of a body of research to guide interventions for addressing atypical sexual arousal in teenaged populations, it makes sense to consider empirically supported and ethically supportable approaches used with parallel populations or parallel problems that are also consistent with the principles of effective prevention. Originally borrowed from Buddhist meditation practices and integrated in Western cognitive therapy approaches, *mindfulness* involves the intentional, accepting, and nonjudgmental focus of one's attention on the emotions, thoughts, and sensations occurring in the present (Kabat-Zinn, 1982; Linehan, 1993). Effective at enhancing attention and focus and reducing anxiety, stress, and depressive symptoms in adults, mindfulness-based strategies have grown considerably in popularity over the past 30 years (Tan & Martin, 2015). More recently, mindfulness approaches have been extended to adolescent populations and have demonstrated utility in enhancing overall mental health and behavior control (increasing self-esteem, mental flexibility, attention, cognitive inhibition, and behavioral regulation) and successfully reducing problems including, anxiety, depression, somatic complaints, and sleep difficulties with youth (Black, Milam, & Sussman, 2009; Burke, 2010; Tan & Martin, 2015). The practice has recently shown value when integrated into interventions for intellectually disabled adults who have offended sexually (Singh et al., 2011).

Mindfulness approaches essentially teach individuals to notice their distressing or unwanted thoughts or urges and, without judgment, monitor their thoughts, feelings, and physiological responses without acting on them. The potential of these strategies for addressing deviant sexual arousal is evident: when applied to the management of sexual arousal, deviant arousal is neither acted upon nor suppressed; rather, it is simply noticed by the client and experienced until it inevitably subsides. Worling (2012) notes that the practice is actually not new to treatment programs for adolescents who have offended sexually, and its adaptation for this particular population has been described in at least one recent publication (Jennings, Apsche, Blossom, & Bayles, 2013). While the practice of mindfulness for addressing atypical sexual arousal in adolescents certainly needs to be evaluated, there are indications that these methods—devoid of aversive conditioning procedures, therapist-directed masturbation, and other elements likely to make engagement in treatment difficult for anyone—hold promise for this population.

Consistent with a strengths-based perspective, an accompanying approach for addressing atypical sexual interests would be to build skills for healthy sexuality. Sexual arousal patterns in adolescence have been observed to be quite fluid and dynamic (Bancroft, 2006; Powell, 2010), and therefore there is good reason to expect that—at least for some adolescents—healthy, nondeviant interests can be strengthened if the youth see the possibility of forming healthy emotionally and sexually intimate relationships in their futures (Worling, 2012). As discussed above,

Association for the Treatment of Sexual Abusers (2014). *Talking about prevention.* Beaverton, OR: Author. Retrieved September 10, 2014, from http://www.atsa.com/pdfs/Prevention/TalkingABoutPrevention.pdf

Bancroft, J. (2006). Normal sexual development. In H. E. Barbaree & W. L. Marshall (Eds.), *The juvenile sex offender* (2nd ed., pp. 19–57). New York, NY: Guilford Press.

Banyard, V. L., Moynihan, M. M., & Plante, E. G. (2007). Sexual violence prevention through bystander education: An experimental evaluation. *Journal of Community Psychology, 35*(4), 463–481.

Beier, K. M., Ahlers, C. J., Goecker, D., Neutze, J., Mundt, I. A., Hupp, E., & Schaefer, G. A. (2009). Can pedophiles be reached for primary prevention of child sexual abuse? First results of the Berlin Prevention Project Dunkelfeld (PPD). *Journal of Forensic Psychiatry and Psychology, 20*, 851–867.

Beier, K. M., Grundmann, D., Kuhle, L. F., Scherner, G., Konrad, A., & Amelung, T. (2015). The German Dunkelfeld project: A pilot study to prevent child sexual abuse and the use of child abusive images. *Journal of Sexual Medicine, 12*, 529–542.

Black, D. S., Milam, J., & Sussman, S. (2009). Sitting-meditation interventions among youth: A review of treatment efficacy. *Pediatrics, 124*, 532–541.

Borowsky, I. W., Hogan, M., & Ireland, M. (1997). Adolescent sexual aggression: Risk and protective factors. *Pediatrics, 100*, 1–8.

Bradford, J. M. W., & Federoff, P. (2006). Pharmacological treatment of the juvenile sex offender. In H. E. Barbaree & W. L. Marshall (Eds.), *The juvenile sex offender* (2nd ed., pp. 358–382). New York: Guilford Press.

Burke, C. A. (2010). Mindfulness-based approaches with children and adolescents: A preliminary review of current research in an emergent field. *Journal of Child and Family Studies, 19*, 133–144.

Caldwell, M. F. (2002). What we do not know about juvenile sexual reoffense risk. *Child Maltreatment, 7*, 291–302.

Caldwell, M. F. (2007). Sexual offense adjudication and sexual recidivism among juvenile offenders. *Sexual Abuse, 19*, 107–113.

Caldwell, M. F. (2010). Study characteristics and recidivism base rates in juvenile sex offender recidivism. *International Journal of Offender Therapy and Comparative Criminology, 54*, 197–212.

Caldwell, M. F., Skeem, J., Salekin, R., & Van Rybroek, G. (2006). Treatment response of adolescent offenders with psychopathy-like features. *Criminal Justice and Behavior, 33*, 571–596.

Caldwell, M. F., & Van Rybroek, G. (2013). Effective treatment programs for violent adolescents: Programmatic challenges and promising features. *Aggression and Violent Behavior, 18*, 571–578.

Carpentier, J., Leclerc, B., & Proulx, J. (2011). Juvenile sexual offenders: Correlates of onset, variety, and desistance of criminal behavior. *Criminal Justice and Behavior, 38*, 854–873.

Catalano, R. F., Berglund, M. L., Ryan, J. A. M., Lonczak, H. S., & Hawkins, J. D. (1998). *Positive youth development in the United States: Research findings on evaluations of positive youth development programs.* Seattle, WA: Social Development Research Group, University of Washington School of Social Work. Retrieved March 20, 2015, from http://aspe.hhs.gov/HSP/PositiveYouthDev99/index.htm

Centers for Disease Control and Prevention. (2004). *Sexual violence prevention: Beginning the dialogue.* Atlanta, GA: Author.

Chaffin, M. (2008). Our minds are made up—don't confuse us with the facts: Commentary on policies concerning children with sexual behavior problems and juvenile sex offenders. *Child Maltreatment, 13*(2), 110–121.

Chaffin, M. (2011). The case of juvenile polygraphy as a clinical ethics dilemma. *Sexual Abuse, 23*, 314–328.

Chaffin, M., Letourneau, E., & Silovsky, J. F. (2002). Adults, adolescents, and children who sexually abuse children: A developmental perspective. In J. E. B. Myers & L. Berliner (Eds.), *The APSAC handbook on child maltreatment* (2nd ed., pp. 205–232). Thousand Oaks, CA: Sage.

Chasan-Taber, L., & Tabachnick, J. (1999). Evaluation of a child sexual abuse prevention program. *Sexual Abuse, 11*, 279–292.

Child Welfare Information Gateway. (2013). *Long-term consequences of child abuse and neglect.* Washington, DC: U.S. Department of Health and Human Services, Children's Bureau. Retrieved August 20, 2014, from http://www.childwelfare.gov/pubPDFs/long_term_consequences.pdf

Coleman, D. L., & Rosoff, P. M. (2013). The legal authority of mature minors to consent to general medical treatment. *Pediatrics, 131*, 786–793.

Cook-Craig, P. (2012, September). *Youth sexual violence prevention.* Harrisburg, PA: VAWnet, a project of the National Resource Center on Domestic Violence. Retrieved September 20, 2014, from http://www.vawnet.org/applied-research-papers/print-document.php?doc_id=3386&find_type=Prevention

Curwen, T., Jenkins, J. M., & Worling, J. R. (2014). Differentiating children with and without a history of repeated problematic sexual behavior. *Journal of Child Sexual Abuse, 23*, 462–480.

Cutajara, M. C., Mullena, P. E., Ogloff, J. R. P., Thomas, S. D., Wells, D. L., & Spataro, J. (2010). Psychopathology in a large cohort of sexually abused children followed up to 43 years. *Child Abuse & Neglect, 34*, 813–822.

Daleiden, E. L., Kaufman, K. L., Hilliker, D. R., & O'Neil, J. N. (1998). The sexual histories and fantasies of youthful males: A comparison of sexual offending, nonsexual offending, and non-offending groups. *Sexual Abuse, 10*, 195–209.

DeGue, S., Simon, T. R., Basile, K. C., Yee, S. L., Lang, K., & Spivak, H. (2012). Moving forward by looking back: Reflecting on a decade of CDC's work in sexual violence prevention, 2000–2010. *Journal of Women's Health, 21*(12), 1211–1218.

DeGue, S., Valle, L. A., Holt, M. K., Massetti, B. M., Matjasko, J. L., & Tharp, A. T. (2014). A systematic review of primary prevention strategies for sexual violence perpetration. *Aggression and Violent Behavior, 19*, 346–362.

DeWalt, T. A. (2008). Primary prevention of sexual violence against adolescents and the Community Readiness Model. *Graduate Journal of Counseling Psychology, 1*(1), 26–49.

Donovon Rice, D., Hafner, J. A. H., & Pollard, P. (2010). Stop it now! In K. L. Kaufman (Ed.), *The prevention of sexual violence: A practitioner's sourcebook* (pp. 275–282). Holyoke, MA: NEARI Press.

Dykman, R., McPherson, B., Ackerman, P., Newton, J., Mooney, D., Wherry, J., & Chaffin, M. (1997). Internalizing and externalizing characteristics of sexually and/or physically abused children. *Integrative Physiological and Behavioral Science, 32*, 62–74.

Fanniff, A. M., & Becker, J. V. (2006). Specialized assessment and treatment of adolescent sex offenders. *Aggression and Violent Behavior, 11*, 265–282.

Finkelhor, D., Ormrod, R., & Chaffin, M. (2009). *Juveniles who commit sex offenses against minors* (NCJ 227763). Washington, DC: U.S. Department of Justice Office of Justice Programs, Office of Juvenile Justice and Delinquency Prevention, 1–11.

Foshee, V. A., Bauman, K. E., Ennett, S. T., Linder, G. F., Benefield, T., & Suchindran, C. (2004). Assessing the long-term effects of the safe dates program and a booster in preventing and reducing adolescent dating violence victimization and perpetration. *American Journal of Public Health, 94*, 619–624.

Foshee, V. A., McNaughton Reyes, H. L., Agnew-Brune, C. B., Simon, T. R., Vagi, K. J., Lee, R. D., & Suchindran, C. (2014). The effects of the evidence-based Safe Dates dating abuse prevention program on other youth violence outcomes. *Prevention Science, 15*, 907–916.

Foshee, V. A., McNaughton Reyes, H. L., Ennett, S. T., Cance, J. D., Bauman, K. E., & Bowling, J. M. (2012). Assessing the effects of families for safe dates, a family-based teen dating abuse prevention program. *Journal of Adolescent Health, 51*(4), 349–356.

Freund, K. (1991). Reflections on the development of phallometric method of assessing erotic preferences. *Annals of Sex Research, 4*, 221–228.

Freyd, J. J., Putnam, F. W., Lyon, T. D., Becker-Blease, K. A., Cheit, R. E., Siegel, N. B., et al. (2005). The science of child sexual abuse. *Science, 308*(5721), 501.

Grabell, A. S., & Knight, R. A. (2009). Examining childhood abuse patterns and sensitive periods in juvenile sexual offenders. *Sexual Abuse, 21*, 208–222.

Groth, A. N., Longo, R. E., & McFadin, J. B. (1982). Undetected recidivism among rapists and child molesters. *Crime & Delinquency, 28*, 450–458.

Hanson, R. K., & Morton-Bourgon, K. E. (2005). The characteristics of persistent sexual offenders: A meta-analysis of recidivism studies. *Journal of Consulting and Clinical Psychology, 73*, 1154–1163.

Harrison, C., Albersheim, S., Arbour, L., Byrne, P., Laxer, R., et al. (2004). Treatment decisions regarding infants, children and adolescents. *Paediatrics & Child Health, 9*(2), 99–103.

Hartinger-Saunders, R. M., Rine, C. M., Wieczorek, W., & Nochajski, T. (2012). Family level predictors of victimization and offending among young men: Rethinking the role of parents in prevention and interventions models. *Children and Youth Services Review, 34*, 2423–2432.

Hartinger-Saunders, R. M., Rittner, B., Wieczorek, W., Nochajski, T., Rine, C. M., & Welte, J. (2011). Victimization, psychological distress and subsequent offending among youth. *Children and Youth Services Review, 33*(11), 2375–2385.

Hunter, J. A., Figueredo, A. J., Malamuth, N. M., & Becker, J. V. (2003). Juvenile sex offenders: Toward the development of a typology. *Sexual Abuse, 15*, 27–48.

Hutchison, E. (1993). Mandatory reporting laws: Child protective case findings gone awry. *Social Work, 38*, 56–62.

Jennings, J. L., Apsche, J. A., Blossom, P., & Bayles, C. (2013). Using mindfulness in the treatment of adolescent sexual abusers: Contributing common factor or a primary modality? *International Journal of Behavioral Consultation and Therapy, 8*, 17–22.

Johnston, L., Ward, T., & Hudson, S. M. (1997). Deviant sexual thoughts: Mental control and the treatment of sexual offenders. *Journal of Sex Research, 34*, 121–130.

Kabat-Zinn, J. (1982). An outpatient program in behavioral medicine for chronic pain patients based on the practice of mindfulness meditation: Theoretical considerations and preliminary results. *General Hospital Psychiatry, 4*, 33–47.

Klein, V., Rettenberger, M., Yoon, D., Köhler, N., & Briken, P. (2015). Protective factors and recidivism in accused juveniles who sexually offended. *Sexual Abuse, 27*(1), 71–90.

Knight, R. A., & Prentky, R. A. (1993). Exploring characteristics of classifying juvenile sex offenders. In H. E. Barbaree, W. L. Marshall, & S. M. Hudson (Eds.), *The juvenile sex offender* (pp. 45–83). New York, NY: Guilford Press.

Krug, E., Dahlberg, L., Mercy, J., Zwi, A., & Lozano, R. (2002). *World health report on violence and health*. Geneva: World Health Organization.

Kumpfer, K. L., & Alvarado, R. (2003). Family-strengthening approaches for the prevention of youth problem behaviors. *American Psychologist, 58*, 457–465.

Laws, D. R. (2000). Sexual offending as a public health problem: A North American Perspective. *Journal of Sexual Aggression, 5*, 30–44.

Laws, D. R. (2008). The public health approach: A way forward? In D. R. Laws & W. T. O'Donohue (Eds.), *Sexual deviance: Theory, assessment, and treatment* (2nd ed., pp. 611–628). New York, NY: Guilford Press.

Laws, D. R., & Marshall, W. L. (1990). A conditioning theory of the etiology and maintenance of deviant sexual preference and behavior. In W. L. Marshall, D. R. Laws, & H. E. Barbaree (Eds.), *Handbook of sexual assault: Issues, theories and treatment of the offender* (pp. 209–229). New York, NY: Plenum.

Letourneau, E. J. (2014, November). *Help wanted: Young people living with sexual attraction to younger children*. Plenary address at the 33rd Annual Conference of the Association for the Treatment of Sexual Abusers, San Diego, CA.

Letourneau, E. J., & Borduin, C. M. (2008). The effective treatment of juveniles who sexually offend: An ethical imperative. *Ethics and Behavior, 18*(2–3), 286–306.

Letourneau, E. J., Eaton, W. W., Bass, J., Berlin, F., & Moore, S. G. (2014). The need for a comprehensive public health approach to preventing child sexual abuse. *Public Health Reports, 129*(3), 222–228.

Linehan, M. M. (1993). *Cognitive behavioral therapy of borderline personality disorder*. New York, NY: Guilford Press.

Mackaronis, J. E., Byrne, P. M., & Strassberg, D. S. (2014). Assessing sexual interest in adolescents who have sexually offended. *Sexual Abuse*. doi: 10.1177/1079063214535818.

Malone, L. (2014, August 10). You're 16. You're a pedophile. You don't want to hurt anyone. What do you do now? *Matter*. Retrieved September 12, 2014, from https://medium.com/matter/youre-16-youre-a-pedophile-you-dont-want-to-hurt-anyone-what-do-you-do-now-e11ce4b88bdb

Mannes, M., Benson, P. L., Scales, P. C., Sesma, A., Jr., & Rauhouse, J. (2010). Positive youth development: Theory, research, and application to sexual violence prevention. In K. L. Kaufman (Ed.), *The prevention of sexual violence: A practitioner's sourcebook* (pp. 85–106). Holyoke, MA: NEARI Press.

Marshall, W. L., & Laws, D. R. (2003). A brief history of behavioral and cognitive behavioral approaches to sexual offender treatment: Part 2. The modern era. *Sexual Abuse, 15*, 93–120.

Marshall, W. L., & Marshall, L. E. (2010). Attachment and intimacy in sexual offenders: An update. *Sexual and Relationship Therapy, 25*, 1–5.

Mathews, B., & Kenny, M. C. (2008). Mandatory reporting legislation in the United States, Canada, and Australia: A cross-jurisdictional review of key features, differences, and issues. *Child Maltreatment, 13*, 50–63.

McCann, K., & Lussier, P. (2008). Antisociality, sexual deviance, and sexual reoffending in juvenile sex offenders: A meta-analytical investigation. *Youth Violence and Juvenile Justice, 6*, 363–385.

McGrath, R., Cumming, G., Burchard, B., Zeoli, S., & Ellerby, L. (2010). *Current practices and emerging trends in sexual abuser management: The Safer Society 2009 North American survey*. Brandon, Vermont: Safer Society Press.

McGrath, S. A., Nilsen, A. A., & Kerley, K. R. (2011). Sexual victimization in childhood and the propensity for juvenile delinquency and adult criminal behavior: A systematic review. *Aggression and Violent Behavior, 16*, 485–492.

Meraviglia, M. G., Becker, H., Rosenbluth, B., Sanchez, E., & Robertson, T. (2003). The expect respect project: creating a positive elementary school climate. *Journal of Interpersonal Violence, 18*(11), 1347–1360.

Miller, E., Tancredi, D. J., McCauley, H. L., Decker, M. R., Virata, M. C. D., Anderson, H. A., et al. (2012). "Coaching boys into men": A cluster-randomized controlled trial of a dating violence prevention program. *Journal of Adolescent Health, 51*(5), 431–438.

Moffitt, T. E. (1993). Adolescence-limited and life-course-persistent antisocial behavior: A developmental taxonomy. *Psychological Review, 100*(4), 674–701.

Moffitt, T. E. (2003). Life-course-persistent and adolescence-limited antisocial behavior: A 10-year research review and a research agenda. In B. Lahey, T. E. Moffitt, & A. Caspi (Eds.), *Causes of conduct disorder and juvenile delinquency* (pp. 49–75). New York, NY: Guilford Press.

Mohnke, S., Müller, S., Amelung, T., Krüger, T. H. C., Ponseti, J., Schiffer, B., … Walter, H. (2014). Brain alterations in paedophilia: A critical review. *Progress in Neurobiology, 122*, 1–23.

Morrison, S., Hardison, J., Mathew, A., & O'Neil, J. (2004). *An evidence-based review of sexual assault preventive intervention programs. Technical Report*. Washington, DC: National Institute of Justice. Retrieved March 20, 2015, from https://www.ncjrs.gov/pdffiles1/nij/grants/207262.pdf

Nation, M., Crusto, C., Wandersman, A., Kumpfer, K. L., Seybolt, D., Morrissey-Kane, E., et al. (2003). What works in prevention: Principles of effective prevention programs. *American Psychologist, 58*, 449–456.

Nation, M., Keener, D., Wandersman, A. & DuBois, D. (2005). *Applying the principles of prevention: What do prevention practitioners need to know about what works?* Retrieved September 20, 2014, from http://www.mentoring.org/downloads/mentoring_4.pdf

National Child Traumatic Stress Network (2005). *Understanding child traumatic stress*. Los Angeles, CA: National Center for Child Traumatic Stress. Retrieved August 30, 2014, from http://www.nctsnet.org/sites/default/files/assets/pdfs/understanding_child_traumatic_stress_brochure_9-29-05.pdf

National Institute of Mental Health (2013). *Helping children and adolescents cope with violence and disasters: For parents of children exposed to violence or disaster*. Bethesda, MD: Author. Retrieved August 30, 2014, from http://www.nimh.nih.gov/health/publications/helping-children-and-adolescents-cope-with-violence-and-disasters-parents-trifold/Helping-Children-and-Adolescents-Cope-with-Violence-and-Disasters-What-Parents-Can-Do_146810.pdf

Nunes, K. L., Hermann, C. A., Malcom, J. R., & Lavoie, K. (2013). Childhood sexual victimization, pedophilic interest, and sexual recidivism. *Child Abuse & Neglect, 37*, 703–711.

Oetting, E. R., Plested, B. A., Edwards, R. W., Thurman, P. J., Kelly, K. J., Beauvais, F., ... Stanley, L. R. (2014). *Community readiness for community change* (2nd ed.). Tri-Ethic Center for Prevention Research, Colorado State University. Retrieved September 20, 2014, from http://triethniccenter.colostate.edu/docs/CR_Handbook_2015.pdf

Ogas, O., & Gaddam, S. (2012). *A billion wicked thoughts*. New York, NY: Plume.

Oliver, B. E. (2005). Thoughts on combating pedophilia in non-offending adolescents [Letter to the editor]. *Archives of Sexual Behavior, 34*, 3–5.

Oxnam, P., & Vess, J. (2008). A typology of adolescent sexual offenders: Millon Adolescent Clinical Inventory profiles, developmental factors, and offence characteristics. *Journal of Forensic Psychiatry & Psychology, 19*, 228–242.

Powell, K. M. (2010). Therapeutic relationships and the process of change. In G. Ryan, T. Leversee, & S. Lane (Eds.), *Juvenile sexual offending* (3rd ed., pp. 253–262). Hoboken, NJ: John Wiley & Sons.

Prentky, R. A., & Righthand, S. (2003). *Juvenile Sex Offender Assessment Protocol-II (J-SOAP-II) manual*. Bridgewater, MA: Justice Resource Institute.

Putnam, F. W. (2003). Ten-year research update review: Child sexual abuse. *Journal of the American Academy of Child and Adolescent Psychiatry, 42*(3), 269–278.

Rasmussen, L. A. (1999). Factors related to recidivism among juvenile sexual offenders. *Sexual Abuse, 11*(1), 69–85.

Reitzel, L. R., & Carbonell, J. L. (2006). The effectiveness of sexual offender treatment for juveniles as measured by recidivism: A meta-analysis. *Sexual Abuse, 18*, 401–421.

Rothman, D. B., & Letourneau, E. J. (2013, October). *Adolescents who have engaged in abusive sexual behaviors: Empirically & ethically supported practice guidelines*. Invited Pre-Conference Seminar presented at the 32nd Annual Conference of the Association for the Treatment of Sexual Abusers, Chicago, IL.

Salter, D., McMillan, D., Richards, M., Talbot, T., Hodges, J., Bentovim, A., ... Skuse, D. (2003). Development of sexually abusive behaviour in sexually victimized males: A longitudinal study. *Lancet, 361*, 471–476.

Santtila, P., Mokros, A., Hartwig, M., Varjonen, M., Patrick Jern, P., Witting, K., ... Sandnabba, N. K. (2010). Childhood sexual interactions with other children are associated with lower preferred age of sexual partners including sexual interest in children in adulthood. *Psychiatry Research, 175*, 154–159.

Schaefer, G. A., Mundt, I. A., Feelgood, S., Hupp, E., Neutze, J., Ahlers, C. J., ... Beier, K. M. (2010). Potential and Dunkelfeld offenders: Two neglected target groups for prevention of child sexual abuse. *International Journal of Law and Psychiatry, 33*(3), 154–163.

Senn, T. E., Carey, M. P., & Vanable, P. A. (2008). Childhood and adolescent sexual abuse and subsequent sexual risk behavior: Evidence from controlled studies, methodological critique, and suggestions for research. *Clinical Psychology Review, 28*, 711–735.

Seto, M., & Lalumiere, M. (2010). What is so special about male adolescent sexual offending? A review and test of explanations through meta-analysis. *Psychological Bulletin, 136*(4), 526–575.

Seto, M. C., Lalumiere, M. L., & Blanchard, R. (2000). The discriminative validity of a phallometric test for pedophilic interests among adolescent sex offenders against children. *Psychological Assessment, 12*, 319–327.

Shingler, J. (2009). Managing intrusive risky thoughts: What works? *Journal of Sexual Aggression, 15*, 39–53.

Silverman, A. B., Reinherz, H. Z., & Giaconia, R. M. (1996). The long-term sequelae of child and adolescent abuse: A longitudinal community study. *Child Abuse & Neglect, 20*(8), 709–723.

Singh, N., Lancioni, G., Winton, A., Singh, A., Adkins, A., & Singh, J. (2011). Can adult offenders with intellectual disabilities use mindfulness procedures to control their deviant sexual arousal? *Psychology Crime and Law, 17*, 165–179.

Snyder, H. (2002, November). Juvenile Arrests 2000. *OJJDP Juvenile Justice Bulletin* (Cooperative Agreement No. 1999- JN-FX-K002). Washington, DC: Office of Juvenile Justice and Delinquency Prevention, U.S. Department of Justice.

Spice, A., Viljoen, J. L., Latzman, N. E., Scalora, M. J., & Ullman, D. (2012). Risk and protective factors for recidivism among juveniles who have offended sexually. *Sexual Abuse, 25*, 347–369.

Spoth, R., & Redmond, C. (2000). Research on family engagement in preventive interventions: Toward improved use of scientific findings in primary prevention practice. *Journal of Primary Prevention, 21*, 267–284.

St. Amand, A., Bard, D. E., & Silovsky, J. F. (2008). Treatment of child sexual behavior problems: Practice elements and outcomes. *Child Maltreatment, 13*, 145–166.

Stop It Now! (2000). *Four-year evaluation: Findings reveal success of Stop It Now! Vermont* (Report No. 5). Northampton, MA: Author. Retrieved September 20, 2014, from http://www.stopitnow.org/sites/default/files/old_site_files/webfm/green/FinalEvalSum2000.pdf

Stop It Now! (2008). *Signs that a child or teen may be at-risk to harm another child*. Northampton, MA: Author. Retrieved September 10, 2014, from http://www.stopitnow.org/sites/default/files/documents/files/signs_child_adolescent_risk_harm_child.pdf

Tan, L., & Martin, G. (2015). Taming the adolescent mind: A randomised controlled trial examining clinical efficacy of an adolescent mindfulness-based group programme. *Child and Adolescent Mental Health, 20*, 49–55.

Taylor, J. F. (2003). Children and young people accused of child sexual abuse: A study within a community. *Journal of Sexual Aggression, 9*, 57–70.

Tharp, A. T., DeGue, S., Valle, L. A., Brookmeyer, K. A., Massetti, G. M., & Matjasko, J. L. (2012). A systematic qualitative review of risk and protective factors for sexual violence perpetration. *Trauma, Violence & Abuse, 14*(2), 133–167.

van Wijk, A., Mali, S. R. F., & Bullens, R. A. R. (2007). Juvenile sex-only and sex-plus offenders: An exploratory study on criminal profiles. *International Journal of Offender Therapy and Comparative Criminology, 51*(4), 407–419.

Viljoen, J. I., Elkovitch, N., Scalora, M. J., & Ullman, D. (2009). Assessment of reoffense risk in adolescents who have committed sexual offenses: Predictive validity of the ERASOR, PCL:YV, YLS/CMI, and Static-99. *Criminal Justice and Behavior, 36*, 981–1000.

Wanklyn, S. G., Ward, A. K., Cormier, N. S., Day, D. M., & Newman, J. E. (2012). Can we distinguish juvenile violent sex offenders, violent non-sex offenders, and versatile violent sex offenders based on childhood risk factors? *Journal of Interpersonal Violence, 27*(11), 2128–2143.

Worling, J. R. (2004). The Estimate of Risk of Adolescent Sexual Offense Recidivism (ERASOR): Preliminary psychometric data. *Sexual Abuse, 16*, 235–254.

Worling, J. R. (2006). Assessing sexual arousal with adolescent males who have offended sexually: Self-report and unobtrusively measured viewing time. *Sexual Abuse, 18*, 383–400.

Worling, J. R. (2012). The assessment and treatment of deviant sexual arousal with adolescents who have offended sexually. *Journal of Sexual Aggression, 18*, 36–63.

Worling, J. R. (2013). What were we thinking? Five erroneous assumptions that have fueled specialized interventions for adolescents who have sexually offended. *International Journal of Behavioral Consultation and Therapy, 8*, 80–88.

Worling, J. R., Bookalam, D., & Littlejohn, A. (2012). Prospective validity of the Estimate of Risk of Adolescent Sexual Offense Recidivism (ERASOR). *Sexual Abuse, 24*, 203–223.

Worling, J. R., & Curwen, T. (2001). *Estimate of risk of adolescent sexual offense recidivism (Version 2.0)*. Toronto, Canada: Ontario Ministry of Community and Social Services.

Worling, J. R., & Langstrom, N. (2006). Assessing risk of sexual reoffending. In H. E. Barbaree & W. L. Marshall (Eds.), *The juvenile sex offender* (2nd ed., pp. 219–247). New York, NY: Plenum.

Worling, J. R., & Langton, C. M. (2015). A prospective investigation of factors that predict desistance from recidivism for adolescents who have sexually offended. *Sexual Abuse, 27*, 127–142.

Worling, J. R., Littlejohn, A., & Bookalam, D. (2010). 20-year prospective follow-up study of specialized treatment for adolescents who offended sexually. *Behavioral Sciences and the Law, 28*, 46–57.

Zolondek, S., Abel, G., Northey, W., & Jordan, A. (2001). The self reported behaviors of juvenile sexual offenders. *Journal of Interpersonal Violence, 16*(1), 73–85.

Chapter 10
Community Control of Sex Offenders

Jill S. Levenson

Evolution of Contemporary Sex Offender Management Policies

There are perhaps no crimes that instill fear and rage in society like sexual offenses. Over the past several decades, in response to a number of highly publicized and heinous sexually motivated abductions and murders, lawmakers have responded to the public's demands for protective legislation. In October 1989, while riding his bike with his brother and a friend in St. Joseph, Minnesota, 11-year-old Jacob Wetterling was abducted by an unknown male assailant. Few suspects were identified, and to date, Jacob remains missing and no arrests have ever been made. The Wetterlings became advocates for more effective laws to aid in the recovery of missing children and recommended that known sex offenders be required to register their addresses with police in order to identify potential suspects in such cases. In 1994, the US Congress passed the Jacob Wetterling Crimes Against Children and Sexually Violent Offender Registration Act, requiring all 50 states to create laws mandating that sex offenders register their addresses with local law enforcement agencies so that their whereabouts are known ("Jacob Wetterling Crimes Against Children and Sexually Violent Offender Registration Act," 1994).

In July 1994, a 7-year-old New Jersey girl named Megan Kanka was lured into the home of a convicted sex offender, sexually assaulted, and strangled. Megan's parents were horrified to learn that her killer was a sex offender living nearby and said that if they had been aware, they would not have allowed their child to play outside unsupervised. In 1996, the Wetterling Act was amended to states to make registry data available to the public, and states were later required to create publicly

J.S. Levenson, Ph.D., L.C.S.W. (✉)
Barry University, 11300 NE 2nd Ave, Miami Shores, FL 305-899-3923, USA
e-mail: jlevenson@barry.edu

© Springer International Publishing Switzerland 2016
D.R. Laws, W. O'Donohue (eds.), *Treatment of Sex Offenders*,
DOI 10.1007/978-3-319-25868-3_10

accessible Internet registries by 2003. About half of the states assigned offenders to risk levels and notify the public differentially according to the offender's threat to public safety. Other states employ broad community notification, publicizing the location of all sex offenders without regard to their risk. The goal of community notification is to increase the public's ability to protect itself by making potential victims aware that a convicted sex offender lives in the vicinity.

In 2006, Congress passed the Adam Walsh Act (named for a Florida child who was abducted from a shopping mall and murdered), which standardized the federal sex offender registration and notification (SORN) guidelines so that laws would be more uniform across all 50 states. The Adam Walsh Act (AWA) created guidelines for states to implement a 3-tier offense classification system with concordant registration frequencies and durations, along with increased penalties for sex offenders who failed to properly register. Currently, 17 states are compliant with AWA federal guidelines.

The constitutionality of community notification statutes has been challenged. In 2003, the US Supreme Court upheld the constitutionality of a Connecticut statute allowing sex offenders to be placed on an Internet registry without first holding a hearing to determine their danger to the community ("Connecticut Dept. of Public Safety v. Doe," 2003). In an Alaska case, the US Supreme Court ruled that registration and notification of sex offenders sentenced before the passage of the law could not be characterized as ex post facto punishment ("Smith v. Doe," 2003). These decisions empowered the national movement toward more inclusive sex offender policies, including increased disclosure of information on public registries and broad dissemination rather than risk assessment-based notification.

Sex offender registration and community notification originally emerged as distinct policies with different goals. Registration was designed as a tool to assist law enforcement agents to track sexual criminals and apprehend potential suspects. Notification was initiated to increase public awareness and arm communities with information which might help them to avoid contact with sex offenders and thus prevent victimization. As state and federal initiatives have moved inevitably toward Internet-based registries, however, registration and notification have become intertwined and even interchangeable.

The Makeup of Registries and How They Work

According to the National Center for Missing and Exploited Children (NCMEC), in June of 2015, approximately 843, 260 registered sex offenders (RSO) resided in the USA. About one-third of RSOs are not listed on public registries, because they have been determined by their state's sex offender management risk assessment process to pose a low risk for future offending (Ackerman, Harris, Levenson, & Zgoba, 2011). Among RSOs on public registries, about 14 % nationally have been designated by states to be high risk, predator, or sexually violent (Ackerman et al., 2011). Over 97 % of RSOs are male, and the average age is about 45 years old. About 85 %

have only one sex offense conviction, approximately 90 % of registered sex offenders have had a minor victim, and about one-third have had victims under 10 years old. Most (87–89 %) victims (adult and minor) are female (Ackerman et al., 2011; Finkelhor et al., 2008). Minorities (especially blacks) are overrepresented on sex offender registries.

A 20-year analysis of sex crimes reported to the National Incident-Based Reporting System in the USA (over 800,000 incidents in 37 states) revealed similar characteristics about sexual perpetrators (Williams & Bierie, 2014). Most of the offenders were white (73 %), and the average age was about 30. Most victims (88 %) were female, and the reports involved an average of one victim per incident; approximately 25 % involved a reported injury to the victim and less than 2 % involved a kidnapping or homicide. About two-thirds of the reports involved minor victims (66 %) and about 34 % involved prepubescent victims (Williams & Bierie, 2014).

The purpose of SORN laws is to improve public awareness about sex offenders living among us so that concerned citizens and parents can take protective action to prevent sexual victimization (Anderson & Sample, 2008; Kernsmith, Comartin, Craun, & Kernsmith, 2009). Furthermore, sex offender registration policies provide a system by which law enforcement agents can track the whereabouts of these criminals and potentially identify a pool of local suspects when new crimes are committed. Though public perception surveys have found very high support for sex offender registries (Levenson, Brannon, Fortney, & Baker, 2007; Pickett, Mancini, & Mears, 2013), few people seem to utilize registries with any regularity (Beck & Travis, 2004; Kernsmith et al., 2009). In one study of sexual assault cases from a victim advocacy center, it was found that less than 4 % of the abusers would have been found on a registry prior to the abusive incident (Craun, Simmons, & Reeves, 2011).

Sex offender laws have been inspired by the common belief that sex crime recidivism rates are exceedingly high (Fortney, Levenson, Brannon, & Baker, 2007; Meloy, Boatwright, & Curtis, 2012; Sample & Kadleck, 2008; Zgoba, 2004). Research indicates, however, that sex offense recidivism rates are lower than commonly believed (Bureau of Justice Statistics, 2003; Hanson & Bussiere, 1998; Hanson, Harris, Helmus, & Thornton, 2014; Hanson & Morton-Bourgon, 2005; Helmus, Hanson, Thornton, Babchishin, & Harris, 2012) and they are lower than recidivism rates in other crime categories (Bureau of Justice Statistics, 2002; Sample & Bray, 2006). As well, recent longitudinal research has found that sex offender recidivism risk decreases substantially over time as individuals remain in the community sex offense-free; after 16.5 years in the community without a new sex crime arrest, even high-risk sexual offenders are no more likely to be arrested for a new sex offense than nonsexual criminals, and low-risk sex offenders commit new sex crimes at rates similar to general criminal offenders (Hanson et al., 2014; Harris & Hanson, 2012).

Despite the pervasive fear of sex offenders, the reality is that sex crimes, like other crimes, have decreased by about 34 % over the past several decades (Finkelhor & Jones, 2006; Uniform Crime Report, 2012). Though the exact causes for the decrease in crime rates are difficult to identify, experts suggest that a number of societal factors have contributed to the change. These include longer prison sentences, more aggressive policing, enhancements in technology and surveillance, the economic stability of the 1990s and early 2000s, changing demographics with the aging of the US population, and other social dynamics related to norms and values (Finkelhor & Jones, 2006; Uggen & McElrath, 2013; Zimring, 2006). Nevertheless, concerns about recidivistic sexual violence have fueled the popularity of sex offender policies.

As stakeholders have become more aware of sex offenders living in our communities, ancillary laws aimed at preventing repeat victimization have also been implemented, such as residential restrictions, enhanced probationary supervision, and mandatory minimum sentencing (LaFond, 2005; Lamade, Gabriel, & Prentky, 2011; Levenson & D'Amora, 2007; Tabachnick & Klein, 2011; Zgoba, 2004). A crucial question is the extent to which sex offender policies in general, and SORN laws more specifically, have achieved their goal of reducing sex offense recidivism. Most studies thus far have not detected a significant decline in sexual reoffending that can be attributed to the enactment of such policies.

Effectiveness of Sex Offender Registration and Notification Policies

At this time, due to the relatively recent implementation of these laws, the empirical research is still in a nascent stage. Moreover, there are many methodological complexities faced by researchers when conducting sex crime policy analysis. For example, low recidivism base rates, the confound of multiple types of sex offender policies enacted within short time frames, challenges obtaining valid recidivism data, and the need for long follow-up periods all contribute to the challenges of determining the impact of these laws. Moreover, though national guidelines exist, the SORN policy in each state is idiosyncratic, complicating efforts to conduct national sex offender policy research (Harris, 2011).

About two dozen studies have been conducted to evaluate the impact of SORN, and most involve one of two methodologies: group comparisons of sex offenders required to register and those who are not and trend analyses of sex crime rates over time. Two studies that have detected reductions in sex crime recidivism as a result of SORN were conducted in Minnesota and Washington (Duwe & Donnay, 2008; Washington State Institute for Public Policy, 2005). Importantly, both states use empirically derived risk assessment instruments to classify offenders, and they limit public notification only to those who pose the greatest threat to community safety. In Minnesota, the sexual rearrest rate of the notification group (5 %) was significantly lower than both the prenotification group (35 % of those matched on risk but released before the law went into effect) and the nonnotification group (13 % of lower-risk offenders not subject to disclosure) (Duwe & Donnay, 2008). After controlling for generally decreasing crime trends, researchers in Washington found a significant decline in sex offense recidivism (from 5 to 1 %) after 1997 when SORN laws were passed in that state (Washington State Institute for Public Policy, 2005).

While the authors acknowledged that they were unable to account for other possible explanations for this reduction (e.g., more severe sentencing guidelines, or improved probationary supervision), they concluded that community notification has likely contributed in some way to reductions in sexual reoffending.

Most research, however, has not detected significant decreases in sex crime rates that can be attributed to SORN policies. In South Carolina, 6064 sex offenders convicted between 1990 and 2004 were followed while controlling for time at risk, and registration status did not predict sexual recidivism (Letourneau, Levenson, Bandyopadhyay, Sinha, & Armstrong, 2010). In New Jersey, researchers compared 250 sex offenders released before Megan's Law went into effect with 300 sex offenders released after the passage of the law, and no significant differences were found in sex offense recidivism, the time it took for sex offenders to reoffend, or the number of victims (Zgoba, Veysey, & Dalessandro, 2010). The authors followed up with a trend analysis, and though a significant decrease was seen in aggregated sexual offense recidivism, they cautioned that variations in different county rates precluded a conclusion that statewide reductions were attributable to Megan's Law implementation (Veysey, Zgoba, & Dalessandro, 2008). Though SORN status was not a significant predictor of sexual recidivism in New Jersey, sex offenders scoring as high risk on risk assessment instruments were more likely to commit future criminal offenses, including sex offenses, and to do so more quickly following release from prison, suggesting that empirically based risk assessment tools are a valuable component of sex offender management (Tewksbury, Jennings, & Zgoba, 2012).

Multistate studies have produced mixed results, as variations in research methodologies and SORN policy characteristics can contribute to different results reported across studies. A time-series analysis investigated the impact of SORN laws on sexual assault rates in ten states (Vasquez, Maddan, & Walker, 2008), with California showing a significant increase in rape rates following implementation of registration, while Hawaii, Idaho, and Ohio had significant decreases in rape rates, and the remaining six states (Arkansas, Connecticut, Nebraska, Nevada, Oklahoma, and West Virginia) showed nonsignificant trends toward reductions in sex crime. The authors concluded that SORN policies did not appear to systematically reduce sex crime rates.

An analysis examining data from over 300,000 sex crimes in 15 states found that while registration appeared to decrease the rate of recidivistic sex offenses, public notification did not (Prescott & Rockoff, 2011). Using Uniform Crime Report (UCR) data from 1985 to 2003, Agan (2011) did not find a significant decline in arrest rates of rape or sexual abuse after registration was implemented, or after public Internet access to registry information was allowed. Agan also examined Bureau of Justice Statistics (BJS) data tracking individual sex offenders after their release from prison in 1994 and determined that having to register as a sex offender did not lead to significant reductions in sex offense recidivism (Agan, 2011). Using UCR data for the years 1970–2002, Ackerman, Sacks, and Greenberg (2012) investigated the impact of SORN legislation and reported that these laws have not resulted in dramatic declines in forcible rapes. Several scholars have concluded that the accumulation of empirical evidence strongly suggests that the fiscal and social costs of these laws outweigh their benefits (Ackerman, Sacks & Greenberg, 2012; Zgoba, Witt, Dalessandro, & Veysey, 2009).

Other recent investigations have raised questions about the utility and validity of the federally mandated Adam Walsh Act tier system. In Florida, New Jersey, Minnesota, and South Carolina (Zgoba et al., 2012) and in New York (Freeman & Sandler, 2010), the AWA classification categories did a poor job of identifying potential recidivists, and researchers concluded that empirically derived procedures (such as Static-99) were better for screening sex offenders into relative risk categories to establish monitoring requirements. When AWA was implemented in Ohio and Oklahoma, the retroactive reclassification process redistributed a significant majority of registrants from lower tier levels to higher ones, contradicting empirical evidence suggesting that the highest risk of sexual reoffense is concentrated among a much smaller group of offenders (Harris et al., 2010).

Finally, the latest research on long-term sex offense recidivism has indicated that risk is highest during the first few years after release and declines substantially over time as individuals live in the community offense-free (Hanson et al., 2014). The findings suggested that after about 16.5 years in the community without a new sex crime arrest, even high-risk sexual offenders (defined by Static-99R scores) are no more likely to be arrested for a new sex offense than nonsexual criminals, and sex offenders scoring below zero on the Static-99R had sexual rearrest rates that were slightly lower than those of nonsexual criminals (Harris & Hanson, 2012). Thus, policies 25-year or lifetime registration requirements are not evidence based and may be unnecessary for many offenders, and resources might be better spent on more intensive supervision and reintegration assistance in the early years of reentry (Hanson et al., 2014).

Residence Restriction Policies and Their Effectiveness

Public access to registries has made citizens more aware of sex offenders living in communities, inciting a cascade of residential housing restrictions. These laws prevent sex offenders from living within close proximity to places where children are likely to be found. There are currently 30 state laws designating where sex offenders can live (Meloy, Miller, & Curtis, 2008). The first state law, passed in 1995 in Florida and applying only to sex offenders on probation and with minor victims, created 1000 ft buffer zones around schools, parks, playgrounds, daycare centers, and other places where children congregate. By 2004, there were 15 state statutes, but within 2 years of the 2005 murder of 9-year-old Jessica Lunsford by a convicted sex offender in Florida, the number of states with housing restrictions doubled. The most common exclusion zones are 1000–2000 ft around venues such as schools, parks, playgrounds, and daycare centers. Some laws include other facilities such as arcades, amusement parks, movie theaters, youth sports facilities, school bus stops, and libraries (Meloy et al., 2008).

Too abundant to count are municipal ordinances passed by cities, towns, and counties which restrict where sex offenders can live. The first local ordinance in the

USA was passed in Miami Beach in June 2005, modeled after zoning laws that prohibit adult establishments (e.g., strip clubs and adult bookstores) from operating within a certain distance from schools. Similar ordinances can be found in most states, even those without statewide laws, and often expand restricted areas to 2500 ft (almost a half mile) surrounding places frequented by children. When one municipality enacts such a law, a domino effect often follows, with surrounding towns and counties passing similar ordinances to avert exiled sex offenders from migrating to their communities.

Sex offender residence restrictions (SORR) are based on the ostensibly logical hypothesis that by requiring child molesters to live far from places where children congregate, the probability of repeat sex crimes can be lowered. The extant research, however, finds no support for the proposition that sex offenders who live close to child-oriented settings are more likely to reoffend. In fact, research indicates that where sex offenders live is not a significant contributing factor to reoffending behavior.

Residential proximity to schools and daycares is not empirically associated with recidivism. Zandbergen, Levenson, and Hart (2010) mapped the locations of recidivists and non-recidivists ($N = 330$) relative to schools and daycares in Florida. Those who lived closer to schools or daycare centers did not reoffend more frequently than those who lived farther away. There was no significant correlation between sexual recidivism and the number of feet the offender lived from school. The recidivists and non-recidivists were matched on relevant risk factors (prior arrests, age, marital status, predator status), and after controlling for risk, proximity variables were not significant predictors of recidivism (Zandbergen et al., 2010). Similarly, in Colorado, the addresses of sex offense recidivists and non-recidivists were found to be randomly distributed within the geographical area with no evidence that recidivists lived closer to schools or daycare centers (Colorado Department of Public Safety, 2004).

In Jacksonville, Florida, researchers investigated the effects of a 2500 ft SORR law on sex crime rates and sex offense recidivism (Nobles, Levenson, & Youstin, 2012). Using a quasi-experimental design, recidivism rates were compared before and after the SORR law was passed, and no significant differences were found. As well, a trend analysis revealed no significant changes in sex crime arrest patterns over time. The authors concluded that the city's residence restriction ordinance had no meaningful effect on sex crime rates or sex offender recidivism and that these laws did not appear to be a successful strategy for preventing repeat sexual violence.

The Iowa Department of Criminal and Juvenile Justice Planning studied the effect of Iowa's 2000 ft residence restriction law that went into effect in August of 2005 (Blood, Watson, & Stageberg, 2008). The researchers did not observe a downward trend in the number of sex offenses following the passage of the law and concluded that Iowa's residence law "does not seem to have led to fewer charges or convictions, indicating that there probably have not been fewer child victims" (Blood et al., 2008, p. 10). Notably, an analysis of 224 recidivistic sex offenses in Minnesota led researchers to conclude that residential restriction laws would not have prevented even one reoffense (Duwe, Donnay, & Tewksbury, 2008). Most of the cases involving minors were committed not by strangers but by individuals who were well acquainted with their victims, such as parents, caretakers, paramours, babysitters, or friends of the family. The repeat offender was a neighbor of the victim in only about 4 % of the cases. Predatory assaults that occurred within a mile of the offender's residence typically involved adult victims, and none of the crimes took place in or near a school, daycare center, or park.

Other scholars concurred that the majority (67 %) of New Jersey offenders met victims in private locations while relatively few (4.4 %) met victims in the types of locations normally identified as off-limits by residential restriction laws (Colombino, Mercado, Levenson, & Jeglic, 2011). Not surprisingly, sex offenders rarely encountered their victims in public locations where children congregate, and the authors pointed out that policies emphasizing residential proximity to schools and parks ignore the empirical reality of sexual abuse patterns. It was found, however, that offenders who had met their index victim in a restricted or child-oriented venue were more likely to commit a repeat sex crime. In other words, those who met their victims at bus stops, parks, camps, carnivals, boardwalks, and hospitals were significantly more likely to sexually reoffend (although only eight offenders recidivated) and seemed more prone to engage in predatory patterns designed to seek out children with whom they were not previously acquainted. Since residence restrictions regulate only where an offender sleeps at night, alternative policies such as loitering laws might be especially helpful for such offenders. Restricting their ability to visit places where vulnerable victims may be present would be a more useful strategy than restricting their residential proximity to such venues, which fails to address their ability to travel to an offense location (Colombino et al., 2011).

In summary, the research literature provides no support for the assumption that sexual reoffending can be prevented by prohibiting sex offenders from residing near places where children commonly congregate. For the minority of sex offenders who display predatory patterns of seeking out minor victims in public settings, laws or case management strategies that forbid such offenders to visit such locations might be more effective than laws designating where they can live. Sex offenders do not abuse children because they live near schools, but rather they take advantage of opportunities to cultivate trusting relationships with children and their families to create opportunities for sexual abuse to take place.

Unintended Consequences of Sex Offender Management Policies

The challenges encountered by criminal offenders when they reenter communities after incarceration are even more pronounced for registered sex offenders. The unique stigma of SORN and the ways these laws can obstruct community reintegration and adjustment are well documented. Sex offenders in many different states report employment obstacles, housing disruption, relationship loss, threats and harassment, physical assault, and property damage (Levenson & Cotter, 2005a; Levenson, D'Amora, & Hern, 2007; Mercado, Alvarez, & Levenson, 2008; Sample

& Streveler, 2003; Tewksbury, 2004, 2005; Tewksbury & Lees, 2006; Zevitz & Farkas, 2000). Psychosocial stressors such as shame, embarrassment, isolation, depression, and hopelessness were also commonly reported by sex offenders as byproducts of public registration. A survey of 584 family members of registered sex offenders across the USA revealed that they too were profoundly impacted by these laws (Levenson & Tewksbury, 2009; Tewksbury & Levenson, 2009). Employment problems experienced by the RSO and resulting financial hardships were identified as the most pressing issue for family members. Family members living with an RSO also reported threats and harassment by neighbors, and some children of RSOs revealed stigmatizing behavior by teachers and classmates.

The US Supreme Court upheld SORN laws in Alaska and Connecticut in 2003, ruling that the laws were not punitive, but regulatory, and that they did not represent ex post facto punishment. Over the past 10 years, however, as laws have been enhanced both at the federal level (Adam Walsh Act) and by states, they have tied to registration an expanding set of restrictions around employment, travel, and housing and an increased number of complex requirements for compliance. As well, penalties for registration violations are severe and can carry a prison term of up to 10 years.

Since the literature points to criminality and self-regulation deficits as robust predictors of both sexual and nonsexual recidivism (Hanson & Morton-Bourgon, 2005), it might seem reasonable for lawmaker to assume that failure to register (FTR) reflects an antisocial orientation which could increase the threat of subsequent sexual and nonsexual criminal behavior. It has been pointed out, however, that most sex offenders arrested for FTR are not willful violators and that they are easily located and have not absconded (Duwe & Donnay, 2010; Harris, Levenson, & Ackerman, 2012; Levenson, Ackerman, & Harris, 2013; Levenson, Letourneau, Armstrong, & Zgoba, 2010; Levenson, Sandler, & Freeman, 2012; Zgoba & Levenson, 2012). Some sex offenders might indeed be inclined to purposely abscond to avoid the stigma and collateral consequences of sex offender registration. Most, however, may carelessly disregard their duty to update registration information or violate their requirements inadvertently, but remain in their known locations despite their lapse. The registration process and its rules have become increasingly complex, and Duwe and Donnay (2010) noted that lower education was associated with a greater likelihood of FTR, suggesting that complicated reporting requirements may be challenging for offenders with limited intellectual resources.

Residential restrictions, which are usually tied to registration status, create particularly profound barriers to offender reintegration and also create unintended consequences for communities (Levenson, 2008; Levenson, Ackerman, Socia, & Harris, 2013). Surveys revealed that housing restriction laws frequently forced sex offenders to relocate, that they were unable to return to their homes after incarceration, that they were not permitted to live with family members, or that they experienced a landlord refusing to rent to them or to renew a lease (Levenson, 2008; Levenson & Cotter, 2005b; Levenson & Hern, 2007; Mercado et al., 2008). Many indicated that affordable housing is less available due to limits on where they can live and that they are forced to live farther away from employment, public transportation, social services, and mental health treatment. Young adults seemed to be especially impacted by these laws; age was significantly inversely correlated with being unable to live with family and having difficulties securing affordable housing (Levenson, 2008; Levenson & Hern, 2007). Family members of RSOs also reported that residential restriction laws created housing disruption for them; larger buffer zones led to an increased chance of a housing crisis (Levenson & Tewksbury, 2009).

Homelessness and transience are other problems that result from residence restrictions. A compelling body of evidence illustrates how residential restrictions can diminish housing options for sex offenders. In Orlando Florida, it was found that 99 % of all residential dwellings are located within 2500 ft of schools, parks, daycare centers, or school bus stops (Zandbergen & Hart, 2006). The vast majority of residential territory in Nebraska and New Jersey is also located within 2500 ft of a school (Bruell, Swatt, & Sample, 2008; Chajewski & Mercado, 2009; Zgoba, Levenson, & McKee, 2009). Affordable housing is especially impacted, since less affluent areas tend to be more densely populated, and therefore, homes are in closer proximity to places frequented by children (Levenson, Ackerman, Socia et al., 2013). Of nearly one million residential parcels studied in Miami-Dade County, Florida, only about 4 % of residential units were compliant with overlapping state laws and local ordinances, and only 1 % had a monthly rental cost of $1250 or less (Zandbergen & Hart, 2009). In Nebraska, average home values were significantly lower within a buffer zone of 2000 ft than outside the buffer zone (Bruell et al., 2008), and in Ohio, compliant addresses were also more likely to be located in less affordable census tracts (Red Bird, 2009).

Researchers studied the entire population of registered sex offenders living in the community in Florida ($n = 23,523$) and found significantly higher proportions of transient sex offenders in counties with residential proximity zones (Levenson, Ackerman, Socia et al., 2013). It was the combination of extensive buffer zones, higher population density, and more costly rental prices that created a "perfect storm" for sex offender transience (p. 20). Sex offenders were more likely than the general population in Florida to become homeless, and the researchers cautioned that when implementing sex offender management policies, lawmakers should consider transience as an unintended negative consequence that undermines the very purpose of sex offender registries (Levenson, Ackerman, Socia et al., 2013).

When prisoners are released from incarceration, they often seek lodging with relatives, but strict housing laws can preclude such options for sex offenders. Unable to reside with family members and without the financial resources to pay for security deposits and rent payments, some sex offenders face homelessness. Ironically, housing instability is consistently associated with criminal recidivism and absconding, and transient sex offenders are more likely to abscond from registration than probation (Levenson, Ackerman & Harris, 2013). In Georgia, every time a parolee moved, the risk of rearrest increased by 25 % (Meredith, Speir, & Johnson, 2007). Residential instability was a robust predictor of absconding in a study of California parolees (F. P. Williams, McShane, & Dolny, 2000), and in a national sample of 2030 offenders, those who moved multiple times during probation were almost twice as likely as stable probationers to have some sort of disciplinary hearing (Schulenberg, 2007). In New Zealand, unstable housing, unemployment, and limited social support were found to predict sexual recidivism (Willis & Grace, 2009; Willis & Grace, 2008). Some prosecutors and victim advocates have publicly denounced residence restrictions, cautioning that the transience created by housing restrictions undermines the validity of sex offender registries and makes it more difficult to track and supervise sex offenders (Iowa County Attorneys Association, 2006; NAESV, 2006).

A final concern about SORR laws is that they may cause offenders to cluster in the few locations where compliant housing is available. Clustering is defined as a disproportional number of sex offenders in a small geographical area. For instance, a task force in Broward County, Florida, found that 8 % of the county's sex offenders lived within a one-square mile area (less than 1 % of the county's land), raising concerns about the safety of children living in that neighborhood (Broward County Commission, 2009). According to Socia (2011), when clustering was measured as the rate of RSOs compared to the population in upstate New York, RSO clustering was associated with modest increases of recidivistic sex crimes, but only for sex offenders with adult victims. On the other hand, in Indianapolis, the number of RSOs in an area was not predictive of a higher number of reported sex crimes (Stucky & Ottensmann, 2014). RSOs tend to cluster in impoverished neighborhoods with lower degrees of social control and higher levels of social disorganization, creating concerns that such communities are less able to provide protective measures for vulnerable children (Socia & Stamatel, 2012; Tewksbury & Mustaine, 2008; Tewksbury & Mustaine, 2006). Whether the result of residence restrictions, the limited ability for offenders to find affordable and available housing elsewhere, or because residents are simply unable to keep RSOs out, the dense clustering of RSOs in limited areas does not appear to be a desirable policy outcome.

Implications for Evidence-Based Sex Offender Management Policy

It is estimated that there are currently about three quarters of a million registered sex offenders in the USA (Ackerman et al., 2011; Ackerman, Levenson, & Harris, 2012; National Center for Missing and Exploited Children, 2012). As those numbers continue to grow and more sex offenders are publicly identified within online registries, law enforcement resources are spread thin, and the ability of the public to distinguish truly dangerous offenders is diluted. Enormous resources are needed to enforce registration compliance and track violators, despite evidence suggesting that failing to register as a sex offender is not predictive of sexual reoffending (Duwe & Donnay, 2010; Levenson, Ackerman & Harris, 2013; Levenson et al., 2010).

Public registries, if used, should be reserved for high-risk offenders. In this way, the public can be better informed specifically about pedophilic, predatory, repetitive, or violent sex offenders likely to commit new sex crimes. At the same time, collateral consequences could be minimized for lower-risk offenders reintegrating into society and attempting to become productive, law-abiding citizens. The use of empirically derived assessments based on factors known to correlate with recidivism should be used to identify those who pose the greatest threat to public safety. The Adam Walsh Act currently requires states to implement an offense-based classification system even though empirically derived risk assessment has demonstrated better utility than AWA tiers in identifying offenders who are likely to reoffend (Freeman & Sandler, 2009; Zgoba et al., 2012).

As more people are placed on registries for long durations (25 years or life) with few mechanisms available for removal from the registry, the average age of registered sex offenders will continue to increase. This anticipated trend contradicts research indicating that risk declines with age for all criminals (including most sex offenders) and sex offense recidivism is especially rare with advanced age (Hanson, 2002; Helmus, Thornton, Hanson, & Babchishin, 2011; Thornton, 2006). Over time the sex offender population will include an increasing proportion of elderly individuals who probably pose quite a low risk for reoffense. Furthermore, registration durations of 25 years to life contradict empirical evidence that risk declines significantly with increased time spent in the community offense-free and that low-risk sex offenders are no more likely to be arrested for a new sex crime than general criminal offenders (Hanson et al., 2014; Harris & Hanson, 2012; Harris, Phenix, Hanson, & Thornton, 2003). Thus, the emphasis on registration compliance over longer registration periods will likely create an inefficient distribution of resources without contributing meaningfully to community safety.

Sex offenders do not molest children because they live near schools. They are able to abuse children by cultivating relationships with youngsters and their families, gaining trust and familiarity which creates opportunities for sexual assault. Thus far, there is no empirical support at all for residential restriction policies, and in fact, a growing body of literature strongly demonstrates a negative impact on housing availability when residence restrictions are in effect. Housing instability exacerbates risk factors for recidivism, and therefore, residence restrictions are apt to create many more problems than they solve. Though intuitively sensible, they regulate only where sex offenders sleep at night and do nothing to prevent sex offenders from frequenting child-oriented venues during the day. For this reason, jurisdictions should consider "loitering zones" in lieu of residence restrictions, which would more effectively prevent sex offenders from hanging around in places where children congregate.

Sex offender management policies are expensive, and lawmakers should invest in evidence-based policies rather than those that demonstrate negligible public safety benefit. Sexual assault is a prevalent social problem, and prevention strategies should reflect not only public opinion but empirical demonstration of effectiveness. Resources spent on policies that fail to enhance community safety take funding away from more promising programs as well as services for victims and prevention initiatives. A paradigm shift toward evidence-based case management might prove more efficient than one-size-fits-all policies in achieving the important goal of preventing repeat sexual violence.

American social policies have been largely reactive to problems of child maltreatment, strongly emphasizing the role of offender punishment and child placement rather than primary prevention. There is a compelling research literature indicating that children who experience early adversity are at increased risk for polyvictimization and subsequently for more pervasive trauma symptoms (Finkelhor, Turner, Hamby, & Ormrod, 2011). As well, children who experience chronic maltreatment and family dysfunction are more likely than non-abused youngsters to become the addicts and criminal offenders of the future (DeHart, 2009; DeHart, Lynch, Belknap, Dass-Brailsford, & Green, in press; Harlow, 1999; Mersky, Topitzes, & Reynolds, 2012; Topitzes, Mersky, & Reynolds, 2012; Widom & Maxfield, 2001). There is little resistance to funding criminal justice initiatives, yet prevention programs and social services are generally among the first to be cut from American legislative budgets. However, it is crucial for victims of child maltreatment to receive therapy and counseling, for abusive parents to receive intervention services, and for the criminal justice community to recognize that sexual and general self-regulation problems in adulthood are often symptomatic of childhood adversity (Baglivio et al., 2014; Levenson, Willis, & Prescott, 2014). Investing in a comprehensive array of prevention and early intervention services for abused children and at-risk families is an important step in halting the cycle of interpersonal violence in our communities (Anda, Butchart, Felitti, & Brown, 2010; Baglivio et al., 2014; Levenson et al., 2014).

Sociologist Robert Merton (1936) cautioned that social policies, even when well intentioned, can sometimes lead to paradoxical results to which he referred as the "law of unintended consequences." Merton observed that when communities overreact to a perceived threat and seek to curtail that threat by drastically altering the social order, unexpected outcomes can inevitably result. As they endeavor to achieve desired goals, advocates of social change may fail to anticipate the potential negative consequences of a law. Collective values also play a role in social movements, which are often motivated by popular concepts of good and evil that can obscure the more detrimental effects of change (Merton, 1936). For all of these reasons, the unintended consequences facilitated by sex offender policies are likely to be ignored by lawmakers and citizens hoping to prevent repeat sexual violence. Those who point out counterproductive effects, especially as they relate to the reintegration of sex offenders, are often dismissed as offender advocates who are unconcerned about the safety of children.

Some scholars have opined that sex offender policies are designed to accomplish both instrumental and symbolic objectives and that understanding both is essential in the continuing dialogue about SORN laws and prevention of sexual violence (Sample, Evans, & Anderson, 2011). While most empirical investigations have not detected instrumental effects such as reduced reoffending (Ackerman, Sacks & Greenberg, 2012; Agan, 2011; Letourneau et al., 2010; Sandler, Freeman, & Socia, 2008; Vasquez et al., 2008; Zgoba, Witt et al., 2009) or increased community protection behaviors (Anderson & Sample, 2008; Kernsmith et al., 2009), SORN policies do accomplish important symbolic goals. Policy enactment can serve to inspire and reinforce social solidarity by uniting against a common enemy (Roots, 2004). These laws send a clear message that sexual victimization will not be tolerated and that politicians are willing to address public safety concerns (Sample et al., 2011;

Sample & Kadleck, 2008). Sample et al. (2011) speculated that symbolic policies might achieve instrumental effects over time—perhaps measured by a wider range of positive outcomes beyond recidivism—and that in the cost/benefit analysis, the symbolic expression of zero tolerance for sexual violence will always outweigh offender rights, fiscal considerations, and empirical testing.

But policy analysis requires a continuous process of evaluation that measures progress toward intended goals as well as unanticipated outcomes that might prove contrary to the best interests of the community. Levenson and D'Amora (2007) opined that ignoring evidence is analogous to Hans Christian Andersen's story of the *Emperor's New Clothes* in which the king paraded through town nude, fooled by gypsies into wearing invisible clothes that purportedly could be seen by only an enlightened few. Similarly, in the absence of compelling evidence indicating that these policies reduce sexual reoffending, attention should be paid to mounting evidence of reintegration obstacles fostered by these laws. In fact, the unintended consequences of these laws might undermine their very purpose, which is to track and monitor sex offenders.

Social policies should be based on scientific data and are most likely to be successful when they incorporate research findings into their development and implementation. A more reasoned approach (Tabachnick & Klein, 2011) to sex offender policies would utilize empirically derived risk assessment tools to create classification systems that apply more aggressive monitoring and tighter restrictions to those who pose the greatest threat to public safety. In this way, laws could more efficiently identify and target higher-risk offenders, resulting in a more cost-effective allocation of fiscal and personnel resources. As well, in the absence of an empirical relationship between residential location and reoffending, sex offender residence restrictions should be abolished as an untenable approach to sex offender management. By tailoring application of these laws to risks and needs, collateral consequences of community protection policies could be minimized, and sex offenders could be better enabled to engage in a law-abiding and prosocial lifestyle. Most sex offenders will ultimately be returned to the community, and when they are, it behooves us to facilitate a reintegrative approach that relies on empirical research to inform community protection strategies. After all, when people have nothing to lose, they begin to behave accordingly.

References

Ackerman, A. R., Harris, A. J., Levenson, J. S., & Zgoba, K. (2011). Who are the people in your neighborhood? A descriptive analysis of individuals on public sex offender registries. *International Journal of Psychiatry and Law, 34*, 149–159.

Ackerman, A. R., Levenson, J. S., & Harris, A. J. (2012). How many sex offenders really live among us? Adjusted counts and population rates in five U.S. states. *Journal of Crime and Justice,* doi:10.1080/0735648X.2012.666407.

Ackerman, A. R., Sacks, M., & Greenberg, D. F. (2012). Legislation targeting sex offenders: Are recent policies effective in reducing rape? *Justice Quarterly, 29*(6), 858–887.

Agan, A. Y. (2011). Sex Offender Registries: Fear without Function? *Journal of Law and Economics, 54*(1), 207–239.

Anda, R. F., Butchart, A., Felitti, V. J., & Brown, D. W. (2010). Building a framework for global surveillance of the public health implications of adverse childhood experiences. *American Journal of Preventive Medicine, 39*(1), 93.

Anderson, A. L., & Sample, L. (2008). Public awareness and action resulting from sex offender community notification laws. *Criminal Justice Policy Review, 19*(4), 371–396.

Baglivio, M. T., Epps, N., Swartz, K., Huq, M. S., Sheer, A., & Hardt, N. S. (2014). The Prevalence of Adverse Childhood Experiences (ACE) in the Lives of Juvenile Offenders. *Journal of Juvenile Justice, 3*(2), 1–23.

Beck, V. S., & Travis, L. F. (2004). Sex offender notification and protective behavior. *Violence and Victims, 19*(3), 289–302.

Blood, P., Watson, L., & Stageberg, P. (2008). *State legislation monitoring report*. Des Moines, IA: Criminal and Juvenile Justice Planning.

Broward County Commission. (2009). *Final Report: Sexual offender & sexual predator residence task force*. Fort Lauderdale, FL: Broward County Commission.

Bruell, C., Swatt, M., & Sample, L. (2008). *Potential consequences of sex offender residency restriction laws: Housing availability and offender displacement*. Paper presented at the American Society of Criminology, St. Louis, MO.

Bureau of Justice Statistics. (2002). Recidivism of prisoners released in 1994 (NCJ 193427). Retrieved from Washington, DC.

Bureau of Justice Statistics. (2003). *Recidivism of sex offenders released from prison in 1994*. Washington, DC: U.S. Department of Justice.

Chajewski, M., & Mercado, C. C. (2009). An Evaluation of Sex Offender Residency Restriction Functioning in Town, County, and City-Wide Jurisdictions. *Criminal Justice Policy Review, 20*(1), 44–61.

Colombino, N., Mercado, C. C., Levenson, J. S., & Jeglic, E. L. (2011). Preventing sexual violence: Can examination of offense location inform sex crime policy? *International Journal of Psychiatry and Law,* doi:10.1016/j.ijlp.2011.04.002.

Colorado Department of Public Safety. (2004). *Report on safety issues raised by living arrangements for and location of sex offenders in the community*. Denver, CO: Sex Offender Management Board.

Connecticut Dept. of Public Safety v. Doe, (01-1231) (U.S. Supreme Court 2003).

Craun, S. W., Simmons, C. A., & Reeves, K. (2011). Percentage of named offenders on the registry at the time of the assault: Reports from sexual assault survivors. *Violence Against Women, 17*(11), 1374–1382.

DeHart, D. (2009). *Polyvictimization among girls in the juvenile justice system: Manifestations and associations to delinquency (Report No 22860)*. Washington, DC: US Department of Justice.

DeHart, D., Lynch, S., Belknap, J., Dass-Brailsford, P., & Green, B. (in press). Life history models of female offending: The roles of serious mental illness and trauma in women's pathways to jail. *Psychology of Women Quarterly,* doi:10.1177/0361684313494357

Duwe, G., & Donnay, W. (2008). The impact of Megan's Law on sex offender recidivism: The Minnesota experience. *Criminology, 46*(2), 411–446.

Duwe, G., & Donnay, W. (2010). The effects of failure to register on sex offender recidivism. *Criminal Justice and Behavior, 37*(5), 520–536.

Duwe, G., Donnay, W., & Tewksbury, R. (2008). Does residential proximity matter? A geographic analysis of sex offense recidivism. *Criminal Justice and Behavior, 35*(4), 484–504.

Finkelhor, D., & Jones, L. (2006). Why have child maltreatment and child victimization declined? *Journal of Social Issues, 62*(4), 685–716.

Finkelhor, D., Hammer, H., & Sedlak, A. J. (2008). *Sexually assaulted children: National Estimates and Characteristics*. Retrieved from Washington, DC.

Finkelhor, D., Turner, H. A., Hamby, S. L., & Ormrod, R. (2011). *Polyvictimization: Children's exposure to multiple types of violence, crime, and abuse*. Des Moines, IA: US Department of Justice, Office of Justice Programs, Office of Juvenile Justice and Deliquency Prevention.

Fortney, T., Levenson, J. S., Brannon, Y., & Baker, J. (2007). Myths and facts about sex offenders: Implications for practice and public policy. *Sex Offender Treatment, 2*(1), 1–17. Retrieved from http://www.sexual-offender-treatment.org/53.0.html.

Freeman, N. J., & Sandler, J. C. (2009). The Adam Walsh Act: A false sense of security or an effective public policy initiative? *Criminal Justice Policy Review, Online First,* doi:10.1177/0887403409338565, http://cjp.sagepub.com.

Freeman, N. J., & Sandler, J. C. (2010). The Adam Walsh Act: A false sense of security or an effective public policy initiative? *Criminal Justice Policy Review, 21*(1), 31–49.

Hanson, R. K. (2002). Recidivism and age: Follow-up data from 4,673 sexual offenders. *Journal of Interpersonal Violence, 17*(10), 1046–1062.

Hanson, R. K., & Bussiere, M. T. (1998). Predicting relapse: A meta-analysis of sexual offender recidivism studies. *Journal of Consulting and Clinical Psychology, 66*(2), 348–362.

Hanson, R. K., Harris, A. J., Helmus, L., & Thornton, D. (2014). High-risk sex offenders may not be high risk forever. *Journal of Interpersonal Violence,* doi:0886260514526062.

Hanson, R. K., & Morton-Bourgon, K. (2005). The characteristics of persistent sexual offenders: A meta-analysis of recidivism studies. *Journal of Consulting and Clinical Psychology, 73*(6), 1154–1163.

Harlow, C. W. (1999). *Prior abuse reported by inmates and probationers.* Rockville, MD: U.S. Department of Justice.

Harris, A. J. (2011). SORNA in the post-deadline era: What's the next move? *Sex Offender Law Report, 12*(6), 81–86.

Harris, A. J. R., & Hanson, R. K. (2012, October). *When is a sex offender no longer a sex offender?* Paper presented at the 31st Annual Research and Treatment Conference of the Association for the Treatment of Sexual Abusers, Denver, CO.

Harris, A. J., Levenson, J. S., & Ackerman, A. R. (2012). Registered sex offenders in the United States: Behind the numbers. *Crime and Delinquency,* doi:10.1177/0011128712443179.

Harris, A. J. R., Phenix, A., Hanson, R. K., & Thornton, D. (2003). *Static-99 coding rules.* Retrieved October 10, 2008, from http://www.static99.org/pdfdocs/static-99-coding-rules_e.pdf.

Harris, A. J., Lobanov-Rostovsky, C., & Levenson, J. S. (2010). Widening the Net: The effects of transitioning to the Adam Walsh Act classification system. *Criminal Justice and Behavior, 37*(5), 503–519.

Helmus, L., Hanson, R. K., Thornton, D., Babchishin, K. M., & Harris, A. J. (2012). Absolute Recidivism Rates Predicted By Static-99R and Static-2002R Sex Offender Risk Assessment Tools Vary Across Samples A Meta-Analysis. *Criminal Justice and Behavior, 39*(9), 1148–1171.

Helmus, L., Thornton, D., Hanson, R. K., & Babchishin, K. M. (2011). Improving the predictive accuracy of static-99 and static-2002 with older sex offenders: Revised age weights. *Sexual Abuse: Journal of Research and Treatment,* doi:10.1177/1079063211409951

Iowa County Attorneys Association. (2006). *Statement on sex offender residency restrictions in Iowa.* Des Moines, IA: Author.

Kernsmith, P. D., Comartin, E., Craun, S. W., & Kernsmith, R. M. (2009). The relationship bewteen sex offender registry utilization and awareness. *Sexual Abuse: A Journal of Research and Treatment, 21*(2), 181–193.

LaFond, J. Q. (2005). *Preventing sexual violence: How society should cope with sex offenders.* Washington, DC: American Psychological Association.

Lamade, R., Gabriel, A., & Prentky, R. (2011). Optimizing risk mitigation in management of sexual offenders: A structural model. *International Journal of Law and Psychiatry, 34*(3), 217–225.

Letourneau, E., Levenson, J. S., Bandyopadhyay, D., Sinha, D., & Armstrong, K. (2010). Effects of South Carolina's sex offender registration and notification policy on adult recidivism. *Criminal Justice Policy Review, 21*(4), 435–458.

Levenson, J. S. (2008). Collateral consequences of sex offender residence restrictions. *Criminal Justice Studies, 21*(2), 153–166.

Levenson, J. S., Ackerman, A. R., Socia, K. M., & Harris, A. J. (2013). Where for art thou? Transient sex offenders and residence restrictions. *Criminal Justice Policy Review,* doi:0887403413512326.

Levenson, J. S., Ackerman, A. R., & Harris, A. J. (2013). Catch me if you can: An analysis of fugitive sex offenders. *Sexual Abuse: Journal of Research and Treatment*, doi:10.1177/1079063213480820).

Levenson, J. S., Brannon, Y., Fortney, T., & Baker, J. (2007). Public perceptions about sex offenders and community protection policies. *Analyses of Social Issues and Public Policy, 7*(1), 1–25.

Levenson, J. S., & Cotter, L. P. (2005a). The effect of Megan's Law on sex offender reintegration. *Journal of Contemporary Criminal Justice, 21*(1), 49–66.

Levenson, J. S., & Cotter, L. P. (2005b). The impact of sex offender residence restrictions: 1,000 feet from danger or one step from absurd? *International Journal of Offender Therapy and Comparative Criminology, 49*(2), 168–178.

Levenson, J. S., & D'Amora, D. A. (2007). Social policies designed to prevent sexual violence: The emperor's new clothes? *Criminal Justice Policy Review, 18*(2), 168–199.

Levenson, J. S., D'Amora, D. A., & Hern, A. (2007). Megan's Law and its impact on community re-entry for sex offenders. *Behavioral Sciences & the Law, 25*, 587–602.

Levenson, J. S., & Hern, A. (2007). Sex offender residence restrictions: Unintended consequences and community re-entry. *Justice Research and Policy, 9*(1), 59–73.

Levenson, J. S., Letourneau, E., Armstrong, K., & Zgoba, K. (2010). Failure to register as a sex offender: Is it associated with recidivism? *Justice Quarterly, 27*(3), 305–331.

Levenson, J. S., Sandler, J. C., & Freeman, N. J. (2012). Failure-to-register laws and public safety: An examination of risk factors and sex offense recidivism. *Law and Human Behavior*, doi:10.1037/b0000002.

Levenson, J. S., & Tewksbury, R. (2009). Collateral damage: Family members of registered sex offenders. *American Journal of Criminal Justice, 34*(1), 54–68.

Levenson, J. S., Willis, G., & Prescott, D. (2014). Adverse childhood experiences in the lives of male sex offenders and implications for trauma-informed care. *Sexual Abuse: A Journal of Research and Treatment*. doi:10.1177/1079063214535819.

Meloy, M., Miller, S. L., & Curtis, K. M. (2008). Making sense out of nonsense: The deconstruction of state-level sex offender residence restrictions. *American Journal of Criminal Justice, 33*(2), 209–222.

Meloy, M., Boatwright, J., & Curtis, K. (2012). Views from the top and bottom: Lawmakers and practitioners discuss sex offender laws. *American Journal of Criminal Justice*, pp. 1–23.

Mercado, C. C., Alvarez, S., & Levenson, J. S. (2008). The impact of specialized sex offender legislation on community re-entry. *Sexual Abuse: A Journal of Research and Treatment, 20*(2), 188–205.

Meredith, T., Speir, J., & Johnson, S. (2007). Developing and implementing automated risk assessments in parole. *Justice Research and Policy, 9*(1), 1–21.

Mersky, J. P., Topitzes, J., & Reynolds, A. J. (2012). Unsafe at any age: Linking childhood and adolescent maltreatment to delinquency and crime. *Journal of Research in Crime and Delinquency, 49*(2), 295–318.

Merton, R. K. (1936). The unanticipated consequences of purposive social action. *American Sociological Review, 1*(6), 894–904.

NAESV. (2006). Community management of convicted sex offenders: Registration, electronic monitoring, civil commitment, mandatory minimums, and residency restrictions. Retrieved April 2, 2006, from www.naesv.org.

National Center for Missing and Exploited Children. (2012). *Registered sex offenders in the United States*. Retrieved July 30, 2012, from http://www.missingkids.com/en_US/documents/sex-offender-map.pdf.

Nobles, M. R., Levenson, J. S., & Youstin, T. J. (2012). Effectiveness of residence restrictions in preventing sex offense recidivism. *Crime and Delinquency, 58*(4), 491–513.

Pickett, J. T., Mancini, C., & Mears, D. P. (2013). Vulnerable victims, monstrous offenders, and unmanageable risk: Explaining public opinion on the social control of sex crime. *Criminology, 51*(3), 729–759.

Prescott, J. J., & Rockoff, J. E. (2011). Do sex offender registration and notification laws affect criminal behavior? *Journal of Law and Economics, 54*, 161–206. Retrieved from http://ssrn.com/abstract=1100663.

Red Bird, B. (2009). *Assessing housing availability under Ohio's sex offender residency restrictions*. Columbus, OH: Ohio State University.

Roots, R. I. (2004). When laws backfire: Unintended consequences of public policy. *American Behavioral Scientist, 47*(11), 1376–1394.

Sample, L. L., Evans, M. K., & Anderson, A. L. (2011). Sex offender community notification laws: Are their effects symbolic or instrumental in nature? *Criminal Justice Policy Review, 22*(1), 27–49.

Sample, L. L., & Bray, T. M. (2006). Are sex offenders different? An examination of rearrest patterns. *Criminal Justice Policy Review, 17*(1), 83–102.

Sample, L. L., & Kadleck, C. (2008). Sex offender laws: Legislators' accounts of the need for policy. *Criminal Justice Policy Review, 19*(1), 40–62.

Sample, L. L., & Streveler, A. J. (2003). Latent consequences of community notification laws. In S. H. Decker, L. F. Alaird, & C. M. Katz (Eds.), *Controversies in criminal justice* (pp. 353–362). Los Angeles, CA: Roxbury.

Sandler, J. C., Freeman, N. J., & Socia, K. M. (2008). Does a watched pot boil? A time-series analysis of New York State's sex offender registration and notification law. *Psychology, Public Policy, and Law, 14*(4), 284–302.

Schulenberg, J. L. (2007). Predicting noncompliant behavior: Disparities in the social locations of male and female probationers. *Justice Research and Policy, 9*(1), 25–57.

Jacob Wetterling Crimes Against Children and Sexually Violent Offender Registration Act, Public Law 103-322 (1994).

Smith v. Doe, (01-729) (U.S. Supreme Court 2003).

Socia, K. M. (2011). The policy implications of residence restrictions on sex offender housing in Upstate NY. *Criminology and Public Policy, 10*(2), 351–389.

Socia, K. M., & Stamatel, J. P. (2012). Neighborhood characteristics and the social control of registered sex offenders. *Crime and Delinquency, 58*(4), 565–587.

Stucky, T. D., & Ottensmann, J. R. (2014). Registered sex offenders and reported sex offenses. *Crime and Delinquency*, doi:10.1177/0011128714556738

Tabachnick, J., & Klein, A. (2011). *A reasoned approach: Reshaping sex offender policy to prevent child sexual abuse*. Beaverton, OR: Association for the Treatment of Sexual Abusers.

Tewksbury, R. (2004). Experiences and attitudes of registered female sex offenders. *Federal Probation, 68*(3), 30–34.

Tewksbury, R. (2005). Collateral consequences of sex offender registration. *Journal of Contemporary Criminal Justice, 21*(1), 67–82.

Tewksbury, R., & Lees, M. (2006). Consequences of sex offender registration: Collateral consequences and community experiences. *Sociological Spectrum, 26*(3), 309–334.

Tewksbury, R., & Levenson, J. S. (2009). Stress experiences of family members of registered sex offenders. *Behavioral Sciences & the Law, 27*(4), 611–626.

Tewksbury, R., & Mustaine, E. E. (2006). Where to find sex offenders: An examination of residential locations and neighborhood conditions. *Criminal Justice Studies, 19*(1), 61–75.

Tewksbury, R., & Mustaine, E. (2008). Where registered sex offenders live: Community characteristics and proximity to possible victims. *Victims and Offenders, 3*(1), 86–98.

Tewksbury, R., Jennings, W. G., & Zgoba, K. M. (2012). A longitudinal examination of sex offender recidivism prior to and following the implementation of SORN. *Behavioral Sciences & the Law, 30*(3), 308–328.

Thornton, D. (2006). Age and sexual recidivism: A variable connection. *Sexual Abuse: A Journal of Research and Treatment, 18*(2), 123–135.

Topitzes, J., Mersky, J. P., & Reynolds, A. J. (2012). From child maltreatment to violent offending: An examination of mixed-gender and gender-specific models. *Journal of Interpersonal Violence, 27*(12), 2322–2347.

Uggen, C., & McElrath, S. (2013). Six social sources of the U.S. crime drop. *The Society Pages: Social science that matters*. Retrieved from http://thesocietypages.org/papers/crime-drop/ Retrieved from http://thesocietypages.org/papers/crime-drop/.

Uniform Crime Report. (2012). *Crime in the United States*. Retrieved from Washington, DC

Vasquez, B. E., Maddan, S., & Walker, J. T. (2008). The influence of sex offender registration and notification laws in the United States. *Crime and Delinquency, 54*(2), 175–192.

Veysey, B., Zgoba, K., & Dalessandro, M. (2008). A preliminary step towards evaluating the impact of Megan's Law: A trend analysis of sexual offenses in New Jersey from 1985 to 2005. *Justice Research and Policy, 10*(2), 1–18.

Washington State Institute for Public Policy. (2005). Sex offender sentencing in Washington State: Did community notification influence recidivism? Retrieved from Olympia.

Widom, C. S., & Maxfield, M. G. (2001). *An update on the "Cycle of Violence"*. Des Moines, IA: US Department of Justice, Office of Justice Programs, National Institute of Justice.

Williams, K. S., & Bierie, D. M. (2014). An incident-based comparison of female and male sexual offenders. *Sexual Abuse: A Journal of Research and Treatment*, doi:1079063214544333.

Williams, F. P., McShane, M. D., & Dolny, M. H. (2000). Predicting parole absconders. *Prison Journal, 80*(1), 24–38.

Willis, G., & Grace, R. C. (2008). The quality of community reintegration planning for child molesters: Effects on sexual recidivism. *Sexual Abuse: A Journal of Research and Treatment, 20*(2), 218–240.

Willis, G., & Grace, R. (2009). Assessment of community reintegration planning for sex offenders: Poor planning predicts recidivism. *Criminal Justice and Behavior, 36*(5), 494–512.

Zandbergen, P., & Hart, T. C. (2006). Reducing housing options for convicted sex offenders: Investigating the impact of residency restriction laws using GIS. *Justice Research and Policy, 8*(2), 1–24.

Zandbergen, P., & Hart, T. (2009). Availability and spatial distribution of affordable housing in Miami-Dade County and implications of residency restriction zones for registered sex offenders. Retrieved September 9, 2009, from http://www.aclufl.org/pdfs/SORRStudy.pdf

Zandbergen, P., Levenson, J. S., & Hart, T. (2010). Residential proximity to schools and daycares: An empirical analysis of sex offense recidivism. *Criminal Justice and Behavior, 37*(5), 482–502.

Zevitz, R. G., & Farkas, M. A. (2000). Sex offender community notification: Managing high risk criminals or exacting further vengeance? *Behavioral Sciences & the Law, 18*, 375–391.

Zgoba, K. (2004). Spin doctors and moral crusaders: The moral panic behind child safety legislation. *Criminal Justice Studies, 17*(4), 385–404.

Zgoba, K., & Levenson, J. S. (2012). Failure to register as a predictor of sex offense recidivism: The Big Bad Wolf or a Red Herring? *Sexual Abuse: A Journal of Research and Treatment, 24*(4), 328–349.

Zgoba, K., Levenson, J. S., & McKee, T. (2009). Examining the Impact of Sex Offender Residence Restrictions on Housing Availability. *Criminal Justice Policy Review, 20*(1), 91–110.

Zgoba, K., Veysey, B., & Dalessandro, M. (2010). An analysis of the effectiveness of community notification and registration: Do the best intentions predict best practices? *Justice Quarterly, 27*, 667–691.

Zgoba, K., Miner, M., Knight, R. A., Letourneau, E., Levenson, J. S., & Thornton, D. (2012). *A multi-state recidivism study using Static99R and Static2002 risk scores and tier guidelines from the Adam Walsh Act*. Retrieved from https://www.ncjrs.gov/pdffiles1/nij/grants/240099.pdf.

Zgoba, K., Witt, P., Dalessandro, M., & Veysey, B. (2009). *Megan's Law: Assessing the practical and monetary efficacy*. Retrieved from http://www.ncjrs.gov/pdffiles1/nij/grants/225370.pdf

Zimring, F. E. (2006). *The great American crime decline*. Oxford: Oxford University Press.

Chapter 11
The Best Intentions: Flaws in Sexually Violent Predator Laws

Kresta N. Daly

Sexually violent predator laws allow states to deprive individuals of their liberty using a civil commitment process. While the civil commitment process has evolved to offer many of the constitutional protections afforded a criminal defendant such as the right to counsel, the right to subpoena witnesses and evidence, and the right to a speedy and public jury trial, the fundamental flaw with the civil commitment process is that it is used in place of the criminal system, thereby circumventing the legal process as envisioned in the constitution. The goals behind sexually violent predator laws are laudable; such restraints are intended to protect the public. The argument made by prosecutors and accepted by courts is these civil commitments are regulatory not punitive. The regulatory argument essentially states these laws are not intended to punish individuals with mental disorders or defects who are considered likely to commit future crimes because of mental disorders or defects.

The passage of sex offender laws began in the 1930s in this country. Originally those laws were known as "sexual psychopath laws." Almost as soon as the sexual psychopath laws were adopted, lawmakers began making changes to those laws. Since the 1930s, the law in this area has continually been changing. At the current point in the evolutionary continuum, most states have some form of sexually violent predator [SVP] laws.

Beginning in the 1980s and continuing into the 1990s, the United States saw the abolition of indeterminate sentencing for criminal defendants. Indeterminate sentencing varied from state to state but generally gave judges the freedom to sentence a person to a span of years, i.e., 7–12 years. In such case the defendant could not be released in fewer than 7 years nor imprisoned more than 12 years. The courts or probation could recommend release if the defendant had proved he or she was deserving of release.

K.N. Daly (✉)
Barth Daly LLP, 431 I Street, Suite 201, Sacramento, CA 95814, USA
e-mail: kdaly@barth-daly.com

© Springer International Publishing Switzerland 2016   243
D.R. Laws, W. O'Donohue (eds.), *Treatment of Sex Offenders*,
DOI 10.1007/978-3-319-25868-3_11

SVP laws were passed in large part to fill the gap for recidivists. These laws contain requirements that invite psychologists and psychiatrists to opine about the mental health diagnosis of individuals and speculate about whether their mental health is likely to cause future criminality. Judges and juries are then required to weigh this speculation in trying to decide whether or not a civil commitment is warranted under the law. There is no empirical evidence supporting an argument that SVP laws have made society safer. In the meantime the jurisprudence in this area has allowed increasingly vague diagnoses to form the basis for civil commitments.

On two occasions, the United States Supreme Court has considered the constitutionality of sexually violent predator laws. In both of those instances, the Court has upheld the constitutionality of these laws and, in so doing, fundamentally lowered the burden for prosecutors. This chapter will consider the two Supreme Court cases holding sexually violent predator laws constitutional: *Kansas v. Hendricks* (1999) 521 U.S. 346 and *Kansas v. Crane* (2003) 534 U.S. 407. These cases allow future courts and juries to assume anyone suffering from a paraphilia by definition suffers from a serious mental disorder notwithstanding the fact that there is disagreement among the scientific community that paraphilia *is* a serious mental disorder.

In light of this disagreement and the concerns among some in the legal community, this chapter concludes by recommending, from a legal perspective, the best practices that would lend credibility to both the legal and scientific processes. More specifically, mental health professionals are going to have to be increasingly diligent in regulating their profession. The temptation to make the wrong diagnosis for the right reason, to testify someone meets the criteria for a sexually violent predator to prevent a future harm when the individual does not fit the diagnoses, must be avoided.

History of Laws Targeting Sexual Offenders

In a 30-year period, between 1937 and 1967, more than half of the states passed laws calling for the indeterminate civil commitment of "sexual psychopaths." The cries for such legislation arose in response to a few highly publicized cases that led to a national fervor over a perceived sex crime wave.

The Social Backdrop Preceding Early Civil Commitment Laws

During a period of approximately 6 months in 1937, three cases involving child victims dominated the headlines. In each of those cases, girls, between the ages of 4 and 9, were sexually assaulted and murdered. Literally hundreds of magazine and newspaper articles discussing these three cases were published across the country. Estelle B. Friedman, "Uncontrolled Desires: The Response To The Sexual Psychopath", 74 J. Am. Hist. 83, 88 (1987). By July 1947, J. Edgar Hoover published an article in the *American* arguing that sexual offenders were committing crimes every 43 min in the United States (J. Edgar Hoover, How Safe Is Your Daughter?, Am.Mag., July 1947, at 32).

During the same time frame, academic journals published an ever-increasing number of articles related to sex crimes. Between 1921 and 1932 approximately six articles were published. Between 1933 and 1941 the numbers jumped by as many as five times. Between 1942 and 1951, there were more than 100 articles published on the subject (Tamara Rice Lave, "Only Yesterday: The Rise and Fall of Twentieth Century Sexual Psychopath Laws", 69 La. Law. Rev. 549, 551).

The public was outraged at this perceived upswing in violent sexual offenses and demanded something must be done. Whether or not there was a sufficient basis for the public's fear remains the subject of some debate. While many law enforcement agencies, including the FBI, reported increased sex crimes in the relevant time frame, those reports have been criticized for decades because of sloppy data collection and imprecise and unclear definitions. Regardless of the legitimacy of the public's reaction, legislators and law enforcement began to take action. For example, the New York City Police Department began compiling a list of "known degenerates." Known degenerates included anyone in the city who had been charged but not necessarily convicted with a sex crime over the past two decades. Police Making List of Sex Criminals, N.Y. Times, Aug. 13, 1937, at 19. Across the country in Los Angeles, the chief of police created a bureau of sex offenses that included low-level sex offenses under the theory that low-level sexual offenders were major sex offenders in waiting.

The Rise of Civil Commitment Laws

In the mid-1930s Michigan passed one of the nation's first "civil commitment" laws. Defendants and criminal defense attorneys have long decried the nomenclature of these laws. The court-ordered detention of an individual against their will in a setting that both looks and feels like a prison is hardly "civil." Legislators labeled both sexual psychopath laws and sexually violent predator laws "civil" to avoid triggering the numerous constitutional protections afforded to a criminal defendant including the protection of the ex post facto clause (i.e., the constitutional prohibition against laws making illegal an act that was legal when committed, increasing penalties for breaking the law after the act was committed, or changing the rules of evidence to make conviction easier)—no such protections are afforded a civil defendant. Among the earliest litigation involving civil commitment laws and the quasi-criminal consequences of such laws involves the case of George Frontczak.

On April 19, 1937, George Frontczak pled guilty to the crime of gross indecency in Detroit, Michigan. Precisely what conduct Mr. Frontczak engaged in is unclear from the records. The current definition of gross indecency in Michigan requires an individual to engage in a "sex act with another person or in an act of masturbation in a public or private place. Michigan Criminal Law 750.338, 750.338a and

750.338b. The conduct can occur between consenting adults and still be considered a felony. For his conduct Mr. Frontczak was sentenced to not less than 30 days and not more than 5 years (People v. Frontczak (1938) 281 N.W. 534, 534–35).

During the time Mr. Frontczak was incarcerated, Act No. 196 came into effect. Act No. 196 is representative of a majority of the sexual psychopath laws passed across the country. It stated, in part:

> When a person convicted of *** indecent exposure, *** gross indecency, *** shall, though not insance [sic], feeble-minded or epileptic, appear to be psychopathic, or a sex degenerate, or a sex pervert, with tendencies dangerous to public safety, the trial court before pronouncing sentence shall institute and conduct a thorough examination and investigation of such person, and of all the facts and circumstances, shall call two or more reputable physicians including one psychiatrist and other credible witnesses***. If it is proved to the satisfaction of said judge or a jury that such person is psychopathic, or a sex degenerate, or a sex pervert, possessed of mental tendencies inimical to society and that, because thereof, such person is a menace to the public safety, then the court, in pronouncing sentence, shall so adjudge: Provided, however, That upon such examination and investigation, such person shall be entitled to a jury hearing. If a prison or jail term is imposed, the court shall include in the commitment an order that upon expiration of such prison or jail term, *** said person be removed and committed to such suitable state hospital or state institution as the court may designate in such commitment, to remain in such state hospital or state institution until said court shall adjudge that such person has ceased to be a menace to the public safety because of said mental condition. (People v. Frontczak 281 N.W. 534, 535)

The Michigan Court that considered this law found it unconstitutional because of the Act's failure to follow the dictates of criminal procedure and secure the constitutional rights of the accused (People v. Frontczak 281 N.W. 534, 537). The dissent in *Frontczak* would have upheld the constitutionality of the Act because of the purported civil nature of the commitment.

The sexual psychopath laws passed by 26 other states and the District of Columbia around the same time as Michigan's Act No. 196 were similar in many regards. Most states required the individual be convicted of specific sex crimes before being subjected to civil commitment proceedings although a few states required only the conviction of any crime. Five jurisdictions did not require any criminal conviction at all—those states would allow for a civil commitment if there was cause to believe the individual was a sexual psychopath.

Most of these laws were vague when it came to the criteria to determine an individual was a sexual psychopath. The laws were so broad that any individual who could be considered sexually deviant, but was not necessarily psychopathic or dangerous, was subject to an indeterminate civil commitment. At this time a civil commitment was civil in name only. In reality individuals who were detained under a civil commitment were housed in prisons with other inmates. Most of them received little or no treatment for the cause of their alleged sexual psychopathy. Sexual psychopath laws came under increasing scrutiny from jurists and mental health professionals alike.

Between 1975 and 1981 approximately half of the sexual psychopath laws on the books nationwide were repealed. The demise of these statutes has been attributed to four factors:

1. The growing influence of the feminist movement which opposed the "medicalization" of rape
2. The 1977 report from the Committee on Forensic Psychiatry of the Group for the Advancement of Psychiatry which referred to the sexual psychopath statutes as a failed experiment that lacked redeeming social value
3. Increasing scrutiny by the courts on the lack of both procedural and substantive due process rights afforded mental health patients
4. Increased social disapproval of the manner in which sexual offenders received, or didn't receive, treatment (Eric S. Janus and Robert A. Prentky, "Sexual Predator Laws: A Two Decade Retrospective", 21 Fed. Sent. R.2.)

From the 1980s until the early 1990s, there was little to no change in sexual psychopath laws. However, the nation was, once again, about to be gripped by several high profile and this time fantastic allegations about sexual abuse. These high-profile sex abuse cases were part of a national hysteria and also coincided with the so-called war on drugs, a time when criminal laws were tightened and the length of prison terms rose at an unprecedented rate.

The Adoption of Sexually Violent Predator Laws in the Latter Portion of the Twentieth Century

The next bout of sexual hysteria began when Judy Johnson, mother of a preschooler in southern California, claimed her son was sodomized by her estranged husband and McMartin Preschool teacher Ray Buckey. Johnson's belief that her son had been molested apparently began when he had painful bowel movements. It's unclear whether or not her son denied or confirmed the alleged abuse. Johnson made other accusations including that day care employees had sexual encounters with animals and flew through the air. The police sent a letter to approximately 200 students of the day care informing them of the nature of the allegations and the suspects. Several hundred children were interviewed by Kee MacFarlane using suggestive interview techniques that invited the children to speculate about possible events. The accusations included ritual satanic abuse, seeing witches fly, traveling in hot-air balloons, being led through underground tunnels, orgies at car washes, and children being flushed down toilets to secret rooms to be abused. The investigation began in the early 1980s. Media coverage of the accusations began shortly after charges were announced in March 1984. The story was consistently in the news until all charges against all defendants were dropped in 1990 after 6 years of criminal trials.

The national reaction to the McMartin case was initially one of horror and fear. The case monopolized national attention. The McMartin case coincided with then President Reagan's highly publicized war on drugs. Alongside stories of the McMartin case were images of street gang warfare and crack babies. In 1986 Congress passed the Anti-Drug Abuse Act which fundamentally changed the penological paradigm on which federal criminal laws were based. The federal system had largely been a rehabilitative system, but after 1986 it became a punitive system. Federal drug statutes contained a myriad of mandatory minimums and increased sentences for many crimes. For nearly 30 years federal judges were largely divested of their sentencing discretion because of the mandatory federal sentencing guidelines. State governments shortly began to follow suit. While federal judges regained portions of their sentencing discretion in 2004 following the United States Supreme Court's decision in *United States v. Booker* (2005) which declared the sentencing guidelines advisory and not mandatory, judges are still constrained by mandatory minimums. In many states state court judges continue to be constrained by mandatory minimums and sentencing schemes that give them little to no ability to fashion a sentence that is appropriate based on the individual characteristics of the defendant.

There was a third force at work which formed the current sexually violent predator laws. The Civil Rights Movement promoted a switch from indeterminate to determinate criminal sentencing. The argument was based on the notion that determinate sentencing would promote sentencing uniformity and therefore promote equality before the law. Among the initial flaws of early determinate sentencing schemes was the failure to account for individuals who had lengthy criminal records. Previously courts had far more discretion in crafting lengthy prison sentences for individuals who were likely to re-offend, including sex offenders. Determinate sentencing laws set maximums, often relatively short maximums, for violent crimes such as rape. Sexually violent predator laws began being passed as a response to the gaps created by early determinate sentencing laws. Alongside the passage of sexually violent predator statutes, legislators began setting high mandatory minima in many cases and adopting new and more stringent indeterminate sentencing schemes for many classes of crimes.

It was against this backdrop the next generation of sexual psychopath laws was passed. Regardless of the nomenclature, the purpose of these laws was to fill the gaps created by the determinate sentencing schemes that were adopted in the past decade. This time labeled sexually violent predator laws, their popularity gained rapidly starting in the early 1990s. Between 1990 and 1999 17 states passed SVP laws. The federal version was added as an amendment to the 2006 Adam Walsh Act in which neither the United States Sentencing Commission nor the House or Senate Committee on the Judiciary was consulted prior to passage of the amendment. Since the passage of the Adam Walsh Act, there have been limited efforts by any state to pass additional SVP legislation. For the reasons referenced above, the passage of the Adam Walsh Act has been harshly criticized by both lawyers and judges. New York was among the most recent states to pass an SVP law when it did so in 2007.

SVP statutes require an individual suffer a prior conviction in order to trigger SVP proceedings. Common among the list of triggering crimes are rape, spousal rape, any of a number of child molest crimes, kidnapping, and assault with intent to commit any of the aforementioned crimes. Some states allow the use of prior convictions when an individual was a juvenile. While each SVP law is slightly different, they all share some common features:

1. An individual must have some mental disease, disorder, or abnormality that causes or is associated with risk of future sexual dangerousness.
2. The commitment of such an individual must be for the purpose of treatment.

These common features pose significant problems for mental health professionals who are called on to testify about the likelihood of future dangerousness, as well as for lawyers and judges who often have little familiarity with mental diseases, disorders, and abnormalities. The causation requirement, the requirement that the mental disorder be the cause of future dangerousness, invites speculation among both the legal and mental health professions. SVP laws have made the opinions and the testimony of mental health professionals of paramount importance in these proceedings. The findings of these evaluators are often the main evidence on which a finding of "sexually violent predator" rests. The American Psychiatric Association has vigorously opposed sexually violent predator statutes (Dangerous Sex Offenders: A Task Force Report of the American Psychiatric Association (1999)).

Among the reasons for the association's opposition is the argument that offenders have already served prison terms for their offenses and further civil detention is nothing more than preventative detention. The Association has also argued that civil commitments violate the constitutional prohibition against double jeopardy, that such detentions may lead to the future detention of other members of groups deemed to have mental disorders, like political dissenters, and that this is an abuse of psychiatry.

The United States Supreme Court has heard three cases on modern SVP laws. In those decisions the Supreme Court rejected the APA's concerns about the ethics or the constitutionality of SVP laws and instead rested their decision. The high court's decisions hinged on the fact that civil commitments were motivated by a regulatory as opposed to punitive intent. If the laws were found to have a punitive intent, they would necessarily violate the double jeopardy clause of the United States Constitution, the prohibition against prosecuting and punishing the same individual for the same crime on more than one occasion. Only criminal or punitive laws are subject to a double jeopardy analysis, so by finding the laws—had a regulatory instead the Court avoided a double jeopardy analysis—an analysis SVP laws could not have survived.

The United States Supreme Court's Validation of Sexually Violent Predator Laws

Facial and As-Applied Constitutional Challenges

Statutes can be challenged on constitutional grounds using two different theories: facial invalidity or as-applied invalidity. An individual arguing facial invalidity claims the statute cannot pass constitutional muster under any circumstance and is therefore always constitutionally void. A successful challenge based on facial invalidity results in a court striking down a statute.

By contrast successful as-applied challenges strike down statutes only in narrow circumstances. As-applied challenges may limit the application of a statute to only certain circumstances or may allow the statute to be applied only under certain conditions.

A Brief History of Constitutional Civil Commitment

Some form or another of civil commitments has long been recognized as socially necessary and constitutionally permissible in this country almost since its inception ("A History of Civil Commitment And Related Reforms In the United States: Lessons For Today", *Developments in Mental Health Law*, Paul S. Appelbaum, 25 Dev.MentalHealthL. 13, January 2006). Civil commitments are recognized as the legitimate use of state and federal police power to protect society from dangerous offenders. In order for civil commitment laws to be constitutionally valid, they must have specific characteristics.

Civil commitment statutes cannot have a punitive intent. In *Foucha v. Louisiana* a statute allowed for the civil commitment of an individual based on an individual's apparent antisocial personality when there was no other evidence of mental illness. Foucha had been charged with a crime but found not guilty by reason of insanity. He was detained in a forensic facility until doctors determined he could be released. Doctors determined Foucha had previously suffered from a drug-induced psychosis but had recovered from that temporary condition. There was evidence he suffered from antisocial personality disorder for which there is no cure (Foucha v. Louisiana, 504 U.S. 71, 73—74 (1992)).

The state sought to prolong Foucha's detention based on his antisocial personality disorder. The Court ruled the state failed in its burden to show by clear and convincing evidence that the individual is both mentally ill and dangerous (Foucha v. Louisiana, 504 U.S. 71, 80–81 (1992)). Here, the court drew a clear line between mental illness and someone suffering from a personality disorder.

Here, in contrast, the State asserts that because Foucha once committed a criminal act and now has an antisocial personality that sometimes leads to aggressive conduct, a disorder for which there is no effective treatment, he may be held indefinitely. This rationale would permit the State to hold indefinitely any other insanity acquittee not mentally ill who could be shown to have a personality disorder that may lead to criminal conduct. The same would be true of any convicted criminal, even though he has completed his prison term. It would also be only a step away from substituting confinements for dangerousness for our present system which, with only narrow exceptions and aside from permissible confinements for mental illness, incarcerates only those who are proved beyond reasonable doubt to have violated a criminal law (Foucha v. Louisiana, 504 U.S. 71, 82 (1992)).

The statute at issue in *Foucha* was facially invalid because the statute was punitive in its intent—the statute punished someone for having a particular personality disorder.

Civil confinements also cannot be indefinite. The confinement has to be for a specific term which can expire. There is no prohibition however against extending the term so long as certain specific procedural safeguards are followed.

The USSC Takes Up Facial Validity of Sexually Violent Predator Statutes

Hendricks

In 1996 the United States Supreme Court first took up the modern SVP laws in the case of *Kansas v. Hendricks*. In 1984 Hendricks was serving a sentence for taking "indecent liberties" with two 13-year-old boys. After serving nearly 10 years in prison, he was slated for release. Before his release the state filed a petition seeking Hendricks' detention as a sexually violent predator. A trial was ultimately held on whether or not Hendricks should be civilly committed. During the trial Hendricks admitted to multiple instances of molesting children. He readily agreed to a state physician's diagnosis that he was a pedophile (Kansas v. Hendricks, 521 US 346, 355 (1997)). The jury found Hendricks was a sexually violent predator, and the judge ordered him civilly committed.

Central to the Supreme Court's conclusion that the SVP statute was a civil statute and lacked a punitive purpose was that the law was regulatory meaning Hendricks was not being "punished" by being civilly committed. His commitment was necessary to treat Hendricks' mental disease or defect and to protect the public while that treatment was in progress. The length of the confinement in *Hendricks'* case, and indeed pursuant to most SVP statutes, was limited to 1-year increments. The fact that confinement could last for the remainder of an individual's life, meted out in 1-year increments, was of no moment to the Court. The Court so concluded because the goal of holding an individual was merely to incapacitate that person until their mental abnormality was treated. The Court stated that treatment, although required by SVP statutes and necessary to a finding that they are constitutional, is incidental. "…[W]e have never held that the Constitution prevents a State from civilly detaining those for whom no treatment is available, but who pose a danger to others" (Kansas v. Hendricks, 521 US 346, 366 (1997)).

Justice Kennedy was the crucial swing vote in *Hendricks*. Kennedy was far more troubled by the system of indeterminate civil commitments:

> The concern is instead whether it is the criminal system or the civil system which should make the decision in the first place. If the civil system is used simply to impose punishment after the criminal system makes an improvident plea bargain on the criminal side, then it is not performing its proper function… We should bear in mind that while incapacitation is a goal common to both the criminal and civil systems of confinement, retribution and general deterrence are reserved for the criminal system alone. (Kansas v. Hendricks, 521 US 346, 372 (1997))

In reaching his concurrence, it was important to Justice Kennedy that the individual at issue, Hendricks, had a serious and highly unusual inability to control his actions, that Hendricks suffered from pedophilia which was accepted by many mental health professionals as a serious mental disorder, and lastly, that Hendricks' pedophilia presented a serious danger to children. While Kennedy was willing to accept the facial validity of SVP statutes, he appeared open to subsequent as-applied challenges.

Seling v. Young

In *Seling v. Young* 501 U.S. 250 (2001), the United States Supreme Court upheld Washington's sexually violent predator commitment scheme. The main significance of *Young* is that the Supreme Court abandoned its statements in *Hendricks* regarding the incidental nature of the requirement that the individual receive treatment. Rather the court indicated that because the sexually violent predator statute at issue was indeed a civil rather than criminal statute, due process required the conditions and duration of commitment bear a reasonable relation to the purpose for which an individual was committed, i.e., treated.

Crane

In 2002 the United States Supreme Court took up a second challenge to SVP statutes in *Kansas v. Crane* 534 U.S. 407, 412 (2002). In *Crane* the High Court clarified that a constitutionally valid SVP statute need not require an individual be wholly unable to control their actions because of their mental disease, defect, or disorder. The Court wrote:

> *Hendricks* underscored the constitutional importance of distinguishing a dangerous sex offender subject to civil commitment 'from other dangerous persons who are perhaps more properly dealt with exclusively through criminal proceedings'. [Citation omitted.] That distinction is necessary lest 'civil commitment' become a 'mechanism for retribution or general deterrence' functions properly those of criminal law, not civil commitment. (*Kansas v. Crane* 534 U.S. 407, 412 (2002))

Crane arguably increased the burden on the state necessary to show a person should be subjected to a civil commitment in an SVP proceeding. While the Supreme Court did not require that an individual be "wholly unable to control" their actions because of their mental disease or disorder, the Court found that the constitution requires the state to prove that the individual lacks control over their behavior. The Court indicated that it is impossible to define "lack of control" such that it would apply in every individual case but that, at a minimum, there must be evidence of a "serious difficulty" in controlling behavior. The Court also required there be a link between the disorder or disease and violent behavior.

Neither *Hendricks* nor *Crane* addressed whether confinement of sex offenders based only on "emotional" impairment was unconstitutional. This opening likely opened the door for the federal SVP statute, contained in the Adam Walsh Act, which allows for commitment when the inability is solely volitional. In *Crane* the Court decided an individual can be civilly committed as long as there is proof of some inability to control the sexually dangerous behavior, whether that inability is due to a volitional or emotional impairment.

Para-What?

The average lawyer operating in the criminal justice system may not have a basic familiarity with paraphilias. The average lay person called on to sit on a jury is in no better position. Yet triers of fact are likely to be called upon to determine whether or not a particular paraphilia or, in some cases, paraphilia not otherwise specified, coupled with other evidence, is sufficient to indefinitely detain an individual. *Crane* in particular opened the door for SVP civil commitments based on the diagnosis of paraphilias so long as the other criteria for an SVP commitment exist.

Any mental health professional about to testify on this issue should be mindful of the history of paraphilias and be prepared to explain to the trier of fact the changing social norms and controversy surrounding the definition and diagnosis of paraphilias. Mental health professionals also need to be prepared to discuss the distinction between paraphilic orientation and an actual paraphilic disorder.

Fifty years ago homosexuality was generally considered a paraphilia. Changing social norms eliminated homosexuality from the list of paraphilias, and the United States Supreme Court's decision in *Lawrence v. Texas* recognized a consenting adult's right to engage in sexual conduct (*Lawrence v. Texas 539 U.S. 558* (2003)). Absent changing social norms constitutionally protected conduct that could have formed the basis for a sexually violent predator classification. In a modern context concern arises because SVP laws permit a civil commitment based on an abnormality and do not require a disorder or a disease. Consider the following and keep in mind that many, if not all, SVP laws do not define what a mental abnormality is: a mental health professional concluded an individual had a paraphilic orientation favoring exhibitionism. The mental health professional concluded the individual had a paraphilic orientation and not a disorder specifically because the paraphilic interest was not disturbing to the individual or others. Under the law a paraphilic orientation can be a mental abnormality. If the same mental health professional was called to testify at an SVP trial that the same individual has a specific paraphilic orientation (aka mental abnormality), that opinion could satisfy one of the requirements for an SVP finding to be made and a civil commitment ordered.

The problem is compounded with the addition of other variables. For example, the reason the mental health professional concluded the paraphilic interest was not disturbing to the individual or others was because the individual never engaged in exhibitionist behavior. A civil commitment based on mere paraphilic orientation with no accompanying conduct is nothing more than committing/punishing people for deviant thoughts.

Consider pedophilia. It's possible for a person to have a pedophilic orientation or have their pedophilia rise to the level of a disorder and not act on their conduct. In an October 6, 2014 op-ed article in the *New York Times*, Margo Kaplan, a professor at Rutgers School of Law, estimated that up to 1 % of the male population may live with pedophilia. Think of a man with pedophilic interests, either an orientation or a disorder, but who has never engaged or attempted to engage in pedophilic conduct. During a messy divorce, the same man attempted to kidnap his children. This man has committed a qualifying offense in most states. He suffers from a disorder or abnormality that is associated with a risk of future dangerousness. It cannot be consistent with notions of due process to confine and attempt to "cure" a person whose disorder or orientation had nothing to do with his underlying crime. Simply being a pedophile is not a criminal offense. A person must act on their pedophilic interests in order to commit a crime, but under SVP laws, a person can be committed/punished even in absence of pedophilic conduct.

While recent efforts have been made to change diagnostic terminology, such efforts appear to have done little more than add fuel to the fire. The distinctions between a disorder and an orientation can become lost when jurors hear terms like "pedophilia." Further concerning from a legal perspective is the criteria for a diagnosis of a paraphilia. To the extent a paraphilia causes harm or endangers children or non-consenting adults, such a paraphilia would be removed from the gamut of this author's concerns. However, since a diagnosis can alternatively be supported by a 6-month period in which the individual experiences distress or other personal problems, it would be ethically and potentially constitutionally infirm to argue if the only person experiencing harm is the individual himself that such a diagnosis should be relied upon for a civil commitment. Yet this is the exact state of affairs *Crane* created.

Lawrence's basic holding is the state has no legitimate interest in criminalizing consensual sexual conduct among adults. While it remains legally untested, logically *Lawrence's* holding would cover any paraphilia involving consenting adults. *Crane* was decided before *Lawrence v. Texas*. To the extent *Crane* opened the door to the inclusion of paraphilias as qualifying disorders for SVP proceedings, it may well have opened the door to individuals being indefinitely confined for engaging in constitutionally protected conduct.

Taken to its extreme, consider the San Francisco night club Power Exchange. It advertises itself as "America's Naughtiest Night Club." Open 7 days a week, public sex acts, bondage, sex acts involving dominance and submission, as well as sadistic and/or masochistic conduct are on display for the price of admission. Among the few limitations on permissible conduct within the club is that all conduct be consensual. On any given night sexual conduct often included in the definition of paraphilia is on display. Under current requirements, nearly every attendee on a given night would exhibit sufficient manifestations of paraphilias to support at least further inquiry into whether a paraphiliac diagnosis is appropriate.

The above example is almost certain to never occur given the current state of sexually violent predator proceedings. SVP proceedings are initiated while individuals are completing their criminal sentences—not attending night clubs. The example underscores the fluid nature of what society considers deviant and the dangers of using paraphilias involving consensual adult conduct in sexually violent predator proceedings.

The constitutional concerns involving paraphilias as the basis for sexually violent predator proceedings are properly raised by lawyers. Mental health professionals face difficult ethical choices in determining whether to offer testimony in such cases. The potential for misuse of paraphilias within the legal system is significant. Commentators and courts alike have commented on the potential for abuse of the civil commitment system in general and the sexually violent predator system in particular. In his concurrence in *Hendricks*, Justice Kennedy wrote:

> If, however, civil confinement were to become a mechanism for retribution or general deterrence, or if it were showed that mental abnormality is too imprecise a category to offer a solid basis for concluding that civil detention is justified, our precedents would not suffice to validate it. (Kansas v. Hendricks, 521 U.S. 346, 373 (1997))

Many paraphilias fall squarely into Justice Kennedy's warnings about imprecise categories that offer potential mechanisms for social retribution. In addition to being prepared to readily acknowledge the controversy surrounding paraphilias to the trier of fact, mental health professionals have to diligently guard against the legal profession's pressure to confine potentially dangerous individuals when those individuals may not accurately fit specific diagnoses.

Expert Opinions About "Likely to Commit" and "Serious Difficulty"

Mental health professionals are often the star witnesses in sexually violent predator trials. Trials are often nothing more than a battle of the experts. While the law struggles to compensate for sentencing changes from the 1980s to 1990s, mental health professionals are asked to express opinions that will lead to determinations about whether a person is indefinitely detained.

When You're Likely to Testify About the Meaning of "Likely"

All state SVP statutes contain the requirement that an individual be likely to commit future acts of sexual violence. The requirements of the federal statute are slightly different—that is, the statute requires that an individual's mental abnormality or disorder make it difficult, if not impossible, for the offender to refrain from future "dangerous behavior." While lawyers and judges will likely spend years arguing the legal significance of these semantic differences, either way it's phrased poses significant real-world difficulties for both legal and mental health practitioners.

"Likely to commit future acts" and "difficult or impossible to refrain from future dangerous behavior" both invite speculation and theoretical discussions on topics such as free will. Theoretical discussions about free will and the ability of law and science to predict a given individual's future conduct are all well and good in an academic setting. Unfortunately given the Supreme Court's lack of guidance, these conversations will take place in courtrooms and will be the basis for decisions about civil liberties and indefinite terms of confinement.

Mental health professionals would likely agree they can identify those people who pose a higher than average likelihood of re-offending—those people who are more "likely" to re-offend. Any person previously convicted of a crime is statistically more likely to re-offend. However, commonly accepted this notion may be, it does little to protect the civil liberties of those individuals facing civil commitment proceedings. Using this logic there, all sex offenders are, at least in theory, similarly situated and therein lies the fault with the law. Among the basic premises on which all sexually violent predator statutes rest is the notion that only the most violent and dangerous sex offenders should be subjected to a civil commitment.

Using the phrase "likely to re-offend" provides no guidance to any mental health practitioner on how to distinguish one offender from another. This subjective standard provides no basis for a forensic mental health practitioner to form a meaningful comparison between offenders. While each state has its own definition of "likely," no definition provides meaningful guidance. California's statute requires "likely that he or she will engage in sexually violent behavior," and the corresponding case law discusses a "serious and well-founded risk." Courts have held that it is erroneous if the risk is defined as over 50 % (People v. Superior Court (Ghilloti), 27 Cal. 4th 888 (2002)). Missouri defines "likely" as "more likely than not to engage in predatory acts of sexual violence," whereas states like Tennessee merely require "likelihood of serious harm."

The problem becomes compounded inside of a courtroom. Jurors are faced with the untenable task of evaluating the testimony of two forensic experts: one testifying the defendant is likely to sexually re-offend and the other testifying the same defendant is unlikely. The typical scientific testimony includes statistical analysis, clinical assessments, and other methodologies for assessing risk. Scientists may argue the benefits of actuarial models versus clinical evaluations—comment on the superiority of either method is beyond the ken of a lawyer. From a legal perspective what is important is how and when these risk assessments are presented to the trier of fact.

What "is likely" is difficult to define, let alone predict. Testifying experts must take care in the presentation of their forensic conclusions. Jurors need the necessary evidence to make informed decisions about the facts of the individual whose case they are deciding. A debate over the merits of phallometric analysis versus psychiatric diagnosis does little to advance the cause of justice and the preservation of civil liberties.

Serious Difficulty Is Probably Just That

Just as no case has specific criteria for "likely," there is little clear guidance regarding "serious difficulty" as required by most states or "volitional control" as discussed in the federal statute. Expert witnesses are required to opine on such issues before juries who come into the court with little background on the causes of criminal recidivism.

Any individual who has committed more than one crime has clearly failed to restrain their criminal urges. However, the causes of a lack of restraint are not necessarily "serious difficulty." The reasons for criminal recidivism are widely varied. It could be someone has never tried to exercise restraint when faced with a choice about committing a crime. In such a case an individual's conduct would not be caused by a serious difficulty in controlling their conduct, rather it would be caused by a lack of effort. It is important therefore to explain to juries that recidivism alone is not necessarily a "serious difficulty." Evidence such as that in *Hendricks*, an individual with a more than 20-year history of sexual offenses against children coupled with admissions that he could not control his conduct, clearly meets the definition of "serious difficulty." There is every reason for experts to provide triers of fact with such hypotheticals such as *Hendricks* to give the trier of fact meaningful comparisons to the evidence before them. That is not to suggest an individual's criminality and mental disorders must rise to the levels displayed in *Hendricks* to render a civil commitment appropriate. Rather expert witnesses are tasked with the duty of educating the jury not just providing an opinion. The diligent performance of that duty requires the expert to provide some background with which to evaluate the expert's opinion. While experts are paid witnesses, they better serve the function of justice if they refrain from acting an advocate inside of the courtroom.

The Future of Sexually Violent Predator Laws

Sexually violent predator laws have received constant criticism since their passage because of their reliance on a so-called civil commitment system. The laws arose in large part to address a gap created by the adoption of determinate sentencing schemes. Some commentators have speculated that the use of sexually violent predator proceedings will decrease due to increasing reinstatement of indeterminate terms in many sex crimes. Many state and federal statutes either carry indeterminate terms for first-time child molesters or sentencing schemes that functionally equate to life sentences. Recidivist sex offenders convicted of crimes that do not involve children also receive substantially longer sentences, often well in excess of 15 or 20 years.

This author does not believe these sentences will bring about the functional if not the actual demise of sexually violent predator proceedings. Both state and federal governments are dealing with the side effects of legislation such as the three-strikes law which has caused rampant prison overcrowding and an aging prison population with skyrocketing medical costs which the public must bear. There is increasing social, political, and financial pressure to address chronic prison overcrowding particularly in light of crime rates that have continually declined over decades. There is ever-mounting attention to the racial sentencing disparities particularly among those who have suffered long prison sentences for relatively minor crimes.

Public sentiment will not support the release of those incarcerated for sex crimes nor will it advocate for changes in how sex offenders are charged, sentenced, or otherwise confined. While legal scholars continue to question the constitutional soundness of civil confinement which looks and feels very much like criminal punishment, the public at large does not appear to share such concerns. Rather the public is increasingly relying on the sciences in general and mental health professionals in particular to dictate the results in the courtroom. The outcomes in criminal trials are influenced more and more by scientific evidence. Because of advances in science and the influence of popular culture, juries have come to expect forensic evidence in every case.

The trier of fact has come to believe science can provide answers to legal questions involving issues of human rights and due process. The more entrenched those beliefs become, the more mental health professionals will find themselves on the witness stand explaining mental diseases and disorders, trying to explain how likely is "likely" and whether or not a person has a "serious difficulty" in controlling their actions. As this process continues mental health professionals, and in particular forensic practitioners, are going to have to be increasingly diligent in regulating their profession. The temptation to make the wrong diagnosis for the right reason, to testify someone meets the criteria for a sexually violent predator to prevent a future harm when the individual does not fit the diagnoses, must be avoided. While it may be argued that society has already begun down the slippery slope toward preventative detention, care must be taken to go no further down the path.

References

Appelbaum, P. S. (2006). A history of civil commitment and related reforms in the United States: Lessons for today. *Developments in Mental Health Law, 25*, 13.

Dangerous Sex Offenders: A Task Force Report of the American Psychiatric Association. (1999).

Foucha v. Louisiana, 504 U.S. 71, 73–74, 80–81, 82. (1992).

Friedman, E. B. (1987). Uncontrolled desires: The response to the sexual psychopath. *Journal of American Histology, 74*, 83–88.

Hoover, J. E. (1947, July). How safe is your daughter? *American*.

Janus, E. S., & Prentky, R. A. Sexual predator laws: A two decade retrospective. 21 *Fed Sent R* 2.

Kansas v. Crane, 534 U.S. 407, 412. (2002).

Kansas v. Hendricks, 521 US 346, 355, 366, 372, 372. (1997).

Lave, T. R. Only yesterday: The rise and fall of twentieth century sexual psychopath laws. *Louisiana Law Review, 69*, 549–551.

Lawrence v. Texas, 539 U.S. 558. (2003).

Michigan Criminal Law 750.338.

Michigan Criminal Law 750.338a.
Michigan Criminal Law 750.338b.
People v. Frontczak. (1938). 281 N.W. 534, 534-3, 535.
People v. Superior Court (Ghilloti). (2002). 27 Cal.4th 888.
Police Making List of Sex Criminals. (1937, August 13). *New York Times*, 19.
Seling v. Young, 501 U.S. 250. (2001).
United States v. Booker 543 U.S. 220. (2005).

Chapter 12
The Shortcomings of Sexual Offender Treatment: Are We Doing Something Wrong?

Pamela M. Yates and Drew A. Kingston

There has been much interest in sexual behaviour, sexual deviance, and the treatment of sexual offenders for more than a century (for reviews see Laws & Marshall, 2003; Marshall & Laws, 2003, and Yates, 2002). Researchers, clinicians, and philosophers have long been intrigued by human sexual behaviour and have offered various theories regarding the origins of, and treatment for, sexual deviance. Indeed, perspectives have been based in psychodynamic theory, behavioural theory, and cognitive-behavioural theory, among many others (Laws & Marshall, 2003; Marshall & Laws, 2003; Yates, 2002, 2003). Moreover, numerous approaches to the treatment of sexual deviance have been proposed and implemented, most without empirical support at the time of implementation. For example, early treatment focussed on medical or pharmacological interventions which, while these seemed promising, were not based on research at the time of implementation. Early behavioural approaches that focussed on extinguishing deviant sexual arousal were not very effective, as these were based on the assumption that addressing deviant sexual arousal was sufficient as a complete intervention on its own (Marshall & Laws, 2003; Yates, 2002). Similarly, early perspectives that viewed sexually deviant behaviour as being based in anger or lack of social skills did not demonstrate anticipated results in terms of outcome.

Over time, cognition came to be recognised as important in understanding sexual deviance and in the treatment of sexual offending, and more comprehensive cognitive-behavioural/social learning approaches were adopted. More recently, the

P.M. Yates, Ph.D. (✉)
Cabot Consulting and Research Services, P.O. Box 590,
Eastern Passage, NS, Canada B3G 1M8
e-mail: pmyates@bellaliant.net

D.A. Kingston, Ph.D., C.Psych.
1804 Highway 2 East, C.P./P.O. Box 1050, Brockville, ON, Canada K6V 5W7
e-mail: drew.kingston@theroyal.ca

© Springer International Publishing Switzerland 2016
D.R. Laws, W. O'Donohue (eds.), *Treatment of Sex Offenders*,
DOI 10.1007/978-3-319-25868-3_12

relapse prevention approach, which was considered the most respected intervention with sexual offenders, (cf. Laws, 1989, 2003), has been discredited due to a number of major shortcomings, not the least of which is its lack of demonstrated effectiveness (see below; Hanson, 1996, 2000; Laws, 2003; Yates, 2005, 2007; Yates & Kingston, 2005). However, although its use in treatment is diminishing, many adherents continue to use this model (McGrath, Cumming, Burchard, Zeoli, & Ellerby, 2010) because of its appeal to clinicians (Laws, 2003; Yates, 2007).

Currently, a multimodal/multiple component model of sexual offender treatment is the norm in most jurisdictions, although again, research support is equivocal. Various researchers have attempted classification systems of sexual offenders (e.g. Knight & Prentky, 1990) and of the sexual offence process (e.g. Ward & Hudson, 1998). While some of this research has proved informative with respect to risk and prevention of reoffending (e.g. Kingston, Yates, & Firestone, 2012; Kingston, Yates, & Olver, 2014), most has not. Newer models such as the good lives model approach (Ward & Stewart, 2003) that have been proposed have not yet been demonstrated in research to influence the ultimate outcome of reduced recidivism and victimisation, despite having been in existence for some time. Furthermore, developments in various jurisdictions, most notably the United States, such as the use of polygraphy, restrictions related to residency, and the containment approach, have similarly not been shown to be effective, despite substantial human and financial investment.

In this chapter, we review and comment upon current approaches to the treatment of sexual offenders. We offer a critical analysis and commentary on current approaches to intervention with sexual offenders, the effectiveness of these approaches, and recommendations for future directions.

Sexual Offender Treatment in Past Practice: Did We Go Wrong Somewhere?

A full review of the history of sexual offender treatment is beyond the scope of this chapter. As such, the interested reader is referred to Laws and Marshall (2003), Marshall and Laws (2003), and the numerous texts available on this topic.

Research and theory regarding the basis of sexual deviance and the best approach to the treatment of sexual offenders is typically described as having evolved considerably over the last 30–40 years. However, when examining the research literature, we submit that this cannot accurately be described in either research or practice as an *evolution*—defined as "a process of change in a certain direction (i.e. unfolding) and "a process of continuous change from a lower, simpler, or worse to a higher, more complex, or better state (i.e. growth; Merriam Webster, 2014). Instead, we argue that a variety of different methods of implementing treatment, based typically on the dominant philosophies, models of behaviour, and/or political influences of the time, have each been attempted as methods of intervention in a relatively random, *ad hoc* manner and/or with a narrow, unidimensional focus on one aspect of sexual offending behaviour. For example, both behavioural interventions and pharmacotherapy were intended to achieve such outcomes via the control of sexual arousal, and these approaches initially showed promise and achieved some of their desired results (Laws & Marshall, 2003; Yates, 2002, 2003). However, it was soon realised that behavioural approaches and pharmacological interventions targeting sexual arousal alone were insufficient as these did not address cognitive and emotional aspects of sexual offending and because deviant sexual interests are present in only a minority of offenders.

Later, with the advent of a feminist perspective on sexual violence, it was thought that sexual offenders were motivated by anger towards women and/or the sociological phenomenon of rape resulting from systemic male privilege (i.e. patriarchy) and women's inequality (see Yates, 1996 for a review). Manuals targeting anger were developed and applied as a model of treatment. However, research and clinical practice is lacking in this area but suggests that the broader target of sexual, emotional, and behavioural self-regulation is more appropriate. In addition, sociological approaches relating to the patriarchy of sexual aggression have not been validated or demonstrated to influence recidivism, and all that remains of this model in actual practice are treatment exercises that attempt to promote understanding and challenging of "rape myths" (Burt, 1980) or, as these are known currently, cognitive distortions. Many other similar examples exist in the treatment literature and upon critical examination of the various treatment programmes available around the world.

One approach to sexual offender treatment where this phenomenon is perhaps most evident is the adoption of the relapse prevention (RP) approach. Originally developed within a medical model to assist alcoholic patients to maintain abstinence following treatment for alcohol addiction (Marlatt, 1982; Marlatt & Gordon, 1985), the RP model assumes that individuals are underregulated with respect to problem behaviours and that they lack adequate coping skills to control behaviour. Treatment within this approach is based on assisting clients to develop an understanding of those situations which place the individual at risk for recurrence of the problem behaviours, developing strategies to avoid these situations, and instilling skills and "adaptive" mechanisms to cope with high-risk situations. Within RP, clients are not viewed as self-directed and are assumed to be continually attempting to abstain from the problem behaviour, to set themselves up to encounter situations which will inevitably lead to failure, and to subsequently experience negative emotional states associated with this failure as a result of deficits in the ability to cope with life events, thereby leading to relapse. Despite this approach not representing the dynamics of sexual offending, its problematic focus on avoidance goals, constructs and methods that are not applicable to many sexual offenders, and lack of empirical support, RP continues to be widely implemented in current interventions. One such example is California's Sex Offender Treatment and Evaluation Project (SOTEP; Marques, Wideranders, Day, Nelson, & van Ommeren, 2005), a programme that was in operation at Atascadero State Hospital between 1985 and 1995 and was subjected to a rigorous outcome evaluation (see below).

To return to the question that is the title of this section, "did we go wrong somewhere?", we submit that the answer is "probably (although not intentionally)". In other words, the manner by which science advances in any field is through trial and error of theoretically based good ideas—methods, approaches, and models that show promise at some level and that are then empirically tested for their effectiveness in practice. So, while we are not prepared to state that earlier efforts were incorrect, we submit that the problem lies in the adherence to models or approaches to intervention that failed empirical testing and the continued application of these approaches in current day intervention. In brief, we have failed to learn lessons from our previous efforts and continue to make the same mistakes. As we discuss below, following a review of the extant treatment outcome literature, this continues to the present day.

What Does the Research Tell Us?

The utility of sexual offender treatment is a contentious issue, and there is considerable debate about how best to evaluate treatment programmes and how effective programmes are in reducing risk for sexual offending (Marshall, Marshall, Serran, & O'Brien, 2011; Rice & Harris, 2003; Seto, 2005).

In one of the first, large-scale narrative reviews regarding the efficacy of sexual offender treatment, Furby, Weinrott, and Blackshaw (1989) examined 42 studies of treated and untreated sexual offenders and concluded that sexual offender treatment has no demonstrable impact on sexual offender recidivism. Researchers have since disputed Furby et al.'s (1989) conclusion and have identified a number of problems with the review (Marshall & Pithers, 1994; Yates, 2002). For example, the interventions were conducted prior to 1980 and, as such, failed to meet contemporary standards of effective intervention. Additionally, very few of the selected studies compared treated and untreated offenders, and, therefore, differences between the studies on issues such as length of follow-up, sample size, and pretreatment levels of risk to reoffend made it difficult to draw firm conclusions (Yates, 2002).

Given the methodological problems inherent in qualitative narrative reviews, several meta-analyses have been conducted to better determine the cumulative effect of treatment outcome studies. Two early meta-analyses (Gallagher, Wilson, Hirschfield, Coggeshall, & MacKenzie, 1999; Hall, 1995) were conducted that examined treated and untreated sexual offenders. Both quantitative reviews reported a positive but small effect of treatment, and, importantly, those certain types of treatment (e.g. cognitive-behavioural) were superior to strictly behavioural interventions. The results of these early quantitative reviews were limited, however, as selected studies incorporated significant bias (e.g. comparing treatment completers versus treatment dropouts). The inclusion of treatment dropouts in the control condition is problematic, and this likely increases this group's recidivism rates, given that such individuals likely possess characteristics related to risk and recidivism.

Not surprisingly, when these biased studies were removed from subsequent analyses, the treatment effect was no longer significant (see Rice & Harris, 2003).

In 1997, the collaborative outcome data project committee was established to organise the existing outcome literature and report on treatment effectiveness. Hanson et al. (2002) conducted a meta-analysis of 43 published and unpublished English language studies on psychosocial treatments comprising 9454 sexual offenders. Results indicated that treated sexual offenders had lower sexual recidivism rates (12.3 %) than sexual offenders in comparison conditions (16.8 %). Studies with the strongest methodological design (i.e. random assignment) showed no effect of treatment, whereas studies described as incidental assignment (i.e. studies with no a priori reason to suspect group differences between treated and untreated sexual offenders) showed a positive effect of treatment. Rice and Harris (2003) have criticised the selection and categorisation of the studies in the Hanson et al. (2002) meta-analysis, and they noted problems ranging from cohort effects to treatment versus control group comparability. After a reanalysis of six studies that met stricter methodological criteria for promoting group comparability, Rice and Harris (2003) concluded that there was no positive effect for treatment and, in fact, that treated sexual offenders had a higher recidivism rate than the comparison group, although this difference was not significant.

Lösel and Schmucker (2005) have since provided the largest and most comprehensive meta-analytic review of sexual offender treatment. Their review consisted of 80 comparisons derived from 69 studies, comprising 22,181 sexual offenders. Overall, results showed that treatment reduced recidivism rates compared to control conditions, but again studies employing more methodologically rigorous designs revealed no group differences in recidivism. Most recently, Långström et al. (2013) conducted a systematic review of psychological, educational, and pharmacological interventions intended to reduce recidivism among sexual offenders against children. Among the original 167 articles selected for review, only eight met minimal methodological quality representing low or moderate risk of bias (three randomised control trials (RCTs) and five controlled observational studies). Results demonstrated some minimal evidence for multisystemic therapy, an intensive approach that targets environmental systems such as schools and families (Borduin et al., 1995), for adolescent sexual offenders (based on one RCT). With regard to adult sexual offenders against children, the authors noted that there was insufficient evidence for medical and psychological interventions from which to draw firm conclusions.

A number of Cochrane reviews have been conducted that focus specifically on RCTs. Briefly, the Cochrane collaboration comprises a number of centres and specific specialities, which conducts systematic reviews on a number of topics and provides access to such reviews within a comprehensive database. The Cochrane collaboration restricts its evidence included in their reviews to RCTs. Most recently, Dennis et al. (2012) conducted a comprehensive search of articles that were published up until 2010. Ten studies were ultimately selected representing 944 sexual offenders. Five studies involved cognitive-behavioural-type interventions, four described behavioural interventions, and one involved psychodynamic treatment. The authors concluded that the evidence for the effectiveness of sexual offender treatment is weak and they advocated for additional RCTs, emphasising methodologies that minimise risk of bias.

In summary, results from meta-analytic reviews of sexual offender treatment have failed to provide strong empirical support for positive treatment outcome. Moreover, effect sizes are generally small but meaningful (see Cohen, 1992), particularly when compared against the effect sizes produced among treatment options for other medical and behavioural disorders (Marshall, 2006). Although there has been some debate about the practical and procedural utility of RCTs (Marshall, 2006), this approach is considered the "gold standard" in programme evaluation, and studies employing this approach have not shown treatment to be associated with reduced recidivism rates. Results from California's Sex Offender Treatment and Evaluation Project (Marques et al., 2005), a programme evaluation in which an RCT was used, failed to show a treatment effect and have often been cited as strong evidence against treatment effectiveness. However, closer inspection of this particular programme demonstrated that, because of the date of implementation, few known criminogenic factors were targeted in treatment. Moreover, finer-grained analyses suggested that there was a certain proportion of offenders (i.e. those who "got it") who may show a greater treatment response than other offenders within the programme. Such findings suggest that perhaps treatment can be effective, but that it must be designed and implemented based on the literature, and continued effort needs to be placed on rigorous evaluations. Specific criteria for establishing evidence-based therapeutic approaches have been provided, which focus on at least two evaluations incorporating appropriate control groups (see Chambless et al., 1998). Such criteria can assist in the implementation and interpretation of outcome evaluations.

Sexual Offender Treatment in Current Practice: Are We Doing Something Wrong?

In response to this question, we submit that, while some progress has been made, the answer is an equivocal "yes".

The most effective approach to sexual offender treatment at present is the risk/need/responsivity (RNR) approach (Andrews & Bonta, 2010), shown to be effective in reducing recidivism among many offender groups, including women, youth, violent offenders, and sexual offenders (Andrews et al., 1990; Dowden & Andrews, 1999a, 1999b, 2000, 2003; Hanson, Bourgon, Helmus, & Hodgson, 2009). This model utilises evidence-based methods to tailor treatment to individual offenders who vary in the risk they pose to reoffend, the factors that lead to offending behaviour, and clients' capacity to respond to our interventions (and our capacity to respond to their needs and individual particularities). It is based on a comprehensive theory based on an empirically based understanding of the reasons for which individuals engage in criminal behaviour (the psychology of criminal conduct; Andrews & Bonta, 2010). The RNR approach demonstrates that treatment is most effective when programmes: (1) target offenders who are at moderate to high risk to reoffend (i.e. the *risk* principle), (2) target changeable risk factors that are empirically linked to recidivism (i.e. the *need* principle), and (3) vary methods of delivery in such a manner as to ensure maximum benefit for individual offenders depending on their own circumstances and capabilities and doing so using a cognitive-behavioural/social learning approach (i.e. the *responsivity* principle). While the RNR also includes the principle of *professional discretion*, we submit that it is this element of the model, for which research support is lacking, to which clinicians most often adhere.

Regrettably, in spite of decades of empirical support, the RNR approach has not been widely adopted in the treatment of sexual offenders. Indeed, research has shown that adherence to RNR principles produces larger and more positive treatment effects among violent offenders (Dowden & Andrews, 2000) and sexual offenders (Hanson et al., 2009) compared to programmes that do not adhere to this model of treatment. Research has also found that delivery of appropriate service (i.e. that which adheres to the RNR) is not more expensive than inappropriate service and is cost-effective. For example, costs for appropriate service for a 1 % reduction in recidivism range from $0.25 to $9.40, compared to the costs of inappropriate service and traditional punishment, costing $19.67 and $40.43, respectively, for a 1 % reduction in recidivism (Romani, Morgan, Gross, & McDonald, 2012). While some jurisdictions explicitly adhere to this model and include it as a matter of policy (e.g. the Correctional Service of Canada), few other organisations and/or jurisdictions utilise this approach. For example, as McGrath et al. (2010) illustrated in their comprehensive survey of sexual offender treatment in North America, use of this model with adult sexual offenders ranges from 0 to 37 % of organisations providing treatment.[1]

The reluctance to implement treatment using such an evidence-based approach is perplexing at best. While criticisms of the RNR model suggest that it is insufficient to engage offenders and to motivate them to explore changing their behaviour (e.g. Ward & Stewart, 2003), these criticisms ignore the substantial body of evidence and the fact that the majority of treatment programmes utilising this model also explicitly take a motivational enhancement approach. (In fact, some clinicians and researchers have mistaken the responsivity construct as constituting wholly or predominantly motivation when it actually encompasses many different internal and external characteristics and circumstances.) In the authors' experience (and according to research), the RNR model applies to treatment regardless of setting (e.g. prison, residential treatment, in the community) and can easily be broadened to include motivational, self-regulation, and positive psychology approaches (Yates, Prescott, & Ward, 2010; Yates & Ward, 2008). As noted earlier, the RNR model has been demonstrated to result in reduced recidivism and can be enhanced via effective

---

[1] One programme area indicated that 50 % of programmes adhered to this model; however, this represented only two programmes of a total of four delivered to adult female offenders.

therapeutic practice. In fact, studies have shown that adherence to the risk, need, and responsivity principles has been associated with a 10, 19, and 23 % difference in recidivism, respectively (Bonta & Andrews, 2007). Among sexual offenders specifically, research indicates that adherence to the principles of the RNR results in incremental effectiveness with adherence to none, one, two, or all three principles (odds ratios of 0.21, 0.63, 0.64, and 1.17, respectively) (Hanson et al., 2009). Given the above, it is perplexing at best how this approach, despite its long-standing existence and empirically demonstrated effectiveness, is absent from the majority of treatment programmes.

Compounding this problem is the continued reliance on implementation approaches that are not supported by research. For example, research has consistently shown that treatment of low-risk offenders (those who are assessed using actuarial measures and determined to be of low risk to reoffend and demonstrating few dynamic risk factors) is, at best, ineffective and, at worst, can have the iatrogenic effect of increasing risk and resulting in increased recidivism. Conversely, appropriate treatment provided to higher-risk offenders has been shown to reduce recidivism while also finding that many programmes continue to provide intensive treatment services to low-risk offenders (Andrews & Bonta, 2010; Hanson & Yates, 2013; Lowenkamp & Latessa, 2002, 2004; Lowenkamp, Latessa, & Holsinger, 2006), yet intensive treatment of these offenders continues at present. Furthermore, substantial sanctions, such as sex offender registries and notification, are utilised with this group of offenders (see Chapter x this volume). Continuing to apply intensive treatment and sanctions, driven by ideology, philosophy, and political factors, can only serve to increase the risk of recidivism and future victimisation. In attempting to understand the rationale for this phenomenon, the authors have found that this appears to be fourfold: (1) denial on the part of clinicians that low-risk offenders actually exist; (2) the belief that low-risk offenders are actually undetected higher-risk offenders; (3) clinicians' and organisations' personal philosophies, such as the belief that all sexual offenders require treatment regardless of risk; and (4) political influence and attendant jurisdictional policies that dictate treatment requirements regardless of research findings (e.g. all offenders must be heavily sanctioned, treated, and managed). It is noted that there is also the potential for loss of livelihood in some cases — for example, in some jurisdictions, clinicians have noted that refusal to treat such offenders would result in financial penalties due to termination of contracts to treat offenders (which also represents a serious ethical concern).

Another approach to which clinicians adhere in spite of the absence of research support is, as noted above, the RP approach. In their survey, McGrath et al. (2010) found that this model continues to be used in as many as 85 % of North American treatment programmes — a figure we find disturbing given research findings that this approach does not address the dynamics of sexual offending and an absence of research demonstrating its effectiveness.

Taken together, the relative absence of adherence to the RNR model, the continued treatment of low-risk offenders, and the high rates of utilisation of RP suggest a strong reluctance, or perhaps an aversion, to applying evidence-based practices to the treatment of sexual offenders.

In addition to the above, various practices are being adopted on a regular basis in the field of sexual offender treatment that are not based on a theory of the causes of sexual offending, research pertaining to effective intervention practices, or research demonstrating effectiveness. As indicated above, while science evolves on the basis of good ideas that are subject to investigation and evaluation, some of these more recent practices (some of which are exceptionally intrusive, not to mention expensive) have not been evaluated or continue to be implemented in spite of early research indicating a lack of effectiveness. Notably, many of these practices, such as the containment approach (a multi-agency collaborative approach that explicitly takes a victim-centred philosophy, that aims to exercise control of risk in the community using treatment, probation, and polygraph, and that does so regardless of the risk level of the offender; English, 1998), sex offender notification and public registries, civil commitment, and the use of the polygraph in treatment, are not driven by research or even theory pertaining to the aetiology of sexual offending behaviour or basic principles of effective therapeutic intervention. In fact, investments continue to be made in these methods, the likely outcome of which is increased recidivism, reduced community safety, and the diversion of scarce treatment resources to these nontherapeutic activities.

What is perhaps most disturbing, in the authors' experience, is the acceptance by organisations and clinicians of such methods as valid clinical practice, with the attendant risk that any hope for the establishment of a therapeutic relationship with clients will be absent or impossible. To provide an example, the use of the polygraph to establish a full sexual history (the value of which is undemonstrated) and/or to evaluate the implementation of therapeutic tasks in the community (i.e. "maintenance" polygraphs) is becoming well entrenched in some jurisdictions, most notably the United States. Recent research, however, does not support the effectiveness of this tool in reducing recidivism and victimisation (Meijer, Verschuere, Merckelbach, & Crombez, 2008; Rosky, 2012) and runs the risk of eventually leading to a deterioration in clinical skills necessary to gather information from clients and to establish an effective working alliance, which is shown in research for various problems to account for a substantial amount of the variance in positive outcome (e.g. Marshall et al., 2003; Witte, Gu, Nicholaichuck, & Wong, 2001). While it is acknowledged that, in some jurisdictions, the use of tools such as polygraphy and containment is a legislative or other requirement for sexual offenders, the extent to which clinicians have adopted and embraced their use as *clinical tools* is disturbing. It is further acknowledged that this is a problem both at the individual clinician level and at the organisational/jurisdictional level, and that organisational or political influence can have a substantial undue impact on clinical practice. It is the authors' hope that clinicians recognise these practices and are provided with appropriate training and opportunity to separate legislative or jurisdictional requirements from clinical practice in the delivery of treatment.

In a related vein, several newer approaches to sexual offender treatment have been proposed, as examples, trauma-informed approaches such as eye movement desensitisation and reprocessing (EMDR; e.g. Ricci & Clayton, 2008; Ricci, Clayton, & Shapiro, 2006), a victim-centred approach (e.g. English, 1998), the self-regulation model (an adaptation of self-regulation theory [Baumeister & Vohs, 2004] to the sexual offence process; Ward & Hudson, 1998), and the good lives model (Ward & Stewart, 2003). In the context of this analysis, it is important to recognise that these approaches have not yet been demonstrated in research to reduce recidivism and victimisation. Yet these have now been in existence for a sufficient period of time that research to assess their impact and effectiveness on ultimate outcome (i.e. recidivism) should have been conducted but has not likely due to reluctance to change on the part of clinicians and organisations. While some research has been conducted on the validity and impact with respect to intermediate treatment targets, such as motivation (e.g. Yates & Kingston, 2006; Yates, Simons, Kingston, & Tyler, 2009), and the extent to which clinicians like the model (in the case of the good lives model; Ware & Bright, 2008), the time has come for the ultimate test of effectiveness (i.e. reduced recidivism). In light of the current status, the authors implore caution in the application and utilisation of these approaches, lest we be destined to repeat the past.

In conclusion, regardless of the specific tool or method or the personal, philosophical, or political approach to sexual offenders, we view as essential to the effectiveness of current and future practice the ability to critically evaluate models and approaches and their application, to do so with a sound understanding of the research basis of each, and to resist practices that will result in the degradation of clinical skills and effective intervention.

Content and Process of Treatment: Have We Got It Right?

Our answer to this question is an unequivocal "no". Treatment of sexual offenders, as indicated above, continues to adhere to models and approaches (new and old) that have not been demonstrated to be effective or that have been demonstrated to be ineffective and to ignore approaches and models that are effective. Nowhere is this more evident than in the examination of the specific content and process of current treatment programmes.

To begin, in many jurisdictions, treatment is delivered entirely without structure or an overarching model and approach based on research and without quality review of adherence to the approach and so of unknown and questionable fidelity, resulting in a lack of information pertaining to content and process of treatment that is implemented with clients. It is no surprise that outcome results are inconclusive and that research is inconsistent given the current state of the field. In this section, we explore a few specific examples as illustrations.

Regrettably, in spite of research to the contrary, many theorists and clinicians continue to insist that treatment manuals create restrictions on clinical practice (Levenson & Prescott, 2013; Marshall, 2009; Gannon & Ward, 2014). It is perplexing and disturbing that our discipline discounts research indicating that the most effective correctional programmes are those that adhere to specific standards, including the use of manuals, which creates consistency, ensures that treatment is evidence based, and ensures treatment integrity and fidelity (Gendreau & Goggin, 1996, 1997; Gendreau, Little, & Goggin, 1996; Hanson et al., 2009; Hanson & Yates, 2004). Those who adhere to this view argue that adherence to treatment manuals is incompatible with the development of an effective therapeutic alliance with clients, a well-established element of treatment in general (e.g. Marshall, Burton, & Marshall, 2013), although research support for this assumption is absent. The notion that structure and content are incompatible with therapeutic process, with the attendant conclusion that content and process are dichotomous constructs that cannot be reconciled, is indeed perplexing. When this argument is presented, reference is ironically made to the work of Andrews and Bonta (2010), in which it is stated that intervention needs to be individualised. What is missing, however, is that this tailoring of treatment must be based on risk, need, and responsivity, as well as structure. However, the reference to the structure of this model, for which there is extensive research support, that involves cognitive-behavioural intervention to target specific criminogenic needs empirically demonstrated to be linked to recidivism, is typically ignored in this argument.

One major problem with current sexual offender treatment is that it is far too long in duration. This appears to be based on the belief that "more is better", as well a negative effect of the amount of time in treatment that is dedicated to factors not demonstrated to be empirically related to sexual offending or recidivism and to the use of extensive exercises of questionable value to treatment (e.g. autobiographies, extensive analyses of the offence process, victim empathy or "clarification" letters, and overcoming denial/minimisation). Admittedly, there is little research evidence pertaining to the effective dosage of treatment required for offenders presenting with varying levels of risk to reoffend and various criminogenic needs or dynamic risk factors. Regarding dosage, recommendations have been made (Bourgon & Armstrong, 2005; Hanson & Yates, 2013), yet treatment in most jurisdictions does not adhere to such risk-based recommendations.

Research has clearly delineated those factors known to be associated with increased risk for recidivism, such as intimacy deficits, sexual and general self-regulation, and the presence of sexual deviance/preference (Hanson, Harris, Scott, & Helmus, 2007). What we are only beginning to learn is how to weight these various factors and their relationship to static risk factors. Regardless and in spite of perplexing academic criticism that these factors have their basis in research (e.g. Gannon & Ward, 2014), factors that place offenders at risk to reoffend, and that can be targeted in treatment, are known and must be targeted if treatment is to be effective. Yet many programmes continue to target treatment goals that are unrelated to recidivism reduction, such as denial, self-esteem, personal distress, empathy, and individual accountability (Hanson & Morton-Bourgon, 2005; Yates, 2009). In the authors' opinion, this continues as a result of individual, societal, and legal values, which emphasise such constructs as remorse and taking responsibility for one's actions. For example, a fundamental premise of the criminal justice system is to hold individuals accountable for their actions, and it is a societal expectation that one experiences remorse when harm to others has been caused. Necessarily, this societal expectation influences organisations and individuals, including clinicians delivering sexual offender treatment. However, while these are laudable goals and are an essential element of punishment (i.e. sentencing) within the criminal justice system, research either does not support their inclusion as treatment targets that will reduce recidivism or the considerable amount of time taken in treatment to address these issues. A similar problem exists with the currently emerging "victim-centred" approach to sexual offender treatment. While it is inarguable that victims' experiences are important and deserving of attention and intervention, their application in the treatment of offenders (e.g. in the form of understanding victims' perspectives and making amends) is undemonstrated. In addition, because the focus is to raise awareness of harm caused (i.e. empathy), this approach is unlikely to influence treatment outcome, thus representing another instance in which treatment continues to absorb practices that are not empirically supported. Clinicians and organisations need to be able to differentiate between the goals of the legal system, societal expectations, and public policy and what works in sexual offender treatment in order to reduce risk and promote community safety.

The above also leads to an artificial dichotomy between protection of the public via reduced recidivism and victimisation and enhancing the psychological and community well-being of the offender. Many treatment programmes and some newer treatment models focus on the well-being of the offender as an essential part of treatment. This is rightfully an important goal of human service providers in all fields—clinicians wish to reduce distress and enhance individuals' lives. However, what is absent is the problematisation of this approach within criminal justice systems and its potential impact on the fundamental human rights and liberty of citizens (which includes offenders). In brief, as a field we need to examine the fundamental ethical violation of incarcerating individuals or applying (sometimes long-term) sanctions such that we may make individuals' lives better. We cannot imagine a profession outside the criminal justice system that would condone restrictions on liberty and freedom in order to improve well-being in the absence of evidence of risk to oneself or others. Despite our legitimate desire to improve people's lives, we do not believe this should be a condition of treatment or a requirement to retain or reacquire freedom in the absence of risk or its reduction, and we view this as unethical.

Much research has been done pertaining to effective therapist characteristics and therapeutic approaches that influence the outcome of treatment (Beech & Fordham, 1997; Marshall et al., 2002; Shingler & Mann, 2006; Yates, 2002, 2014; Yates et al., 2000). Andrews and Kiessling (1980) introduced several dimensions of effective correctional practice, termed core correctional practice, that were intended to promote treatment outcome in offender populations. Arguably, the most important principle was the quality of interpersonal relationships, which denotes the specific therapist characteristics that are associated with treatment success (Dowden & Andrews, 2004). Specific therapist characteristics that have been shown to enhance treatment effectiveness include demonstrating such features as empathy, respect, sincerity, confidence, and interest in the client. Being a prosocial model, being "firm but fair", reinforcing and encouraging clients, creating opportunities for success, dealing appropriately and effectively with resistance, being appropriately challenging without being aggressively confrontational, and creating a secure treatment atmosphere all contribute to treatment outcome (Fernandez, 2006; Marshall et al., 2002). For example, research indicates that establishing a positive therapeutic relationship with the client accounts for a significant proportion of the variance in treatment outcome (Fernandez, Shingler, & Marshall, 2006; Hanson et al., 2009; Witte et al., 2001; Mann, Webster, Schofield, & Marshall, 2004; Marshall et al., 2003).

Behavioural rehearsal and practice, designed to inculcate new skills into individuals' behavioural repertoires, are also essential elements of treatment yet are methods that are insufficiently utilised in current insight-based approaches (Fernandez et al., 2006; Yates et al., 2010). Similarly, using motivational enhancement techniques and creating a positive and safe treatment environment lead to improved compliance with treatment, progress, and enhanced motivation and prevent termination or dropout from treatment (Beech & Fordham, 1997; Kear-Colwell & Pollack, 1997; Marshall, Anderson, & Fernandez, 1999; Prescott, 2009).

Given that research clearly indicates that offenders who do not complete treatment reoffend at significantly higher rates than offenders who complete treatment (Hanson & Bussière, 1998; Hanson et al., 2002), it is essential that treatment is delivered in a manner that is motivating and engaging for clients. However, the authors are aware of few programmes or organisations that explicitly select or screen therapists for such characteristics and that train treatment providers in these effective techniques or that deliberately train service providers to respond to the characteristics of the offenders with whom they work (i.e. attending to responsivity). In fact, unlike other professional practice areas such as psychology, psychiatry, or social work, there are no universally standard professional practice requirements for therapists delivering sexual offender treatment, who range in training and experience from prison officers to probation officers to other professionals with various levels and type of education and training. While there is no research suggesting the superiority of one discipline over another in the delivery of treatment, practice requirements and training are highly variable across jurisdictions, clinicians are not typically preselected for the essential characteristics that enhance treatment success, supervision and quality review of treatment implementation is not consistently utilised, and training received by clinicians is often absent or inconsistent.

As a final note, we note the lack of tolerance for harm reduction in the field of sexual offender treatment, which has long been proposed as having potential as a measure of treatment outcome or success (Laws, 1996). While from a clinical perspective we as a field purport to advocate for the reduction of harm through intervention and treatment, in practice, the goal of sexual offender treatment appears to remain one of complete abstinence (while simultaneously holding the belief that sexual offending is a life-long problem from which one cannot recover). However, if we were working in the area of addictions or general mental health, we as clinicians would be at least minimally satisfied with a level of progress that reduced symptomatology and risk to self or others. If we were treating a patient suffering from depression, we would be satisfied with reducing active suicidal intent, even if the client remained feeling hopeless. In such a case, we would not restrict freedom and liberty (i.e. we would not [and could not legally] commit the patient while we continued to work with the client for depression in the absence of imminent risk of harm). In sexual offender treatment, we do not work this way. To provide a parallel example, sexual offender treatment aims to reduce the potential for sexual victimisation and harm. However, even if we effectively treat the client to manage deviant sexual arousal or to effectively manage risk, if such a client continues to present with deviant sexual fantasy or urges, we continue to incarcerate or otherwise restrict the offender, until he or she is able to demonstrate that such urges no longer exist—an outcome that is impossible to assess and determine definitively, in addition to being an unlikely occurrence.

Sexual Offender Treatment in the Future: Where Do We Go from Here?

In this chapter, we have reviewed current and previous processes of the development and implementation of sexual offender treatment. We have noted that various theories of sexual offending behaviour, models of intervention, and elements of specific practice have been developed in an ad hoc fashion based on good ideas at the time, which may or may not have had a basis in research and theory. We further argued that current approaches to the treatment of sexual offenders apply and retain elements of intervention that are undemonstrated in research to be effective or that have been demonstrated to be ineffective while omitting approaches known to be effective and that this state of affairs is unduly influenced by political, organisational, and personal bias regarding the objectives of sexual offender treatment and the manner in which it should be implemented. While research supporting the effectiveness of sexual offender treatment is equivocal at best, we nonetheless implore those responsible for the delivery of sexual offender treatment to attend to the research basis for the content and structure of treatment, its specific implementation and delivery methods, and the requirements for effective therapy, in order to maximise the probability of success via reduced recidivism and victimisation and increased community safety. We need to do so while continuously examining and challenging our own biases and those of our organisations, jurisdictions, and political circumstances while differentiating between ideology, legal requirements for practice, and political influence, so we can deliver empirically supported interventions in an ethical and effective manner.

References

Andrews, D. A., & Bonta, J. (2010). Rehabilitating criminal justice policy and practice (5th edition). *Psychology, Public Policy, and Law, 16*(1), 39–55.

Andrews, D.A. and Kiessling, J.J. (1980). *Program structure and effective correctional practice: A summary of cavic research.* In R. Ross & P. Gendreau (Eds.), Effective correctional treatment (pp.439–463). Toronto, ON: Butterworths.

Andrews, D. A., Zinger, I., Hoge, R. D., Bonta, J., Gendreau, P., & Cullen, F. T. (1990). Does correctional treatment work? A clinically relevant and psychologically informed meta-analysis. *Criminology, 28*, 369–404.

Baumeister, R. F., & Vohs, K. D. (2004). *Handbook of self-regulation: Research, theory, and applications.* New York, NY: Guilford Press.

Beech, A., & Fordham, A. S. (1997). Therapeutic climate of sexual offender treatment programs. *Sexual Abuse: A Journal of Research and Treatment, 9*, 219–237.

Bonta, J., & Andrews, D. A. (2007). *Risk need model of offender assessment and rehabilitation.* Ottawa, ON: Public Safety Canada.

Borduin, C. M., Mann, B. J., Cone, L. T., Henggeler, S. W., Fucci, B. R., Blaske, D. M., & Williams, R. A. (1995). Multisystemic treatment of serious juvenile offenders: Long-term prevention of criminality and violence. *Journal of Consulting and Clinical Psychology, 63*, 569–578.

Bourgon, G., & Armstrong, B. (2005). Transferring the principles of effective treatment into a "real world" prison setting. *Criminal Justice and Behavior, 32*, 3–25.

Burt, M. R. (1980). Cultural myths and supports for rape. *Journal of Personality and Social Psychology, 39*, 217–230.

Chambless, D. L., Baker, M. J., Baucom, D. H., Beutler, L. E., Calhoun, K. S., Crits-Christoph, P., Woody, S. R. (1998). Update on empirically validated therapies II. *The Clinical Psychologist, 51*, 3–16.

Cohen, J. (1992). A power primer. *Psychological Bulletin, 122*, 155–159.

Dennis, J., Huband, N., Khan, O., Ferriter, M., Jones, H., Powney, M., Duggan, C. (2012). Psychological interventions for adults who have sexually offended or are at risk of offending. *Cochrane Database of Reviews Issue: 12.* doi:10.1002/14651858 CD007507 pub2.

Dowden, C., & Andrews, D. A. (1999a). What works in young offender treatment: A meta-analysis. *Forum on Corrections Research, 11*, 21–24.

Dowden, C., & Andrews, D. A. (1999b). What works for female offenders: A meta-analytic review. *Crime and Delinquency, 45*, 438–452.

Dowden, C., & Andrews, D. A. (2000). Effective correctional treatment and violent offending: A meta-analysis. *Canadian Journal of Criminology and Criminal Justice, 42*, 449–467.

Dowden, C., & Andrews, D. A. (2003). Does family intervention work for delinquents? Results of a meta-analysis. *Canadian Journal of Criminology and Criminal Justice, 45*, 327–342.

Dowden, C., & Andrews, D. A. (2004). The importance of staff practice in delivering effective correctional treatment: A meta-analytic review of core correctional practice. *International Journal of Offender Therapy and Comparative Criminology, 48*, 203–214.

English, K. (1998). The containment approach: An aggressive strategy for the community. *Management of Adult Sex Offenders, Psychology, Public Policy, and Law, 4*, 218–235.

Fernandez, Y. M. (2006). Focusing on the positive and avoiding the negative in sexual offender treatment. In W. L. Marshall, Y. M. Fernandez, L. E. Marshall, & G. A. Serran (Eds.), *Sexual offender treatment: Controversial issues* (pp. 187–197). Hoboken, NJ: John Wiley & Sons.

Fernandez, Y. M., Shingler, J., & Marshall, W. L. (2006). Putting "behaviour" back in cognitive-behavioral treatment. In W. L. Marshall, Y. Fernandez, L. Marshall, & G. Serran (Eds.), *Sexual offender treatment: Controversial issues.* London: Wiley & Sons, Ltd.

Furby, L., Weinrott, M. R., & Blackshaw, L. (1989). Sex offender recidivism: A review. *Psychol Bull, 105*(1), 3–30.

Gallagher, C. A., Wilson, D. B., Hirschfield, P., Coggeshall, M. B., & MacKenzie, D. L. (1999). A quantitative review of the effects of sex offender treatment on sexual reoffending. *Corrections Management Quarterly, 3*, 19–29.

Gannon, T. A., & Ward, T. (2014). Where has all the psychology gone? *Aggression and Violent Behavior, 19*, 435–446.

Gendreau, P., & Goggin, C. (1996). Principles of effective correctional programming. *Forum on Corrections Research, 8*, 38–41.

Gendreau, P., & Goggin, C. (1997). Correctional treatment: Accomplishments and realities. In P. Van Voorhis et al. (Eds.), *Correctional Counseling and Rehabilitation* (pp. 271–279). Cincinnati, OH: Anderson.

Gendreau, P., Little, T., & Goggin, C. (1996). A meta-analysis of the predictors of adult offender recidivism: What works! *Criminology, 34*, 3–17.

Hall, G. C. N. (1995). Sexual offender recidivism: A meta-analysis of recent treatment studies. *Journal of Consulting and Clinical Psychology, 63*, 802–809.

Hanson, R. K. (1996). Evaluating the contribution of relapse prevention theory to the treatment of sexual offenders. *Sexual Abuse: A Journal of Research and Treatment, 8*, 201–208.

Hanson, R. K. (2000). What is so special about relapse prevention? In D. R. Laws (Ed.), *Relapse prevention with sex offenders* (pp. 1–31). New York, NY: Guilford.

Hanson, R. K., Bourgon, G., Helmus, L., & Hodgson, S. (2009). The principles of effective correctional treatment also apply to sexual offenders: A meta-analysis. *Criminal Justice and Behavior, 36*, 865–891.

Hanson, R. K., & Bussière, M. (1998). Predicting relapse: A meta-analysis of sexual offender recidivism studies. *Journal of Consulting and Clinical Psychology, 66*, 348–362.

Hanson, R. K., Gordon, A., Harris, A. J. R., Marques, J. K., Murphy, W., Quinsey, V. L., & Seto, M. C. (2002). First report of the collaborative outcome data project on the effectiveness of psychological treatment for sex offenders. *Sexual Abuse: A Journal of Research and Treatment, 14*, 169–194.

Hanson, R. K., Harris, A. J. R., Scott, T., & Helmus, L. (2007). *Assessing the risk of sexual offenders on community supervision: The Dynamic Supervision Project (User Report No. 2007-05).* Ottawa, ON: Public Safety Canada.

Hanson, R. K., & Morton-Bourgon, K. E. (2005). The characteristics of persistent sexual offenders : A meta-analysis of recidivism studies. *Journal of Consulting and Clinical Psychology, 73*, 1154–1163.

Hanson, R. K., & Yates, P. M. (2004). Sexual violence: Risk factors and treatment. In M. Eliasson (Ed.), *Anthology on interventions against violent men*. Uppsala: Department of Industrial Relations.

Hanson, R. K., & Yates, P. M. (2013). Psychological treatment of sex offenders. *Current Psychiatry Reports, 15*, 1–8.

Kear-Colwell, J., & Pollack, P. (1997). Motivation and confrontation: Which approach to the child sex offender? *Criminal Justice and Behavior, 24*, 20–33.

Kingston, D. A., Yates, P. M., & Firestone, P. (2012). The self-regulation model of sexual offender treatment: Relationship to risk and need. *Law and Human Behavior, 36*, 215–224.

Kingston, D. A., Yates, P. M., & Olver, M. E. (2014). The self-regulation model of sexual offending: intermediate outcomes and post-treatment recidivism. *Sexual Abuse: A Journal of Research and Treatment, 26*, 429–449.

Knight, R.A., & Prentky, R.A. (1990). Classifying offenders. Handbook of sexual assault. *Applied Clinical Psychology*, pp. 23–52.

Långström, N., Enebrink, P., Laurén, E.-M., Lindblom, J., Werkö, S., & Hanson, R. K. (2013). Preventing sexual abusers of children from reoffending: Systematic review of medical and psychological interventions. *British Medical Journal, 347*(f4630).

Laws, D. R. (1989). *Relapse prevention with sex offenders*. New York, NY: Guilford.

Laws, D. R. (1996). Relapse prevention or harm reduction? *Sexual Abuse: A Journal of Research and Treatment, 8*, 243–248.

Laws, D. R. (2003). The rise and fall of relapse prevention. *Australian Psychologist, 38*(1), 22–30.

Laws, D. R., & Marshall, W. L. (2003). A brief history of behavioral and cognitive behavioral approaches to sexual offenders: Part 1. Early developments. *Sexual Abuse: A Journal of Research and Treatment, 15*, 75–92.

Levenson, J., & Prescott, D. S. (2013). Déjà vu: from Furby to Långström and the evaluation of sex offender treatment effectiveness. *Journal of Sexual Aggression, 20*(3), 257–266.

Lösel, F., & Schmucker, M. (2005). The effectiveness of treatment for sexual offenders: A comprehensive meta-analysis. *Journal of Experimental Criminology, 1*, 117–146.

Lowenkamp, C., & Latessa, E. (2002). *Evaluation of Ohio's community based correctional facilities and halfway house programs*. Unpublished manuscript, Division of Criminal Justice, University of Cincinnati, OH.

Lowenkamp, C., & Latessa, E. (2004). Increasing the effectiveness of correctional programming through the risk principle: Identifying offenders for residential placement. *Criminology and Public Policy, 4,* 501–528.

Lowenkamp, C. T., Latessa, E., & Holsinger, A. (2006). The risk principle in action: What have we learned from 13,676 offenders and 97 correctional programs? *Crime & Delinquency, 51,* 1–17.

Mann, R. E., Webster, S. D., Schofield, C., & Marshall, W. L. (2004). Approach versus avoidance goals in relapse prevention with sexual offenders. *Sexual Abuse: A Journal of Research and Treatment, 16,* 65–75.

Marlatt, G. A. (1982). Relapse prevention: A self-control program for the treatment of addictive behaviours. In R. B. Stuart (Ed.), *Adherence, compliance and generalization in behavioral medicine* (pp. 329–378). New York, NY: Brunner/Mazel.

Marlatt, G. A., & Gordon, J. R. (1985). *Relapse prevention: maintenance strategies in the treatment of addictive behaviors.* New York, NY: Guilford.

Marques, J. K., Wideranders, M., Day, D. M., Nelson, C., & van Ommeren, A. (2005). Effects of a relapse prevention program on sexual recidivism: Final results from California's Sex Offender Treatment and Evaluation Project (SOTEP). *Sexual Abuse: A Journal of Research and Treatment, 17,* 79–107.

Marshall, W. L. (2006). Appraising treatment outcome with sexual offenders. In W. L. Marshall, Y. M. Fernandez, L. E. Marshall, & G. A. Serran (Eds.), *Sexual offender treatment: Controversial issues* (pp. 255–273). Chichester: John Wiley & Sons.

Marshall, W. L. (2009). Manualization: A blessing or a curse? *Journal of Sexual Aggression, 15,* 109–120.

Marshall, W. L., Anderson, D., & Fernandez, Y. M. (1999). *Cognitive behavioral treatment of sexual offenders.* Chichester: Wiley.

Marshall, W. L., Burton, D. L., & Marshall, L. E. (2013). Features of treatment delivery and group processes that maximize the effects of offender programs. In J. L. Wood & T. A. Gannon (Eds.), *Crime and crime reduction: The importance of group processes* (pp. 159–174). New York, NY: Routledge.

Marshall, W. L., Fernandez, Y. M., Serran, G. A., Mulloy, R., Thornton, D., Mann, R. E., & Anderson, D. (2003). Process variables in the treatment of sexual offenders: A review of the relevant literature. *Aggression and Violent Behavior, 8,* 205–234.

Marshall, W. L., & Laws, D. R. (2003). A brief history of behavioral and cognitive behavioral approaches to sexual offenders: Part 1. The modern era. *Sexual Abuse: A Journal of Research and Treatment, 15,* 93–120.

Marshall, W. L., Marshall, L. E., Serran, G. A., & O'Brien, M. D. (2011). *Rehabilitating sexual offenders.* Washington, DC: American Psychological Association.

Marshall, W. L., & Pithers, W. D. (1994). A reconsideration of treatment outcome with sex offenders. *Criminal Justice and Behavior, 21,* 10–27.

Marshall, W. L., Serran, G., Moulden, H., Mulloy, R., Fernandez, Y. M., Mann, R. E., & Thornton, D. (2002). Therapist features in sexual offender treatment: Their reliable identification and influence on behaviour change. *Clinical Psychology and Psychotherapy, 9,* 395–405.

McGrath, R. J., Cumming, G. F., Burchard, B. L., Zeoli, S., & Ellerby, L. (2010). *Current practices and emerging trends in sexual abuser management: The Safer Society 2009 North American Survey.* Brandon, VT: Safer Society Press.

Meijer, E. H., Verschuere, B., Merckelbach, H. L., & Crombez, G. (2008). Sex offender management using the polygraph: A critical review. *International Journal of Law and Psychiatry, 31,* 423–9429.

Prescott, D. S. (2009). Motivational interviewing in the treatment of sexual abusers. In D. S. Prescott (Ed.), *Building motivation for change in sexual offenders.* Brandon, VT: Safer Society Press.

Ricci, R. J., & Clayton, C. A. (2008). Trauma resolution treatment as an adjunct to standard treatment for child molesters. *Journal of EMDR Practice and Research, 2,* 42–51.

Ricci, R. J., Clayton, C. A., & Shapiro, F. (2006). Some effects of EMDR on previously abused child molesters: Theoretical reviews and preliminary findings. *Journal of Forensic Psychiatry & Psychology, 17*, 538–562.

Rice, M. E., & Harris, G. T. (2003). The size and sign of treatment effects in sex offender therapy. *Annals of the New York Academy of Sciences, 989*, 428–440.

Romani, C. J., Morgan, R. D., Gross, N. R., & McDonald, B. R. (2012). Treating criminal behavior: Is the bang worth the buck? *Psychology, Public Policy, and Law, 18*, 144–165.

Rosky, J. W. (2012). The (F)utility of post-conviction polygraph testing. *Sexual Abuse: A Journal of Research and Treatment., 25*(3), 259–281.

Seto, M. C. (2005, November). *The evolution of sex offender treatment: Taking the next step.* Paper presented at the 24th Annual Research and Treatment Conference of the Association for the Treatment of Sexual Abusers, Salt Lake City, UT.

Shingler, J., & Mann, R. E. (2006). Collaboration in clinical work with sexual offenders: Treatment and risk assessment. In W. L. Marshall, Y. M. Fernandez, L. E. Marshall, & G. A. Serran (Eds.), *Sexual offender treatment: Controversial issues* (pp. 173–185). Hoboken, NJ: Wiley.

Ward, T., & Hudson, S. M. (1998). The construction and development of theory in the sexual offending area: A metatheoretical framework. *Sexual Abuse: A Journal of Research and Treatment, 10*, 47–63.

Ward, T., & Stewart, C. (2003). Criminogenic needs and human needs: A theoretical model. *Psychology, Crime & Law, 9*, 125–143.

Ware, J., & Bright, D. A. (2008). Evolution of a treatment programme for sex offenders: Changes to the NSW Custody-Based Intensive Treatment (CUBIT). *Psychiatry, Psychology and Law, 15*, 340–349.

Witte, T., Gu, D., Nicholaichuck, T., & Wong, S. (2001). *Working Alliance Inventory (WAI): Prediction in a forensic psychiatric hospital.* Poster presented at the 62nd Annual Convention of the Canadian Psychological Association, Saint-Foy, QC.

Yates, P.M. (1996). An investigation of factors associated with definitions and perceptions of rape, propensity to commit rape, and rape prevention. Doctoral dissertation, Carleton University, Ottawa.

Yates, P. M. (2002). What works: Effective intervention with sex offenders. In H. E. Allen (Ed.), *What works: risk reduction: Interventions for special needs offenders.* Lanham, MD: American Correctional Association.

Yates, P. M. (2003). Treatment of adult sexual offenders: A therapeutic cognitive-behavioral model of intervention. *Journal of Child Sexual Abuse, 12*, 195–232.

Yates, P. M. (2005). *Pathways to the treatment of sexual offenders: Rethinking intervention Forum summer* (pp. 1–9). Beaverton, OR: Association for the Treatment of Sexual Abusers.

Yates, P. M. (2007). Taking the leap: Abandoning relapse prevention and applying the self-regulation model to the treatment of sexual offenders. In D. Prescott (Ed.), *Applying knowledge to practice: The treatment and supervision of sexual abusers.* Oklahoma City, OK: Wood 'n' Barnes.

Yates, P. M. (2009). Is sexual offender denial related to sex offence risk and recidivism? A review and treatment implications. *Psychology Crime and Law Special Issue: Cognition and Emotion, 15*, 183–199.

Yates, P. M. (2014). Treatment of sexual offenders: Research, best practices, and emerging models. *International Journal of Behavioral Consultation and Therapy Special Issues: Current Approaches and Perspectives in the Treatment of Adult and Juvenile Sexual Offending, 8*, 89–95.

Yates, P. M., Goguen, B. C., Nicholaichuk, T. P., Williams, S. M., Long, C. A., Jeglic, E., & Martin, G. (2000). National sex offender programs (moderate, low, and maintenance intensity levels). Ottawa, ON: Correctional Service Canada.

Yates, P. M., & Kingston, D. A. (2005). Pathways to sexual offending. In B. K. Schwartz & H. R. Cellini (Eds.), *The sex offender (volume V)* (pp. 1–15). Kingston, NJ: Civic Research Institute.

Yates, P. M., & Kingston, D. A. (2006). Pathways to sexual offending: Relationship to static and dynamic risk among treated sexual offenders. *Sexual Abuse: A Journal of Research and Treatment, 18*, 259–270.

Yates, P. M., Prescott, D. S., & Ward, T. (2010). *Applying the good lives and self-regulation models to sex offender treatment: A practical guide for clinicians.* Brandon, VT: Safer Society Press. http://www.safersociety.org/safer-society-press/.

Yates, P. M., Simons, D. A., Kingston, D. A., & Tyler, C. (2009). *The good lives model of rehabilitation applied to treatment: assessment and relationship to treatment progress and compliance.* Presented at the 28th Annual Convention of the Association for the Treatment of Sexual Abusers (ATSA), Dallas, TX, October, 2009.

Yates, P. M., & Ward, T. (2008). Good lives, self-regulation, and risk management: An integrated model of sexual offender assessment and treatment. *Sexual Abuse in Australia and New Zealand: An Interdisciplinary Journal, 1*, 3–20.

Chapter 13
Desistance from Crime: Toward an Integrated Conceptualization for Intervention

Patrick Lussier

Introduction

The idea that sexual offending is a symptom of an underlying fixed and stable propensity to commit sexually deviant acts is prevalent among the public, but also among policymakers and practitioners (e.g., Letourneau & Miner, 2005; Simon, 1998). In that context, perhaps, it is not surprising that the topic of desistance from sexual offending is only beginning to emerge and spark interest among scholars and practitioners. In the current criminal justice model, much emphasis has been put over the years on community protection and risk management, including the reliance on actuarial risk assessment and risk prediction with adult sex offenders (Feeley & Simon, 1992). In fact, probably no subgroup of individuals has been affected more by this actuarial justice model than those convicted for a sexual offense (Simon, 1998). The new penology and its emphasis on risk management rather than rehabilitation has had important policy ramifications and implications for the prevention of sexual violence and abuse. Indeed, criminal justice policies have been increasingly focused on community protection (Petrunik, 2002, 2003; Murphy et al., 2009). If the vast majority of individuals convicted for a sexual offense eventually return the community, then issues surrounding their community reentry and community reintegration needs to be on the agenda. Currently, the actuarial-based community protection model, is concerned with the identification of risk factors statistically associated with sexual recidivism and the clinical assessment of these risk factors to make valid and reliable prediction of future offending of individuals (e.g., Quinsey, Rice, & Harris, 1995). Clinical researchers and

P. Lussier, Ph.D. (✉)
School of Social Work (Criminology program), Université Laval,
Pavillon Charles-De Koninck, 1030, Ave. des Sciences-Humaines, Québec City,
QC, Canada G1V 0A6
e-mail: patrick.lussier@svs.ulaval.ca

© Springer International Publishing Switzerland 2016
D.R. Laws, W. O'Donohue (eds.), *Treatment of Sex Offenders*,
DOI 10.1007/978-3-319-25868-3_13

practitioners have raised issues and concerns with this static perspective of risk, and, as a result, the field of sexual violence and abuse has witnessed the gradual introduction of a more dynamic view which includes dynamic risk factors and treatment/intervention needs to guide the case management of offenders and modify the risk of sexual reoffending (Hanson & Harris, 2000, 2001). In spite of the emergence of a more dynamic view of offending, the underlying assumption that this group of individuals always remain at some risk of sexual reoffending, albeit at different level, remains. This probabilistic view is no stranger to the fact that the concept of desistance from sex offending has been relatively absent from the scientific literature in the field of sexual violence and abuse (e.g., Lussier & Cale, 2013). It is telling that risk assessors are routinely assessing the probability of sexually reoffending, yet remain relatively silent about desistance from sex offending (notable exceptions, Laws & Ward, 2011; Robbé, Mann, Maruna, & Thornton, 2014; Worling & Langton, 2014). Yet prospective longitudinal research has repeatedly shown that most, if not all offenders, eventually desist from crime at some point over their life course.

Every time an individual comes into contact with the criminal justice system, their level of service in terms of risk factors and intervention needs increase. This is true especially for young offenders which emphasizes the importance of identifying key desistance factors early on. As a result, and because of the important discontinuity of offending around that period, desistance research has focused mostly on the adolescence–adulthood transition (e.g., Mulvey et al., 2004). This early adulthood age stage is critical given the long-standing age–crime curve perspective that identified a substantial downward trend in prevalence of general offending around this time (e.g., Farrington, 1986). In other words, most youth involved in juvenile delinquency do not go on to pursue an adult criminal career, quite the contrary. Recent studies, however, suggest that this downward trend toward the end of adolescence may not characterize all types of offenders (e.g., Loeber, Farrington, Stouthamer-Loeber, & White, 2008). In other words, the age–crime curve may not be the same for all offenders and offense types (Sampson & Laub, 2003) and desistance from crime may be characterized by different paths (Lussier & Gress, 2014). That said, Mulvey et al. (2004) identified a fundamental limitation when they asserted that previous longitudinal studies have provided minimal understanding and policy guidelines concerning offenders in the "deep end" of the criminal justice system. While research on more serious subgroups of offenders, especially chronic offenders (e.g., Loeber & Farrington, 1998), has dramatically increased in the past two decades with regard to desistance, other subgroups such as those having committed a violent offense (e.g., Corrado, 2002; Tzoumakis, Lussier, Le Blanc, & Davies, 2012) and/or a sexual offense (e.g., Lussier & Blokland, 2014; Lussier, Van Den Berg, Bijleveld, & Hendriks, 2012; McCuish, Lussier, & Corrado, 2015) remain under-researched. The relative absence of research for this subgroup is telling of the underlying assumption that these serious offenders remain at-risk of violent and/or sexual offending over long-time periods. Yet, in their seminal study, Sampson and Laub (2003) concluded that desistance was the norm even among serious and persistent offenders. Their study highlighted that previous offending record had little predictive validity regarding lifelong patterns of offending. In other words, the most criminogenic profiles do not guarantee a lifelong pattern of chronic serious and violent offending. These assertions have several important theoretical, empirical, methodological, and policy implications.

The concept of desistance from crime emerged in the scientific literature in the late 1970s in the writings of criminal career researchers who were concerned with the description and understanding the whole longitudinal sequence of individual offending (e.g., Blumstein, Cohen, Roth, & Visher, 1986; Le Blanc & Fréchette, 1989). For criminal career researchers, the factors responsible for the onset, course, and termination of offending were said to be relatively different. In other words, individuals do not stop offending for the same reasons that they start offending or escalate to more serious forms of crimes. While this concept seems relatively straightforward, scholars have approached desistance differently over the years. Several innovative studies aimed to describe and explain desistance from crime among youth emerging from the corpus of developmental life course paradigm have been conducted. The generalizability of the various desistance hypotheses that have utilized longitudinal data from general and at-risk youth drawn from schools, however, has been questioned. While this research, very importantly, has identified factors associated with desistance around the adolescence–adulthood transition, these findings are not necessarily generalizable to certain subgroups of youth involved in serious, chronic, violent and/or sex offending. Most importantly, the representative samples as well as those based on at-risk youth are not likely to include many chronic juvenile offenders, young murderers, gang members, or juvenile sex offenders. In other words, both theoretically and in policy terms, it is unclear whether the current state of knowledge on desistance is readily generalizable to those youth involved in the most serious forms of crimes or presenting the most serious patterns of offending. More specifically, the current state of knowledge is rather limited regarding these "special categories" of young offenders, therefore limiting the possibility of drawing specific policy recommendations for the most serious juvenile offenders (e.g., Rosenfeld, White, & Esbensen, 2012). In that regard, Cernkovich and Giordano (2001) confirmed that social bonding mechanisms appear to operate on general samples, but not with institutionalized samples of offenders, which includes more serious offenders. Policy recommendations are also significantly limited by the lack of a general consensus between scholars regarding the conceptual definition of desistance. Indeed, researchers have mainly defined desistance from crime as an event or a process. It is unclear, however, whether the conceptualization of desistance either as an event or a process adequately represents the phenomena for all individuals involved in sexual offenses.

The Conceptualization of Desistance from Crime

Among criminologists, there is a lack of a general agreement as to what constitute desistance from crime. According to the Merriam-Webster, to desist refers to someone who ceases something. This term comes from the French word *désister* which refers to someone voluntarily giving up something (e.g., a right, a claim, a legal proceeding). The English term is more behavioral-focused as it implies the termination of a particular behavior, whereas the original French term is focused on a particular decision taken by someone. Whether desistance from offending refers to the decision to stop offending or to a behavioral change implying the termination of offending is an important distinction at the core of much debate between criminologists. Indeed, someone may take the decision to change a particular bad habit, due to certain contingencies, will occasionally repeat this habit for a certain period of time before completely ending this habit. Some researchers have focused their attention to desistance of offending as the termination of offending and this line of work has now been referred to the study of desistance as an event. For others, desistance is a process that starts with the decision to stop offending, but this process can take some time and involve lapses and relapses until complete termination. Among scholars, the debates surrounding the conceptualization of desistance have been characterized by two distinct approaches: (a) those who describe desistance as an event (i.e., to cease offending altogether) and (b) those who define desistance as a process (i.e., a decision to stop offending until complete termination of the behavior) (Table 13.1).

Desistance from Crime as an Event

According to several scholars, desistance is conceptualized as an event involving the relatively abrupt termination of offending. From this standpoint, therefore, desistance is relatively sudden. In the criminal career literature, for example, the term desistance has often been alluded to a burnout representing a key moment in someone life course (Soothill, Fitzpatrick, & Francis, 2013). In the field of correctional psychology, desistance from crime is typically perceived as an event where treatment and intervention play a key role. More specifically, correctional programming, case management, treatment programs and therapeutic interventions aiming to help offenders is built around the idea that desistance is an event.

Table 13.1 Definitions of desistance from crime

Conceptualization	Description	Focus	Measure	Measuring issues
Desistance as an event	Desistance is sudden and abrupt	Identification of the factors/processes associated with the termination of offending	Absence of reoffending	Crime switching and intermittency of offending over time
Desistance as a process	Desistance is gradual and may involves a series of lapses and relapses	Understanding the transition from offending to non-offending	Deceleration of offending until termination	Access to repeated measurements of crime/delinquency over long time periods to capture the dynamic process

The goal is to help offenders stop their offending and participation in a treatment program is the event that can help achieve this goal. Yet it has not been evident that all or even most offenders terminate offending immediately following their last offense or much later. In that context, desistance from offending is conceptualized as a non-offending state and the maintenance of this state. Hence, reoffending, or an offending state, is considered to be the opposite of desistance.

The concept of desistance as an event or a state has raised several criticism stemming stemming from research examining offending patterns over time. The first issue surrounding the conceptualization of desistance as an event is the versatility of offending which characterizes most individual criminal careers. Indeed, persistent offenders tend to be involved in several crime types. Therefore, when examining desistance as an event, researchers have raised concerns over the importance of crime-switching (e.g., Mulvey et al., 2004). Offending is dynamic and can take many forms and shape over time and across criminal careers. An individual involved in a series of burglaries may later be involved in drug-related offenses, while another involved in a series of auto theft may later be involved in a sexual offense. Hence, examining whether or not an individual has committed the same crime type or not over some follow-up time period is too limited and does not take into account what developmentalists refers to as the diversification process of offending (e.g., Le Blanc & Fréchette, 1989). Criminologists, therefore, usually consider a broad definition of reoffending (e.g., a new offense, a new arrest or conviction) to be able to show that termination is not just the result of crime switching.

The second issue related to the conceptualization of desistance as an event has to do with individual offending rates. More specifically, individuals involved in crime do not offend all the time, in fact they do not offend most of the time, making it difficult to pinpoint whether desistance has occurred or not. Sampson and Laub (2005) described individual offending patterns in terms of zigzag criminal careers. In other words, offending patterns are generally characterized by much intermittency which is counterintuitive to the idea of desistance as an abrupt cessation of offending (Piquero, Farrington, & Blumstein, 2003). The intermittency of offending, therefore, may lead to issues of false negative or the false identification of someone as a desister, when in fact, with a longer follow-up period, these individuals do reoffend (Bushway, Thornberry, & Krohn, 2003). As a result, researchers studying desistance as an event somewhat disagree as to how long a significant non-offending state needs to be to be indicative of desistance (e.g., 1, 3, 5, 10 years) (e.g., Shover & Thompson, 1992). Kazemian (2007) argued that desistance from crime unlikely occurs abruptly and that the sole emphasis on termination of offending may overlook important and valuable information on the criminal careers of offenders, particularly for chronic offenders.

There is a now a long tradition of research in the field of sexual violence and abuse about the sexual recidivism of individuals having been convicted for a sexual crime following their release. Studies have shown that the base rate of sexual reoffending is about 10 % for an average follow-up period of 5 years, the base rate increasing to about 20 % when followed for an average of 20 years (Hanson,

Morton, & Harris, 2003). Over the years, these studies have reported the base rate of sexual recidivism among various subgroups of individuals having been convicted for a sexual offense (adolescents, adults, males, females, etc.). These sexual recidivism studies present the same limitations as those observed in desistance research. More specifically, these studies only looks at the offending behavior of the same individuals at two time points (e.g., from the prison release until the end of the follow-up period) and generally over a short follow-up period. It is not unusual, for example, to examine the proportion of offenders having sexually reoffended or not over a 4 or 5 year period. Hence, these sexual recidivism studies are also vulnerable to the issues and offending intermittency and crime switching. These studies have also shown that general recidivism rates are significantly higher than sexual recidivism rates suggesting that there is crime-switching among persistent offenders. In other words, individuals desisting from sexual offending might not entirely desist from crime. For example, a meta-analysis has shown that the general recidivism rate is about five times higher than the sexual recidivism rates among adolescent offenders (Caldwell, 2010). Similar results have been reported for adult offenders (e.g., Hanson & Bussière, 1998).

These findings for sexual recidivism have also shown that, with longer follow-ups, especially with adult offenders, the base rate of sexual recidivism increases (Hanson et al., 2003). This suggests that there is also the presence of offending intermittency among individuals having committed a sexual offense. For example, individuals who may have looked like they had desisted from sexual offending 3 years after being released from prison sexually reoffend a few years later (the case of false negative in risk assessment studies). This intermittency has to be interpreted in the context that the base rate of sexual recidivism are relatively low to begin with. While, from a policy standpoint, it is informative to determine the proportion of individuals being rearrested or reconvicted for a sexual offense within the first 4 or 5 years following their release, it only provides an aggregated snapshot of these individuals' entire offending patterns over life course. The presence or absence of sexual recidivism during some follow-up period may miss important aspects of individual offending pattern over life course (Lussier & Cale, 2013), such as whether offending is more or less serious over time, more or less frequent, as well as more or less specialized and patterned. In other words, these sexual recidivism studies are not well-suited to contextualize desistance for this population. Interestingly, while longitudinal studies overwhelmingly show that most individuals convicted for a sexual offense do not sexually reoffend during the follow-up period examined, the authors rarely speak of *desistance* for those offenders who did not sexually reoffend or did not reoffend at all.

Desistance from Crime as a Process

Whereas the above conceptualizations describe desistance as an abrupt termination of offending, developmental life course criminologists have emphasized desistance as a time-based process toward termination of offending (e.g., Le Blanc & Fréchette,

1989; Loeber & Le Blanc, 1990). This perspective aims to understand the transition from offending to non-offending, rather than non-offending itself. Bushway, Piquero, Broidy, Cauffman, and Mazerolle (2001), for example, defined desistance as the process of reduction in the rate of offending from a nonzero level to a stable rate empirically indistinguishable from zero. In fact, research has shown that *lambda* (i.e., the rate of offending) tends to decrease with age (Piquero et al., 2003). While this specific formulation involves a near mathematical definition of desistance, the theoretical focus is the understanding and specification of risk and protective factors affecting the transition from offending to non-offending. This approach, for example, leads to the important question of whether there are biological, individual, social factors that can trigger the onset of desistance from crime. Indeed, for example, building human and social capital is not immediate, it takes time, and consequently, offending may, as a result, be characterized by intermittent periods of offending (e.g., Sampson & Laub, 2003). In effect, desistance is described as a process involving stages where gradual but not necessarily automatic or consistent reduction of offending occurs prior to the termination of offending. Reoffending lapses, therefore, are expected, but at a gradually and eventually lower rate until termination. When traditional measures of recidivism (e.g., having been arrested for a new offense) are used, persistent offenders and offenders in the process of desisting can be confounded into a single category: the recidivist.[1] Drawing from concepts in developmental psychology, Le Blanc and Fréchette (1989) were among the first to operationalize the various parameters indicative of desistance from offending using multiple offending indicators. According to this model, desistance is a process whereby offending stops progressing (i.e., involvement in less serious offenses), starts decelerating (i.e., offending rate is decreasing) and become more patterned and specialized (i.e., increase tendency to commit fewer different crime types) over time until complete termination of offending.

Comparing Desistance as an Event and a Process

Empirical studies usually conceptualize desistance as an event or as a process but rarely both. Yet both conceptualizations considerably differ and this may lead to different classification of persisters and desisters depending on the operationalization chosen. This idea was first examined in the Bushway et al. (2003) study using self-reported data from the Rochester Youth Development Study on the development of general delinquent behavior among adolescents and young adults.

---

[1] Conversely, intermittent offenders (i.e., active offenders), offenders in the process of desistance, and offenders having completely desisted can be confounded into another misleading category: the non-recidivists. In other words, individuals in a desistance phase may still be involved in crime and continue to have contact with the justice system.

The authors compared and contrasted two definition of desistance. First, to measure the event perspective, desisters were defined as those persons who offended at least once during adolescence but who had entered a non-offending state after turning 18 years old. Second, using sophisticated statistical modeling, the authors examined offending trajectories throughout the study period (from 13 to 22 years age) and identified seven distinct general offending trajectories. The event approach identified about 28 % of the sample as desister, whereas the process approach identified only 8 % of the sample as showing a clear desistance trend. The agreement between the two methods in terms of identifying the same individuals was just shy of 5 %. Similar findings were reported recently by Lussier, Corrado, and McCuish (2015) with a Canadian sample of incarcerated youth followed in early adulthood. Clearly, these two studies highlight that different definition may identify different individuals as desisters. Furthermore, these studies demonstrate that approaching desistance as a process may hold more promise as, not only it informs about termination of offending, it also informs about changes that leads to termination of offending.

Desistance and the Dynamic Aspect of Offending Over Time

Several criminological theories of crime and delinquency generally recognize the importance of both between-individual and within-individual changes to explain longitudinal patterns of offending (e.g., Farrington, 2003; Moffitt, 1993). Desistance research has been typically based on a risk-factor approach that focuses on the identification of between-individual differences associated with desistance from crime. Emerging research on the desistance from sexual offending has also taken this perspective by highlighting possible and promising factors that could trigger desistance from sexual offending (e.g., Robbé et al., 2014). If researchers have gradually accepted the idea that desistance from crime is a process involving gradual changes over time, then the notion of *within-individual changes* should be central to understanding factors responsible for desistance. In spite of growing implementation of longitudinal studies with repeated measurements over time, the study of within-individual changes and desistance from crime has received very limited attention from scholars. These two approaches refers to what scholars describe as variable-oriented and person-oriented approaches (Bergman & Magnusson, 1997; Magnusson, 2003). The variable-oriented approach is concerned with differences between people and the identification of characteristics and processes that operate in a similar fashion for all members in a group. In contrast, the person-oriented approach is concerned with how a group of individuals may function differently than others under the same circumstances. In other words, the person-oriented approach stipulates that there is heterogeneity as to how a particular factor operates in relation to other individual characteristics. These two approaches with respect to the study of desistance from sexual offending are contrasted below.

Variable-Oriented Approach and Between-Individual Differences

The variable-oriented approach has been predominant in criminological research focused on the explanation of desistance from crime and has also been the traditional approach taken by researchers in the field of sexual violence and abuse to distinguish sexual recidivists from non-recidivists. From a variable-oriented viewpoint, researchers are concerned with the identification of factors associated with sexual recidivism with the assumption that individuals presenting this risk factors are all at increased risk of sexually reoffending (e.g., a prior conviction for a sexual offense). Traditionally, research has focused on relatively stable individual differences which can inform about long-term potential for sexual reoffending. These indicators have generally been identified through correlational-type statistical analyses designed to identify linear associations between two or more variables.[2] These empirical studies have combined offenders from different age-groups (i.e., early 20s, mid 40s, late 60s) at different life stages (e.g., young and single; married with children; retired and widow) but also at different stages of their criminal career (i.e., first-time offenders, recidivists, multirecidivists, desisters). From a variable-oriented perspective, aggregating individual characteristics from these persons is not an issue because individual characteristics such as age and criminal history are typically included in statistical analyses as covariates. From a variable-oriented perspective, the following assumptions are key: (a) the risk of reoffending is heterogeneous across offenders; (b) that heterogeneity can be captured by the accumulation (or not) of risk factors statistically related to recidivism; (c) the accumulation of risk factors is linearly related to the risk of reoffending; and (d) between-individual differences in offending are relatively stable over time.

Several qualitative and quantitative reviews have described and discussed the risk factors of sexual recidivism (e.g., Craig, Browne, Stringer, & Beech, 2005; Hanson & Bussière, 1998; Hanson & Morton-Bourgon, 2005; McCann & Lussier, 2008). These studies have highlighted the presence of multiple risk factors empirically associated with sexual recidivism. First, static risk factors are historical characteristics of individuals that cannot be changed through treatment or intervention. The most common static risk factors of sexual recidivism identified through actuarial studies refer to the offender's prior criminal history (e.g., number of prior convictions, prior conviction for a violent offense), prior sexual offending (e.g., prior sexual offense, prior noncontact sexual offense), victimology (e.g., male victim, prepubescent victim), and prior criminal justice intervention outcomes (e.g., treatment noncompletion, revocation of parole). Second, dynamic risk factors are

---

[2] Typically, empirical studies having identified risk factors of sexual recidivism are based on only two time-points: (a) Time 1, measurement of the risk factors, only once, often at prison intake (sometimes just prior to parole hearings or prior to prison release); and (b) Time 2, measurement of sexual recidivism at follow-up.

relatively stable characteristics of the individual and are considered to be changeable through treatment/intervention (e.g., Craissati & Beech, 2003; Hanson & Harris, 2000, 2001). These risk factors are important for case management and treatment planning, given that changes to these risk factors might decrease the risk of reoffending. Dynamic risk factors tend to refer to the psychological functioning of the offender (e.g., sexual self-regulation, poor self-regulation), personality traits or disorders (e.g., antisocial personality disorder, psychopathy), deviant sexual arousal/preferences (e.g., pedophilia), and cognitive distortions or false beliefs supporting sex crimes (e.g., Beech & Ward, 2004). There has been some debate about the relative importance of both types of predictors (e.g., Dempster & Hart, 2002). At the center of this debate is the question of whether or not risk is dynamic and can change over time. If reoffending is associated with risk indicators that are *theoretically changeable* through treatment/intervention, then the risk of reoffending is susceptible to change. There has been limited research, however, testing the so-called dynamic aspect of these risk factors.

Person-Oriented Approach and Within-Individual Changes

Developmental psychologists proposed a person-oriented approach to describe a paradigm that shifts the focus from variables to individuals (Bergman & Magnusson, 1997). The person-oriented approach emphasizes the importance of studying the individual as a whole to better understand processes such as desistance from crime. From a person-oriented perspective, one cannot isolate social factors said to favor desistance such as marriage, work, or education from other individual characteristics such as strengths (e.g., social support, motivation to change, social skills, problem-solving skills) and difficulties (e.g., positive attitudes toward crime, affiliation with antisocial peers, impulsivity). Therefore, the person-oriented approach was proposed to address limitations of the variable-oriented perspective. The variable-oriented approach is based on aggregate data and average series across individuals which can misrepresents individual patterns of development (von Eye & Bogat, 2006). From a variable-oriented approach, for example, research has shown on several occasions that individuals with low attachment to social institutions (e.g., school, work, family) are more likely to persist offending. While these findings are certainly important, they do not inform about whether low social bonding is important in all or most persistent offenders, whether desistance can occur for those characterized by low bonding to social institutions, or about the longitudinal pattern of this association over time. Similarly, ongoing difficulties at work might create a context conducive to sexually violent behavior at home. Having been convicted for a sexual offense might also lead to problems findings a stable and fulfilling job. Only longitudinal data with repeated measurement can help disentangle these effects over time. Furthermore, while the impact between social factors and offending can be reciprocal, it can also change across developmental stage (e.g., adolescence, emerging adulthood, adulthood). Attachment to certain social institutions might be more important at particular developmental stages. For example, school might be more important during adolescence while work might be more important during the adult-entry period. In sum, conclusions from variable-oriented studies might not apply to all or most individual cases and a person-oriented perspective can provide a complementary viewpoint to the process of desistance from crime.

To better account for the heterogeneity of individual development, the person-oriented approach focuses on the disaggregation of information and the identification of individual longitudinal patterns, with the understanding that some patterns occur more often than others (Magnusson, 2003). In that regard, development can be conceptualized as a process characterized by states that can change over time (Bergman & Magnusson, 1997) not unlike the process of desistance from crime. Therefore, repeated measurements become pivotal to the identification of continuity and change and fluctuate as individual age. As such, this perspective needs to account for the diversity of onset and developmental course of the behavior. To this end, nonlinear modeling becomes crucial to detect trends in individual development over time.

Lussier (2015) proposed a developmental process model of sexual offending to help describe and identify developmental patterns of sexual offending. The developmental model recognizes the presence of three developmental stages (a) activation of sexual offending, or the onset and the process by which the age of onset of leads to repetitive, diverse and persistent sexual offending; (b) escalation of sexual offending or the process by which sexual offending becomes chronic and escalate to more serious sexual offenses; and (c) desistance or the process by which offending becomes more patterned and infrequent until complete termination. Each developmental stage also recognizes the presence of heterogeneity by suggesting that some processes are more prevalent than others. For example, this model suggests that most patterns of sexual offending are initiated late (in emerging adulthood/adulthood), that escalation is minimal and desistance from sexual offending is near immediate. At the opposite, it is suggested that there are some instances where sexual offending starts early, escalate to more serious sexual offenses and where desistance is slow and gradual. According to this model, therefore, desistance from sexual offending includes a range of processes that vary from desistance being near immediate to another whereby desistance is slow and gradual over a long-time period. This person-oriented approach, therefore, recognizes the presence of certain developmental patterns, with the understanding that some patterns are more prevalent than others. Hence, configurations of variables, longitudinal data with repeated measurements, nonlinear patterns of continuity, and changes over time best characterizes the person-oriented approach. This is not to say that the person-oriented approach is superior to the variable-oriented approach, but that it provides a different perspective on human development (Bergman & Trost, 2006). This perspective is in sharp contrast to most sexual recidivism studies which only looks at individuals at two time point across the life-course, irrespective of the life stages and the offending stage individuals are at. Sexual recidivism studies have been exclusively based on a variable-oriented approach, and as a result, are not designed to inform about within-individual changes and underlying processes responsible for desistance among all individuals convicted for a sexual offense.

Offending Trajectories and Desistance from Crime

In order to account for the heterogeneity of longitudinal pattern of development and the dynamic aspect of offending over time, researchers theorized that desistance patterns are an integral part of offending trajectories (e.g., Le Blanc & Fréchette, 1989; Moffitt, 1993). Offending trajectories consist of patterns delineating onset, course, and termination of offending over time. This perspective asserts that there are relatively few but rather specific and predictable longitudinal patterns of offending. From a trajectory perspective, desistance from crime is hypothesized to be intrinsically linked to both the age of onset of offending and the course of offending. There is a consensus that age of onset of offending is statistically related to longer criminal careers (e.g., Blumstein et al., 1986; Farrington, 2003; Loeber & Le Blanc, 1990). Hence, researchers have formulated hypotheses regarding desistance from crime based on the age of onset of offending distinguishing early and late starters, with an emphasis on the adolescence–adulthood transition (e.g., Moffitt, 1993). Researchers generally recognize the presence of an early-onset, persistent patterns of general delinquency (also known as life-course persisters) who tend to escalate to the most serious forms of crime and delinquency, such as violent and sexual offenses (Moffitt, 1993; Le Blanc & Fréchette, 1989). Researchers have theorized that late-onset, also known as adolescence-onset offending, is more likely to be associated with a pattern of desistance prior to or immediately during the initial adult transition period than early, childhood-onset of offending. The explanation rests on developmental perspective assertions that late entry into delinquency more typically involves youth who have benefited from prosocial influences and learned the necessary prosocial skills to adjust to the adolescence–adulthood transition prior their delinquency involvement (e.g., Moffitt, 1993). To measure and identify such patterns, advanced statistical techniques have been developed such as group-based modeling (Nagin, 2005) or latent-growth curve modeling (e.g., Duncan & Duncan, 2004) have been utilized by researchers to identify trajectories and patterns of desistance from crime. Very importantly, longitudinal studies conducted by at-risk samples have shown that the adolescent-limited pattern of offending with desistance prior to age 18 is not as common as first believed. For example, the Bushway et al. (2003) study found that a trajectory described as "bell-shape desistors," an offending pattern that resembled the classic age–crime curve where offending is limited and circumscribed to the period of adolescence, comprised only 8.5 % of the sample of at-risk youth. More specifically, for most youth included in this sample, desistance from offending occurred after age 18. The adolescent-limited desistance type has questionable explanatory relevance regarding desistance patterns of more serious patterns of offending, such as chronic, violent and sexual offending.

Offending Trajectories of Individuals Involved in Sexual Offense

The interest for offending trajectories and patterns of desistance among individual having committed a sexual offense has grown in recent years. Researchers have examined general offending among samples of adult offenders (Francis, Harris, Wallace,

Soothill, & Knight, 2014; Lussier, Tzoumakis, Cale, & Amirault, 2010) as well as juvenile offenders (Cale, Smallbone, Rayment-McHugh, & Dowling, 2015; Lussier et al., 2012; McCuish et al., 2015). Researchers have focused on the identification of general offending as opposed to sexual offending trajectories because individuals involved in sexual offenses are first and foremost involved in nonsexual offenses. Focusing on general offending has also the advantage of taking into account and examining the entire criminal activity simultaneously, therefore addressing the above-mentioned issues of intermittency of offending as well as crime-switching.

These longitudinal studies highlighted the presence of distinct general offending trajectories among individuals having been committed a sexual offense (e.g., Francis et al., 2013; Lussier et al., 2010; Lussier et al., 2012). Such research highlight that there not one but multiple offending trajectories among individuals involved in sexual offenses. More specifically, research has found empirical evidence for the presence of the following patterns: (a) a high-rate chronic offending trajectory who mirrors the life-course persistent pattern of offending theorized by Moffitt (1993) and characterizes individuals whose offending is characterized by an early-onset, a high volume of very diverse offenses, continuity in adulthood and gradual slowing down of offending in adulthood; (b) a low-chronic offending trajectory, which characterizes an offending pattern that starts relatively early, which persist over time and continues into adulthood, but offending is not as diverse not as important as the high-rate chronics; (c) a low rate offending trajectory, whose offending is intermittent and occasional if not somewhat limited to sexual offenses; (d) an adolescence-limited offending trajectory where offending is relatively circumscribed to the period of adolescence. Each of the patterns that have been found thus far with samples of individuals involved in sexual offenses mirrors those found with general samples of at-risk youth. These offending trajectories are relatively distinct in terms of the age of onset, the peak of offending, and the rate (and change of rate) of offending across the study period.

Furthermore, these study findings highlight the fact that there are distinct desistance patterns among this population. In fact, the typical age–crime curve (Farrington, 1986) does not represent well the diversity longitudinal offending patterns identified among adolescent and adult offenders. Of the identified general offending patterns found, the findings reiterate the importance of adolescence–adulthood transition has a turning point favoring desistance from crime. For some, desistance appears to start in middle/late adolescence, while for others, such as chronic offenders, the process of desistance occurs around the transition into adulthood (McCuish et al., 2015; Lussier, Corrado & McCuish, 2015). Also, for chronic offenders, the transition to adulthood can involve the initiation of a deceleration process that, in itself, may not be sufficient to both decrease the probabilities of reoffending and create conditions necessary for the maintenance of a non-offending state. In other words, the mechanisms responsible for desistance during the adolescence–adulthood transition may not be sufficient to terminate offending for some individuals. For most individuals, the onset of desistance from general offending is highlighted by a decelerating pattern in the rate of offending. The process of deceleration, though, may be either relatively short and prompt, more gradual over a portion of adolescence or very slow. For others, however, the adolescence–adulthood transition may have a limited impact on deceleration, and consequently has no impact or a limited impact on decreasing the probabilities of reoffending. This group of individuals, characterized by an increase of offending after the adolescence–adulthood transition, not well documented in the criminological literature, may not benefit from the same turning points that others benefit from (Lussier, Corrado & McCuish, 2015).

There has been even more limited theoretical and empirical research on the sexual offending trajectories of adolescent and adult offenders (Lussier et al., 2012; Lussier & Davies, 2011; Tewksbury & Jennings, 2010). The scientific literature suggests the presence of much discontinuity, albeit some continuity, in sexual offending over time (e.g., Lussier & Blokland, 2014). Discussing specifically the presence of sexual offending trajectories among youth, Becker (1998) suggested the presence of three groups: (a) an abstainer group (i.e., nonrecidivist) who do not sexually reoffend; (b) an antisocial group whose sexual offense is part of a general tendency to engage in crime and delinquency), and (c) a sexual group who is more at risk of persistence in sexual offense. The model is clinically intuitive but has not been empirically tested. It does suggest, however, that the sexual group will never desist from sexual offending, which is not supported by the empirical literature. This hypothesis also implicitly states that the antisocial group is not at risk of sexually reoffending, which is counterintuitive with the fact that adolescents whose sexual offending persists in adulthood are more involved in nonsexual offending than those who do not persist (Lussier & Blokland, 2014; Zimring, Piquero, & Jennings, 2007). Furthermore, Becker's (1998) focus on recidivism informs neither about other developmental aspects of offending such as desistance nor about offending trajectories. With the advent of longitudinal studies and the emergence of statistical techniques allowing the modelization of longitudinal patterns of development, researcher have been able to examine and uncover the presence of sexual offending trajectories. The current state of theoretical and empirical knowledge highlight the presence of at least three distinct sexual offending trajectories: (a) the adolescent-limited, (b) the high-rate/slow-desisters, and (c) the adult-onset (e.g., Lussier, 2015; Lussier et al., 2012). It is hypothesized that these trajectories can be distinguished on a series of developmental indicators.

Adolescence-Limited Sexual Offending

The adolescent-limited group are hypothesized to represent the vast majority of adolescents involved in sexual offenses. Their prevalence, however, might not be as important in clinical settings or in the juvenile justice system. This group may share some similarities with the young male syndrome described by Lalumière, Harris, Quinsey, and Rice (2005). This group is unlikely to show sexual behavior problems during childhood and is hypothesized to be characterized by a relatively normal sexual development up to puberty. Their offending is suggested to start between the period of early and mid-adolescence. It is also argued that the growth of their sexual offending will be very limited given that these young persons may offend only once although some of them may repeat their behavior. Persistence, therefore, is possible if the associated risk factors are present and the protective factors are limited. In the context where there is persistence of sexual offending over time, it is argued that the sexual offending behavior will tend to be of the same nature. It is believed that, for this group, the risk factors for sexual offending are transitory and more specific to the period of adolescence (e.g., puberty, peer influence, binge drinking, delinquency involvement, sexual arousal, opportunity). It is also hypothesized that sexual offending may take various shapes (e.g., child abuse, peer abuse) because situational, contextual, and social factors will be pivotal in creating opportunities for illegal sexual behaviors. It is therefore argued that their offending will neither be reflective of overwhelming deviant sexual thoughts, fantasies, or urges, nor of a deviant sexual preference in the making. However, these individuals may show a pattern of non-sexual juvenile delinquency.

The study by Lussier et al. (2012) has shown that desistance from sexual offending is rapid, if not immediate, for most of them and occur in either late adolescence or in emerging adulthood. This pattern was found for those having offending against peers, children or in group. If there is persistence of offending beyond that period, it is expected that offending will be nonsexual in nature. Indeed, emerging research has shown that this group may persist offending in adulthood, but such offending is predominantly nonsexual in nature (Lussier et al., 2012). Indeed, a subgroup of youth involved in adolescence-limited sexual offending, persist their criminal activities in adulthood but such activities are nonsexual in nature. This finding is unclear and may be the result of different processes. It could be hypothesized that sexual offending and the societal response to it may create a general pattern of marginalization through a labeling effect with long-lasting effects. It could also be that juvenile sexual offending was simply opportunistic and part of a general proclivity toward delinquency in general (the antisocial youth as suggested by Becker, 1998). In both cases, focusing intervention solely on sexual offending and desistance from sexual offending would be inappropriate. This group is most likely to be found in community-based samples and therefore reflects trends and observations found in community-based studies. Currently, given the absence of a developmental model to guide clinical assessment and the similarities in terms of offending during adolescence, these adolescents may be misclassified as high-rate/slow-desisters.

High-Rate Slow Desisters

The second sexual offending trajectory found has been described as the high-rate/slow-desisters and they represent a small subgroup of adolescents having committed a sexual offense (Lussier, 2015). This group was initially found by Lussier et al. (2012) in a group of juvenile offenders followed over a twenty-year period. A very similar pattern, referred to as a high-rate limited trajectory found by Francis et al. (2013) with a sample of adult offenders, consists of juvenile-onset offenders who persist in adulthood but their sexual offending gradually decrease until what appears to be termination in their late-30s. The high-rate/slow-desisters are most likely to be found in clinical samples and therefore reflect trends and observations found in clinical studies. This group is unlikely to be found in self-reported, population-based community samples given the overall low prevalence of this developmental pattern. This pattern, however, is more prevalent in criminal justice settings, especially those handling more serious cases and juvenile sexual recidivists (i.e., detention, inpatient treatment programs). It is hypothesized that their onset of sexual offending occurs in childhood, as manifested by the onset of atypical sexual behaviors during childhood, which may precede or co-occur with their sexual offending (Lussier, 2015). This is not suggesting that all children showing atypical sexual behaviors go on to become juvenile sexual offenders, but rather that the atypical sexual behaviors of this group in particular persist beyond childhood due to the presence of other risk factors working in combination with an early onset of atypical sexual behaviors. In other words, this group is at risk of sexual offending during adolescence, especially if the exposure to risk factors of sexual offending persists and continues to overcome the protective factors. The growth of their sexual offending will be gradual and constant without any intervention.

This group is more likely to persist in their sexual offending beyond the period of adolescence. It is argued that these juveniles will eventually desist from sexual offending, but the desistance process is significantly longer due to the long-lasting effect of the multiple risk factors to which they have been exposed to early (Lussier, 2015). They are more likely to be characterized with developmental risk factors related to sexual offending (e.g., childhood sexual victimization, exposure to sexually deviant models). There is little empirical studies examining the factors associated specifically with the persistence or desistance from sexual offending for this particular group. It has been hypothesized that persistence of their sexual offending is reflective of the presence and the role of more stable risk factors and individual differences conducive to the commission of sexual offenses. Lussier et al. (2012) hypothesized that the high-rate/slow-desister group is also the one most likely to show evidence of diversification of sexual offending, which is most likely to occur during adolescence and young adulthood, as well as progressive evidence of specialization in sexual offenses over time until termination of sexual offending.

Adult-Onset Sexual Offending

The term adult-onset sexual offending has been rarely used in the scientific literature given the long held view that sexual deviance starts during childhood or adolescence (for example, see Abel, Osborn, & Twigg, 1993). Longitudinal research, however, does not support the view that all or that most adults involved in sexual offenses were juvenile-onset offenders (for a review, Lussier & Cale, 2013). The lack of longitudinal research on offending trajectories limits conclusions that can be drawn about the adult-onset sexual offending group. Therefore, it remains unclear whether there is one or multiple adult-onset sexual offending trajectories but emerging evidence seems to point to the latter scenario. Prospective longitudinal research with community-based sample has shown that adult-onset sexual offending is sometime part of an escalation process of crime and delinquency. More precisely, youth involved in chronic offending, with no evidence of involvement in sexual offending during adolescence, who failed to desist from crime around the adolescence–adulthood transition escalate their offending behavior to sexual crime in early adulthood (e.g., Lussier & Blokland, 2014; Zimring et al., 2007). The combined observations that these individuals' offending behavior is still progressing an escalating in adult-hood combined with the inability to take advantage of turning points when transitioning in adulthood suggests that this group and the underlying processes for the unfolding of this pattern are different from the adolescent-onset groups. In fact, adult-onset sexual offending is unlikely to be characterized by the same developmental background as the adolescence-onset offenders and emerging research provides preliminary evidence of distinct childhood risk factors for adolescence-onset versus adult-onset sexual offending (Lussier, Blokland, Mathesius, Pardini, & Loeber, 2015). Furthermore, using retrospective data, Knight, Ronis, and Zakireh (2009) reported that adult as opposed to juvenile sexual offending tend to be more strongly associated with evidence of experiences of verbal and sexual abuse during childhood. The examination of longitudinal patterns of sexual offending among adult-onset offenders is particularly important, therefore, as it can uncover additional pathways of desistance specific to this group.

In a study conducted by Francis et al. (2013), three adult-onset sexual offending trajectories were identified in a sample of offenders in a mental health institution. The first trajectory, the late-onset accelerators (about 8 % of the sample), refers to a longitudinal pattern where sexual offending emerges in the 40s with no evidence of desistance thereafter. The two other groups, the high-rate accelerators (12 % of the sample) and the low rate persistent (56 %) show similar longitudinal pattern where the former group sexually offended at a higher rate than the latter. For both groups, sexual offending rapidly peaked in adulthood and show a downward trend thereafter, especially when these individuals were in their 40s. Similar patterns were reported by Lussier and Davies (2011) with a sample of convicted adult offenders. Clearly, the desistance patterns found in the Francis et al. (2014) study suggests the presence of additional desistance patterns when looking more specifically among a group of adult offenders to those observed for adolescent offenders. It is unlikely the context and factors responsible for the desistance process identified for the adolescent-limited pattern are also responsible the desistance among the high-rate slow desisters (or high-rate limited in the Francis et al., 2013 study) and the late-onset accelerators.

In all, if these preliminary findings highlight the presence of some heterogeneity in sexual offending trajectories and desistance patterns, additional research is needed to unveil the whole spectrum of theoretically and clinically relevant sexual offending trajectories across developmental periods. If this line of research is very promising, more research is also needed to identify the factors responsible for desistance from sexual offending and determine whether these factors are specific to sexual offending and this population.

Explanatory Models of Desistance

Several explanations of desistance from offending have been proposed over the years (for reviews, Cusson, 2008; Kazemian, 2014; Laub & Sampson, 2001; Maruna, 2001; Soothill et al., 2013). These explanations and hypotheses have focused on the impact of age and aging, life transitions and developmental stages, the role of social factors, life events and turning points, as well as the impact of formal and informal sanctions (e.g., threats, victimization, arrest, incarceration). It is possible to organize the current state of knowledge around three dimensions (Table 13.2): (a) individual characteristics and the role of internal changes; (b) external factors, pressure and contingencies; and (c) developmental life course perspective. The first dimension emphasizes the person and individual characteristics as key factors promoting desistance. The second dimension puts more emphasis on the role and importance of the social environment to explain the mechanisms of desistance from crime. The final dimension emphasizes the role and importance of person–environment interactions and the sociodevelopmental context in which such interactions take place. These three dimensions and associated issues are presented below.

Individual Characteristics and Internal Changes

Maturation and Aging Out of Crime

The maturation hypothesis is probably one of the first and most widely held view about the causal mechanisms of desistance from crime and delinquency. This hypothesis was initially proposed following observations about the age–crime curve, that is, while delinquency involvement peaks during mid-adolescence, it gradually drops with age, especially past the adolescence–adulthood transition (Glueck & Glueck, 1940). The maturational hypothesis is based broadly on the idea that adolescents typically becoming more emotionally stable, interpersonally more sophisticated and skilled, and intellectually more knowledgeable and more future-oriented with age. These changes, in turn, increases moral reasoning, reduce impulsivity and facilitate more future-oriented goals and planning. Were probably among the first to examine offending as part of a longitudinal cohort study of a large sample of juvenile delinquents. They noticed that participation in crime dropped as youth reach their 20s and 30s and suggested that this age effect was the result of a maturation effect. They argued that, desistance occurs naturally with age and aging, as a result of physical, moral, intellectual and mental changes characterizing a maturation process. This process was the result of a changing environment but reflected internal changes whereby youth became less impulsive, more future-oriented. As a result of this maturation process, crime became less attractive and acceptable. They also argued that this maturation effect was part of a normal process of aging unless youth had been exposed to severe neuropsychological or environmental problems. The maturational hypothesis has regain attention in recent years with emerging research from the field of neuroscience. Research has convincingly shown that the adolescent's brain is different than the child and the adult's brain and part of a natural brain developmental process than influence the person's ability to regulate cognitions, emotions and behavior (Steinberg, 2010). Relatedly, longitudinal research has been able to identify patterns of development with respect to personality characteristics, impulse control, and future-oriented perspective that mirrors that are associated with desistance from offending (e.g., Monahan, Steinberg, Cauffman, &

Table 13.2 Summary of probable explanatory mechanisms of desistance from crime

Focus	Processes and mechanism responsible for desistance	Description	Key factor
1. Individual factors, characteristics and internal changes	(a) Biological impact of aging	The biological consequences of aging on the organism, which in turn impacts participation in a lifestyle conducive to crime	Aging
	(b) Maturation	Age and aging has an indirect impact on offending as a result of biological, emotional, behavioral, social, and moral development associated with age	Brain maturation
	(c) Identity construction and scripts	To desist from crime, individuals need to develop a coherent and prosocial identity for themselves	Self-identity change
2. External factors, pressure and contingencies	(a) Deterrence	Desistance is the result of a particular decision-making process whereby the individual come to the conclusion that the costs of crime outweighs its benefits	Cumulative negative impact of crime participation
	(b) Offending opportunities	With age and aging, interesting and profitable offending opportunities become rare and less attractive. Offenders not adapting to the changing opportunity structure may chose to desist from crime	Limited access to profitable and interesting criminal opportunities
	(c) Social learning	Changing patterns of peer relations and influence participation in crime and delinquency	Cutting ties with negative social influences and developing ties with positive ones
3. Developmental life course	(a) Developmental	Desistance/persistence are bounded to particular developmental experiences and developmental trajectories	Overcoming exposure to early life adversities and the consequences of delinquency participation
	(b) Life events, life transitions, and turning points	Entry into certain social roles such as work, marriage and the military can help knif-off the past, increase informal social controls and promote self-identity changes	Timely access to certain conventional social roles

Mulvey, 2009). In fact, research has shown that there are distinct patterns of personality development that are associated with distinct offending patterns over life course (Morizot & Le Blanc, 2005).

The Inexorable Age Effect

The age–crime curve and the aging out effect were interpreted differently by Hirschi and Gottfredson (1983). They argued that the (a) age–crime curve is invariant across individuals; (b) that the age–crime association is robust across time, place, and social condition; (c) that age has a direct effect on crime, and (d) that conceptualization of the age effect is largely redundant. Hence, unlike the Gluecks and their maturational hypothesis, Hirschi and Gottfredson argued that age has a direct effect on crime and desistance. They later added that, while the propensity to commit crime remains relatively stable throughout life course, offending declines with age due to the inexorable aging of the organism (Gottfredson & Hirschi, 1990). In other words, the desistance from crime is the result of a biological process that need not to be explained further. From this standpoint, aging affects offending participation the same way it affects cognitive performance and memory, performance in sports, scholarly productivity, and other age-dependent behaviors. Hence, they asserted that life events and transitions such as education, employment and marriage have no or little impact on desistance. These assertions, however, have been criticized on various grounds. Farrington (1986), for example, presented data suggesting that the peak of offending in middle adolescence followed by a rapid drop off from middle adolescence to early adulthood was a product of modern society and the emergence of a new developmental stage, that is, adolescence. Greenberg (1985) and Moffitt (1993) also proposed alternative explanations of the age–crime curve. Of importance, Moffitt (1993) as well as Blumstein, Cohen, and Farrington (1988) argued that the age-effect was not invariant across individuals. According to this view, a subgroup of individuals, chronic offenders, did not experience the same drop in offending rate in adulthood as other did. As a result, some suggested that the maturation effect did not appear to be as prevalent among chronic, serious and violent offenders as it appears to be in the general population of juvenile offenders (e.g., Tolan & Gorman-Smith, 1998). Maruna (2001), however, argued that the age-effect is somewhat overstated considering that it is more pronounced for official (e.g., arrest) than self-reported measures of offending. With age, Maruna hypothesized that individuals become more adept at not being caught or they slow down their criminal activity to a level at which they rarely get apprehended and/or they switch to less risky offenses, such as white-collar crimes. If they do get caught, they spend more time incarcerated

Cognitive Changes and Self-Identity Transformation

Another line of research proposes that within-individual subjective changes are key to the process of desistance from crime and delinquency. In this oft-cited study, Shover and Thompson (1992) reported observations collected from a sample of prison inmates, that the probability of desistance from crime increases as expectations for achieving friendship, money, autonomy and happiness via crime decreased. Changes in perceptions such as those noted by Shover and Thompson (1992) has lead researchers to focus more on describing subjective changes through the study of narratives from individuals with a sustained pattern of offending. Maruna (2001), for example, identified distinct cognitive schema or scripts in individuals described as persisters and those described as desisters. Desisters, as opposed to persisters, were characterized by a more positive and optimistic outlook on life. These individuals reported having a certain control over their destiny as opposed to being pessimistic and powerless. Desisters were more likely to describe themselves as decent people wanting to make good. Persisters, on the other hand, felt powerless toward their involvement criminal activities in spite of reporting feeling tired of this lifestyle and their social status. These individuals felt incapable of changing their lifestyle mainly because of their drug/alcohol dependence, their limited of education and professional skills necessary to find a decent job, as well as feeling prejudiced because of their criminal history. This approach stresses the role and importance of significant, dramatic life events (e.g., a friend being killed, a serious accident). Such events may lead to the cognitive transformation of the self or an identity change necessary for desistance to occur, giving these individuals an opportunity to redefine themselves as decent individuals (e.g., Maruna, 2001). Interestingly, the conditions that can trigger the decision to desist from crime are quite similar to those conducive to a reoffense (Zamble & Quinsey, 1997), which may reinforce the idea that the individual's interpretation of these negative events in a given context, more specifically life stages and stages of offending, is more important than these negative life event themselves. Maruna (2001) argues maturation occurs independently of age and leads to subjective self-identity changes essential for desistance from crime to occur.

Similarly, Giordano, Cernkovich, and Rudolph (2002) examined desistance and persistence patterns among a sample of male and female adolescents involved in serious delinquency. Contrary to social control perspective model of desistance (e.g., Laub & Sampson, 2009), their study findings showed that neither marital attachment nor job stability was a significant factor of desistance from offending. As a result, these researchers proposed an alternative explanation using a symbolic interactionist perspective. This model is said to account for (a) the initial attempts to desistance from crime before the person had much chance to accumulate the necessary human and social capital (b) the observations that individuals exposed to opportunities to take advantage of prosocial experience and conventional social roles (e.g., work, marriage) fail to take advantage of them, and (c) subjective, cognitive changes that occur during the desistance phase. According to Giordano et al. (2002), desistance is a transformation process whereby *cognitive shifts* play an integral part. The authors distinguished different cognitive shifts playing an integral part in desistance from crime. The first cognitive shift involves changes in the individual's basic openness and readiness to change. While this openness to change is necessary, it is often not sufficient for desistance to occur. Next, exposure to what the authors refers to a "hooks for change" (i.e., prosocial experiences) as well as a positive attitude toward them are key to promoting transformation. These hooks for change, similar to the concept of turning points (Sampson & Laub, 2003), provide opportunities and reinforcements for a self-identity change. The third cognitive shift characterizing the process of desistance is the individual's ability for identify change and redefine their self, in line with Maruna (2001). Fourth, the authors recognize the role and importance of a shift as to how individuals view crime and delinquency as well as the associated lifestyle itself. The focus of this perspective is on individual–environment interactions, in particular, the ability to change including openness for change as well as the environment providing prochange conditions. Laub and Sampson (2009), in particular have been critical of the importance of such cognitive transformation and identity shifts, as they argue that individuals do desist from crime without making a conscious decision to make good, as Maruna (2001) suggested.

External Factors, Pressure and Contingencies

Rational-Choice Theory and Deterrence

Another set of hypotheses emphasizes the deterrent role and importance of negative formal and informal consequences of crime and delinquency. From this standpoint, desistance from crime is the result of a conscious and rational decision made by an individual. According to this perspective, when the negative consequences outweigh the positive and pleasurable aspects of crime, desistance is more likely to occur. A long held view of desistance as a rational-choice desistance involves an underlying process suggesting that with successive arrests, offenders become more known to the police and criminal justice system officials. This familiarity then results in the increased probability of subsequently of not only being arrested but also receiving more punitive legal sanctions. The increased punitive probabilities is said to deter offender from future criminal involvement. This idea is counterintuitive to the observations that recidivism rates increase over successive arrests (e.g., Wolfgang, Figlio, & Sellin, 1972).

Alternative explanations have been proposed from the study of offender's narratives. Cusson and Pinsonneault (1986) conducted a series of interviews with ex-robbers to determine the context under which these individuals took the decision to give up crime. The ex-robbers reported that their decision was triggered either by a shocking event often occurring during the commission of a crime (e.g., shootout with the police, co-offender killed) or some delayed deterrence effect. Additionally, Shover and Thompson (1992) examined the linked between past criminal success and desistance from offending. The researchers concluded that individuals who managed to escaped detection and apprehension the most were less likely to desist from crime. They added that detection avoidance may promote persistence into crime as it falsely gives individuals a certain illusion that he or she possesses particular skills allowing to avoid detection and get away with it while creating an impression of uncertainty and low risk of detection and sanctions. Cusson (2008) later concluded that desistance was a consequence of formal and informal sanctions resulting from an antisocial lifestyle. He added that three key sanction types typically weigh on the offender's decision to give up crime: (a) increased fear of victims and being victimized on their next offense; (b) fear of apprehension and incarceration; and (c) increased fear of death. In effect, others have argued that the deterrence effect is more of a process by which the negative consequences of crime and the associated lifestyle cumulated over time to a point where they surpass their positive aspects. Cusson (2008), for example, spoke of a delayed deterrent effect of the cumulative impact of formal (e.g., arrest, incarceration) and informal sanctions (e.g., victimization) as well as the negative consequences of the criminal lifestyle (e.g., injuries, fatigue). As a result, the negative consequences of further involvement in crime outweigh the positive or pleasurable aspects of continued offending that moderate the drive to commit a crime.

Opportunity Structure of Crime

Tremblay (1999), on the other hand, argued that desistance from offending could be explained, at least in part by the contingencies characterizing criminal opportunities. According to this hypothesis, with age, individuals gradually desist from crime as a result of the most attractive and profitable criminal opportunities being difficult to access. Therefore, individuals are eventually confronted by the reality that criminal involvement has little payoffs compared to the negative consequences that can results from criminal participation. As Shover and Thomson (1992; p. 91) note, "… growing disenchantment with the criminal life also causes offenders to lower their expectations for achieving success via criminal means." Confronted by the realization of poor prospects resulting from not so profitable offenses, offenders face the dilemma of either opting out of crime or trying to maximize their gain through strategic decisions involving, among others things, selective association and alliance with co-offenders and organized crime (Tremblay, 1999). Similarly, Piliavin, Gartner, Thornton, and Matsueda (1986) reported from their study that the effect of age on persistence in crime was mediated by the individual's belief that expected earnings from crime were greater or equal to expected earnings from a legitimate job. The offender's perception of legal risk has not been shown to be consistently related to the decision to desist from crime. In fact, research suggests that contacts with the criminal justice system may actually lower offenders' perceptions of being caught and convicted for their crime in the future (e.g., Corrado, Cohen, Glackman, & Odgers, 2003; Pogarsky & Piquero, 2003). While this research may suggest the need for a more punitive approach to crime and delinquency, others have raised concerns over such conclusions. For example, Laub and Sampson (2001; p.57) coined the term cumulative continuity to refer a process whereby delinquency involvement mortgages the person's future by *generating negative consequences for the life chances of stigmatized and institutionalized youth*. They argue that arrest and incarceration may in weaken social bonds, spark failure at school/work, cut these individuals off from the most promising life avenues and in turn increase adult crime.

Peer Influence

While criminologists have long recognized the role and importance of peer influence in delinquent activities (e.g., Sutherland, 1947), its interpretation differs across school of thoughts. Control theorists generally argue that peer delinquency is a consequence of individuals seeking the company of others with similar background, interests, lifestyle, and routine activities. In other words, the presence of negative social influences is a consequence rather than a cause of delinquency (e.g., Gottfredson & Hirschi, 1990). This is reinforced by the idea that, especially in adolescence, delinquency is a group-phenomenon where co-offending is common (e.g., Farrington, 2003). Social learning theorists, however, argue that delinquency is learned from others through the acquisition of attitudes supportive to crime and delinquency (Sutherland, 1947) or imitation and reinforcement (Akers & Cochran, 1985), while others argue that the peer-delinquency association is bidirectional (Thornberry et al., 1994)—i.e., association with delinquent peers increase delinquency involvement through reinforcement provided by members of the peer network, while delinquency involvement favor further development of delinquent peer association. Warr (1993) has examined the role of peer influence in the context of desistance from offending. He reported that the amount of time spend with friends, exposure to them and their influence as well as their commitment of friends follows the age–crime curve, that is, it peaks during adolescence at a time where delinquency involvement is most important and it typically drops thereafter. Warr (1998) argued that crucial to desistance from crime are changing patterns of peers relations over life course and significant life transitions may favor such changes. Of importance, marriage appears to discourage crime and delinquency by weakening former criminal associations. Warr's analyses of the National Youth Survey data, a national probability sample of teens including a follow-up until age 24, revealed that time spent with friends changed following marriage and not before, suggesting that these individuals chose to settle not as a result of fractured peer relationships. These findings are intriguing but should be interpreted cautiously as these were observed with samples drawn from the general population which do not necessarily generalize to samples including chronic, violent and sexual offenders. With a highly delinquent sample, Giordano et al. (2003) has shown that while marriage can serve to reduce contact with negative peer influence, it is not inevitable. They stressed that without a strong motivation to change and commitment to the idea of developing a more respectable identity, the person may simply ignore the partner's efforts or even break the relationship altogether.

Developmental, Life Course Explanations

Life Course, Turning Points, and Access to Adult Roles

Life course researchers have stressed the role of social factors and local circumstances to explain human development. Elder (1998), for example, argues that developmental trajectories are altered by social circumstances. This author emphasized the importance of approaching human lives from a dynamic perspective in that human development is not limited to the period of childhood but applies to the life span. More specifically, human lives should be conceived as a succession of life transitions and social roles (e.g., school entry, entry into the labor force, marriage, parenthood). The developmental impact of this succession of life transitions is contingent on when they occur in a person's life. This age-graded perspective of life transitions and social roles proposed by Elder (1998) suggests that a specific life transition occurring too early (e.g., teen pregnancy, high school dropout) or too late can produce a cumulating effects of life disadvantages, such as economic deprivation and loss of education. This social perspective was later applied by criminologists to explain longitudinal patterns of crime and delinquency by focusing on the transition to adulthood and access to adult roles that diminish the acceptability and efficacy of delinquent behaviors. According to Laub and Sampson (2009), when employed, married or in military service, individuals are less likely to commit crimes. Marriage, parenthood, military service, and work are key examples of essential turning points that typically constitute powerful informal social controls that can impact routine activities, criminal opportunities and reduce offender's decisions to continue offending into adulthood (e.g., Laub & Sampson, 2009; Sampson & Laub, 2005). From this perspective, though, it is not solely the presence of these life events and turning points, but their quality and stability involving strong prosocial ties in different contexts (e.g., at home, at work) with prosocial peers that disapprove of deviant behaviors while promoting prosocial ones that influence desistance (e.g., Kazemian & Maruna, 2009). Prospective longitudinal research has shown, for example, that the *same* individuals are more likely to be involved in crime when single or divorced than when married (e.g., Blokland & Nieuwbeerta, 2005). In other words, social factors and local life circumstances are said to influence the decision to participate in crime. In fact, researchers have argued that most adult routine roles (e.g., fatherhood) are inconsistent with a delinquent lifestyle, which usually is characterized by unstructured and unsupervised routines activities. Giordano et al. (2003) have emphasized the importance of the subjective quality of these life experiences and cognitive interpretation of those rather than simply their presence or absence from the individual's life course.

The adult roles, in contrast, involve structured and prosocial expectations that work, intimate relationships, family, and community roles may bring. Once these new adult roles are established, they become valued, and are, therefore, protected and guarded (Mulvey et al., 2004). As with the above hypotheses, there is research that challenges any simple correspondence between the young adulthood stage and the access to prosocial turning points. Unlike life course criminologists, developmental criminologists assert that turning points and life transitions in the initial adulthood stage are more problematic, and even relatively dependent from an individual's developmental history (e.g., Loeber et al., 2008). In other words, latter theorists question whether most, let alone all, older adolescents and young adults either have sufficient access to prosocial adult roles or similarly can necessarily benefit from their influence to desist from crime. Regarding the latter theme, and in line with Elder's (1989) age-graded perspective on life transitions, there is research that indicated that these early stages' entry into work and marriage was not associated with a decrease in offending and, even possibly, contributed to the maintaining of offending. For example, according to Uggen (2000), only after about age 26 did work appeared to become a turning point with respect to desistance. Furthermore, longitudinal research examining the long-term criminal careers show that such age-graded changes in life circumstances only have a modest impact on offending (Blokland & Nieuwbeerta, 2005). Longitudinal research examining the role of work and marriage on offending trajectories and desistance from crime lead researchers to the conclusion that, while social life circumstances do impact offending patterns, the importance of these factors might have been overstated as much of the age effect on crime remains unexplained. For example, research suggests that social factors and life circumstances might be more important for some individuals than others and that chronic, persistent offenders are be less likely to desist from crime as a result their entry into adult roles (e.g., Blokland & Nieuwbeerta, 2005) compare to other individuals involved in crime and delinquency (e.g., occasional offenders).

Furthermore, social control explanations of desistance may work best for young persons that are in life stages that are defined by their dependency. Adulthood, how-ever, characterizes a period or an ever increasing number of experiences, social influences and contexts representing options that were not available at earlier life stages as well as more leverage to choose and influence their course of actions. In that regard, Giordano et al. (2003) suggested that "…even individuals whose lives can be considered quite limited and marginal, *as adults* are exposed to an ever increasing number of experiences, others and contexts." This somewhat larger social and spatial arena of adulthood presents the actor with potential influences and options that were not available earlier on. In addition, adults, compared with chil-dren, have greater behavioral leeway; that is ability to influence the specific course of action they will take. Actors of all ages undoubtedly possess the capacity to make agentic moves, but certain phases of life will tend to facilitate or inhibit this basic capacity to take efficacious individual action. Thus, attention to reflective, inten-tional processes (changing cognitions) seems well suited to a focus on behavioral changes that occur during the adult years (i.e., desistance). While life transitions such as marriage, employment, pregnancy, and parenthood should be considered primary desistance experiences, Giordano et al. (2003) also stressed the presence of secondary processes such as reduced susceptibility to peer pressure and movement toward more prosocial peers even in the absence of a partner/spouse.

Developmental Explanations

Better understanding person–environment interactions throughout life course are much needed to describe the process by which someone desist from crime. Moffitt (1993) offered perhaps one of the most convincing description and explanation of desistance from antisocial behavior using a developmental framework. This frame-work stipulates that the age of onset of antisocial behavior is intrinsically tied to desistance. According to this theory, there are two meta-trajectory of antisocial behavior: the life-course persisters and the adolescent-limited. Life-course persistent antisocial behavior is characterized by a childhood-onset and persistence and aggravation throughout adolescence into adulthood. These individuals are most likely to be multi-problem youth characterized by neuropsychological deficits in conjunction with a criminogenic familial environment. According to her model, it is not so much the neuropsychological deficits or the criminogenic familial environment that are conducive to long-term persistence of offending, but a developmental process by which a vulnerable children with executive function deficits repeatedly interacts with a familial environment that is ill prepared to act and react to the child's difficult and disruptive behavior and such negative reactions can further entrench the child's behavioral and emotional problems. The adolescent-limited group presents a delinquency that is short-lived, transitory, and circumspect to the period of adolescence. Contrary to their life-course persistent counterpart, these youth do not present an early onset of antisocial behavior in spite of their adolescent-limited involved in crime and delinquency. Contrary to Sampson and Laub (2005) assertions, Moffitt (1993) contends that access to adult roles are not independent from individuals' developmental history. On the one hand, the theory asserts that life-course persisters suffer from the cumulative disadvantages or their early and persistent antisocial behavior which can disrupt their school performance, which in turn will impact their educational achievement, and consequently their access to fulfilling, rewarding, and stable jobs. On the other hand, late-onset adolescent-limited antisocial behavior only emerges after youth have accumulated the individual and interpersonal skills and stronger attachments necessary to access adult roles conducive to desistance from crime. In other words, these adolescent-limited offenders did not experience the early-onset of behavioral problems during the formative years that can disrupt the development and create long-last cumulative deficits. Moffitt's theory recognizes that some youth presenting all the characteristics of an adolescent-limited antisocial behavior may be ensnared into adult criminal activities due to the negative consequence of their implications in juvenile delinquency (e.g., teen pregnancy, drug abuse, arrest/conviction). More recently, Stouthamer-Loeber, Wei, Loeber, and Masten (2004) examined the data from the Pittsburgh Youth Study on the development of delinquency and found that youth involved in serious delinquency with gang ties who endorsed an antisocial lifestyle and use hard drugs were more likely to persist offending into adulthood. While Moffitt's original developmental model has received empirical validation (e.g., Piquero & Moffitt, 2005), results suggest that there are additional developmental patterns not accounted by the developmental model.

Common Explanations of Desistance and Sexual Offending

The scientific literature on the theoretical, clinical and empirical factors linked to desistance from sexual offending is in its infancy (Laws & Ward, 2011). Currently, there is little theoretical or empirical work suggesting that factors supporting desistance from sexual offending are distinct or different than those from general offending. It could be reasonably assumed that the same factors responsible for desistance from general offending also by extension favor desistance from sexual offending.

Aging, self-identity, access to social roles, informal social controls, deterrence and negative consequences of offending as well as key developmental factors could theoretically explain desistance from sexual offending the same way these factors are said to explain desistance from offending. At the very least, for a research perspective, the importation of criminological research on desistance from crime and delinquency can be justified on the observation that individuals involved in sexual offenses tend to be involved in other crime types (e.g., Lussier, 2005). Researchers have, for the most part, exported ideas from the criminological literature to examine the factors associated with desistance from sexual offending.

Static Explanations

According to Lussier and Cale (2013), there are two main schools of thought explaining the propensity to sexually reoffend over time. These two schools of thought emerged following controversies and debate surrounding the risk assessment of sexual recidivism and whether or not risk assessors should consider the role of age and aging. While the criminological literature recognizes that the age play a key role on offending over time, whether because of a direct effect and/or indirectly through a maturation effect, it remained unclear whether it also applied to sexual offending. For some researchers, therefore, the age–crime curve does not apply to sexual offending and risk assessment need not to be adjusted for the offender's age at assessment. This perspective is known as the static-propensity approach. Other researchers, however, argued instead that there is an age effect and risk assessors should adjust individual's level of risk according to their age at assessment. In other word, this static-maturational hypothesis impacts the propensity to sexually reoffend over time. These two school of thoughts are presented below.

The static-propensity approach suggests that historical and relatively unchangeable factors are sufficient to identify individuals most likely to sexually reoffend over time. The key assumption here is that the propensity to sexually offend is relatively stable over time and, therefore, risk assessment tools should only be used for measuring the full spectrum of this propensity. For static-propensity theorists, the only age factors that risk assessors should include are those reflecting a high propensity to reoffend, such as an early age of onset and indicators of past criminal activity. For example, Harris and Rice (2007) argued that the effect of aging on recidivism is small. In fact, they argued that age of onset is a better risk marker for reoffending than age at release. In other words, those who start their criminal career earlier in adulthood show an increased risk of reoffending irrespective of age and aging. Therefore, according to the static-propensity hypothesis, older offenders with high actuarial risk scores represent the same risk of sexually reoffending as younger offenders with similar scores (Doren, 2004; Harris & Rice, 2007). Their findings showed that the offender's age-at-release did not provide significant incremental predictive validity over actuarial risk assessment scores (i.e., VRAG) and age of onset. However, this could be explained, in part, by the fact that age of onset and age at release were strongly related, that is, early-onset offenders are more likely to be released younger than late-onset offenders. The high covariance between these two age factors might have limited researchers in finding a statistical age at release effect in multivariate analyses. Furthermore, looking at the predictive validity of the VRAG and the SORAG (Quinsey, Harris, Rice, & Cormier, 1998), Barbaree, Langton, and Blanchard (2007) found that after correcting for age at release, the predictive accuracy of instruments decreased significantly, suggesting that an age effect was *embedded* in the risk assessment score and the risk factors included in such tools (see also, Lussier & Healey, 2009). Indeed, if actuarial tools have been developed by identifying risk factors that are empirically linked to sexual reoffending and the risk of sexually reoffending peaks when offenders are in their 20s, it stands to reason that characteristics of this age group are most likely to be captured and included in actuarial tools. Consequently, scores of risk assessment tools might be more accurate with younger offenders, but might overestimate the risk of older offenders.

The static-maturational perspective refers to the idea that the risk of sexual (re) offending is subject to some maturational effect across the life course (Barbaree et al., 2007; Hanson, 2006; Lussier & Healey, 2009). It is based on the idea that the age–crime curve also applies to sexual offending. The static-maturation hypothesis is based on the assumption of a stable propensity to sexually reoffend, but the risk of reoffending changes with age and aging. In other words, the rank ordering of individuals (between-individual differences) on a continuum of risk to reoffend remains stable, but the offending rate decreases (within-individual changes) in a relatively similar fashion across individuals. For example, Barbaree, Blanchard, and Langton (2003) argued that if the sexual drive is a key component of sexual aggression and this drive is age-dependent, it stands to reasons that an age-effect should characterize sexual aggression across the life course. It was determined that the offender's age at release contributes significantly to the prediction of reoffending, over and above scores on various risk factors said to capture sex offenders' propensity to reoffend. In fact, sexual recidivism studies have reported that, after adjusting for the scores on Static-99, the risk of sexual reoffending significantly decreased for every 1-year increase in age after release (Hanson, 2006; Lussier & Healey, 2009; Thornton, 2006). Clearly, these two perspectives highlight the need for a closer look at age, aging, and sexually offending over the life course.

Age and Aging

Research has shown over and over that only a minority of individuals having been convicted for a sexual offense sexually reoffend following their release (e.g., Hanson et al., 2003; Proulx & Lussier, 2001). In line with the static-maturational hypothesis, one of the key factors associated with the absence of sexual recidivism across individuals and subgroups of offenders has been shown to be the offender's age at the time of release (Barbaree et al., 2003; Doren, 2006; Hanson, 2006; Harris

& Rice, 2007; Lussier & Healey, 2009; Prentky & Lee, 2007; Thornton, 2006; Wollert, 2006; Wollert, Cramer, Waggoner, Skelton, & Vess, 2010). Empirical studies have consistently shown showed an inverse significant relationship between the age at release and sexual recidivism. In fact, a meta-analysis conducted with a large sample of sex offenders showed that the correlation of the individual's age at release was in the low 10s for sexual recidivism and in the mid 20s for nonsexual violent recidivism (Hanson & Bussière, 1998). These results suggest that the age effect might be more pronounced for violent reoffending compared with other types of reoffending which may have to do with the lower base rate of sexual recidivism. Looking more closely at these findings, results show that young adults in their early 20s represent the group most likely to sexually reoffend after their release. In fact, researchers generally include items reflecting the offender's age at the time of assessment in risk assessment instrument to assess the risk of sexual recidivism (e.g., Quinsey et al., 1998; Hanson & Thornton, 2000). However, these actuarial instruments differ as to the cutoff age at which the risk is considered to be higher (i.e., being less than 25, 27, 30 years age, etc.). Research has also shown that older offenders present a very low risk of sexual reoffending. Offenders in their 50s show a significant decline in risk of reoffending compared with offenders in their 20s and 30s (Barbaree et al., 2003). In fact, data indicated that sexual recidivism rates are as low as 2 % over a 5-year period for offenders aged 60 and older (Hanson, 2006; Thornton, 2006; Lussier & Healey, 2009). Indeed, longitudinal studies have demonstrated that the risk of sexual recidivism decreases steadily as the offender's age increases from the time of his release (Barbaree et al., 2003; Barbaree et al., 2007). The linear decrease was found for sexual (Barbaree et al., 2003; Hanson, 2002; Lussier & Healey, 2009; Thornton, 2006; Prentky & Lee, 2007) and violent reoffending (including sexual offenses) (e.g., Fazel, Sjöstedt, Långström, & Grann, 2006).

Although a downward linear trend appears to characterize the risk of reoffending as the offender's age at release increases, other findings suggest that the age–sexual recidivism relationship is more complex. Researchers generally agree on the recidivism rates of the younger adult offenders and older offenders, but there is controversy about the age effect occurring for other offenders. Three main points have been at the core of the debate about the link between aging and reoffending in adult offenders: (a) identification of the age at which the risk of reoffending peaks; (b) how to best represent the trend in risk of reoffending between the youngest and the oldest group; and (c) the possibility of differential age–crime curves of reoffending. One hypothesis states that, when excluding the youngest and oldest group of offenders, age at release and the risk of sexual recidivism might be best represented by a plateau. Thornton (2006) argued that the inverse correlation revealed in previous studies may have been the result of the differential reoffending rates of the youngest and oldest age groups, rather than a steadily declining risk of reoffending. In that regard, one study presented sample statistics suggesting a plateau between the early 20s and the 60s + age groups (Langan, Schmitt, & Durose, 2003). No statistical analyses were reported between the groups, thus limiting possible conclusions for that hypothesis. Another hypothesis suggests there might be a curvilinear relationship between age at release and sexual recidivism, at least for a subgroup of offenders. Hanson (2002) found empirical evidence of a linear relationship between age and recidivism for rapists and incest offenders but a curvilinear relationship was found for extrafamilial child molesters (see also, Prentky & Lee, 2007). Whereas the former two groups showed higher recidivism rates in young adulthood (i.e., 18–24), the group of extrafamilial child molesters appeared to be at increased risk when released at an older age (i.e., 25–35). This led researchers to conclude that, although rapists are at highest risk in their 20s, the corresponding period for child molesters appears to be in their 30s. These results, however, have been criticized on methodological grounds, such as the use of small samples of offenders, the presence of a small base rate of sexual reoffending, the use of uneven width of age categories to describe the data, the failure to control for the time at risk after release, and the number of previous convictions for a sexual crime (Barbaree et al., 2003; Lussier & Healey, 2009; Thornton, 2006). More recent research, however, with a large sample of individuals convicted for a sexual offense shows that the age-invariance effect is present across individuals, irrespective of their static risk of sexual recidivism (Wollert et al., 2010).

The aging effect has been examined differently in the context of the unfolding of offending activities over time. Amirault and Lussier (2011) examined the predictive value of a past conviction in a sample of incarcerated adult males all convicted at least once for a sexual offense. Rather than comparing the sexual recidivism rates of individual with and without a prior conviction, these researchers looked at the offender's age at the time of each past conviction. The results were in line with those reported by Kurlychek, Brame, and Bushway (2006) as well as those by Bushway, Nieuwbeerta, and Blokland (2011) with general samples. Amirault and Lussier (2011) found that older past conviction lost their predictive value for general, violent as well as sexual recidivism. Furthermore, only recent past charges and convictions were predictive of recidivism in this sample of adult offenders. In other words, not recognizing whether past convictions are recent or date far back might overestimate or underestimate the risk of reoffending for this population. More recently, Nakamura and Blumstein (2015) analyzed the hazard and survival probability of a group of individuals who were arrested for the first time as adults in New York in 1980, 1985, or 1990. The results demonstrated that, in terms of the recidivism for any offense, sex offenders tend to have a lower risk of general recidivism than other subtypes of offenders (see also, Sample & Bray, 2003). Furthermore, the risk of sexual recidivism reported for this sample was much smaller than the risk of recidivism for any offense due to the low prevalence of sexual offending (about 2 % of all rearrests). When these researchers compared to the risk of sex offense arrest for sexual offenders to that of the general population, the sex offenders' risk of recidivism remains higher during the 10-year follow-up. Although sex offenders' sexual recidivism did not seem to become comparable to the risk of general population, the concept of risk tolerance was not examined in this study. While evidence of redemption is emerging from longitudinal study, it remains unclear what are the underlying factors promoting desistance in this population.

Individual and Social Factors

The growing consensus among scholars of the presence of an age effect on sexual offending combined to the relatively low sexual recidivism rates has generated interest for factors explaining desistance from sexual offending. While the field of research on desistance from crime has been focused on contextual factors (e.g., turning points, developmental stages and life transitions) and those factors that are external to the offenders, the field of sexual violence and abuse has somewhat limited the scope to those that are internal (e.g., age, aging). The rationale for this different focus is unclear but it implicitly suggests that sexual offending is driven by a specific propensity for sexual crimes that can be measured through individual differences. Farmer, Beech, and Ward (2012) conducted a qualitative study in order to describe the process of desistance using a very small sample child sexual abusers ($n = 10$) in a sex offender treatment program in the United Kingdom. They compared a group of five potentially active sexual offenders to a group of five potentially desisters using cognitive-based themes identified by Maruna (2001). Desistance was operationalized using "self-narratives," by detecting the presence of five different themes, that is, redemption, generativity, agency, communion, and contamination. Both groups were identified using a semi-structured clinical judgment conducted by therapists. The study findings show that, on the one hand, individuals in the desisting group identified treatment as being a turning point in their lives and reported a better sense of personal agency and an internalized locus of control. On the other hand, individuals in the persistent group were more likely to blame external factors for their life difficulties. Potential desisters reported the importance and significance of belonging to a social group or being part of a social network while the group identified as potentially active described feeling socially isolated. Similarly, Harris (2014) examined and compared three theoretical perspectives on desistance from offending: (1) natural desistance, in other words aging out of crime; (2) cognitive transformation of the self; and (3) informal social control. Using qualitative data collected from 21 men convicted of sexual offenses who returned to the community and were taking part in a treatment program, the study findings provided mixed support for these three theories. Notably, concerning informal social controls, many participants addressed the obstacles to having a relationship or an employment and the consequences of the stigma associated to being a convicted sex offender.

Kruttschnitt, Uggen, and Shelton (2000) were among the first to report about the social factors of desistance from sexual offending. While they used the term desistance from sexual offending, their conceptualization and operationalization of desistance was no different than those used in the past 50 years of research on sexual recidivism (Hanson et al., 2003). While their measure of desistance as an event was subject to the limitations raised earlier (e.g., vulnerable to the intermittency of offending), this study was nonetheless important as it provided a first look at indicators of formal and informal social controls and its role of persistence/desistance. Indeed, following the work of Sampson and Laub (1995), Kruttschnitt et al. (2000) examined the impact of formal (e.g., criminal justice sanctions) and informal (e.g., family, employment) social control mechanisms on recidivism among 556 sex offenders placed on probation in Minnesota in 1992. Desistance was operationalized in various ways such as the absence of a new arrest for any crime, personal crime, as well as sex crimes over a period of about 5 years. Using a series of survival analyses, the authors found that most individuals on probation did not sexually reoffend within 5 years after the start of the follow-up period. When looking at desistance from any crime, findings showed that job but not marriage stability was related to desistance from crime during the study period. In fact, those with stable employment at the time of sentencing were approximately 37 % less likely to be rearrested for any crime. The same effect was reported for personal crimes but not sexual crimes. In other words, contrary to Sampson and Laub (2003) assertions, job stability was not associated with lower risk of sexually reoffending during the study period. What the study showed, however, was that participation in a court-ordered sex offender treatment program more specifically for those showing employment stability was associated with desistance from sexual offending. In other words, individuals with stable work histories receiving a sex offender treatment program were significantly less likely to sexually reoffend. This could be interpreted as suggesting that desistance from sexual offending is most likely to occur when formal (i.e., court-ordered treatment) and informal (i.e., work) social control mechanisms are present and operating. It could also reflect Giordano et al. (2002) hypothesis of cognitive shifts in the presence of hooks (i.e., prosocial experience) for change.

More recently, Blokland and van der Geest (2015) used data from the Criminal Career and Life Course Study (CCLS), a longitudinal study of a cohort of individuals who had their a criminal case adjudicated in 1977 in the Netherlands. The study, has allowed researchers to map out the entire criminal history of these individuals up to age 72. This is perhaps one of the most complete analyses of the criminal activity of individuals convicted for a sexual offense. From this group, Blokland and van der Geest (2015) examined the desistance pattern of the entire population of individuals whose 1977 criminal case pertained to a sexual crime (about 4 % of the entire sample; $n = 500$). During the entire 25 year-follow period, about 30 % of the population were reconvicted for a sexual offense which is congruent with the scientific literature for such a long follow-up period (e.g., Hanson et al., 2003). While historical factors such as having a prior sexual offense was related to sexual recidivism, life course social circumstances were not. Similar to the Kruttschnitt et al. (2000) study findings, being employed as well as not having alcohol/drug issues in 1977 were not related to desistance. They did not examine, however, the presence of an interaction effect between participation in a sex offender treatment program and employment. Furthermore, individuals who were married had lower sexual recidivism rates, again, contrary to what had been reported in the Kruttschnitt et al. (2000) study. Of importance, sexual recidivism rates were not different across subtypes of offenders. The contradictory findings between the Blokland and the Kruttschnitt study raise several issues. For example, the Kruttschnitt et al. study is more vulnerable to the issue of offending intermittency compared to the Blokland and van der Geest (2015) study which examined desistance over a 25-year period. In light of the Blokland et al. findings, the Kruttschnitt et al. study findings might simply be reflective of temporary conformity for those individuals subject to increased social controls. But as those social controls mechanisms erode, offenders could revert back to old patterns and sexually reoffend. Clearly, more research is needed with repeated measurement of life circumstances over time. If anything, these studies highlight the urgent needs of additional research to examine the role of individual and social factors on desistance from sexual offending.

For adolescents involved in sexual offenses, the period of *emerging adulthood* appears to be a critical turning point where most youth desist from sexual offending (Lussier et al., 2012; Lussier & Blokland, 2014; Lussier, Blokland et al., 2015). Emerging adulthood (18–25 years) is described as a transition period between adolescence and adulthood. During this period, individuals are relatively independent from parents, yet are still in the process of obtaining education and training for a long-term adult occupation, and while they may cohabit with an intimate partner, they are unmarried or not in a common-law relationship and have yet to have established a stable residence and to have children (Arnett, 2000). Interestingly, work, marriage and parenthood have all been described by life-course criminologists as key factors leading to desistance from crime (e.g., Sampson & Laub, 2003). Therefore, it is unlikely that such social factors play a role in the desistance process of these youth as desistance from sexual offending appears to occur earlier than entry into these social roles. In western countries, it is suggested that emerging adults are more concerned about accepting responsibility for their actions, deciding on one's beliefs and values, establishing an equal relationship with their parents, and becoming financially independent, and less concerned with thinking about their career, marriage, and parenthood (Arnett, 2000). In effect, in contrast with Gottfredson and Hirschi's (1990) general theory of crime, the number of plausible life directions during this period of emerging adulthood is greater than for any other developmental period (Arnett, 2000; Giordano et al., 2002). Given the number of possible directions, it is unlikely that all juvenile offenders go through this developmental stage experiencing these changes or experiencing these changes the same way. While discontinuity of sexual offending is important in adolescent offenders, the role of transitioning into emerging adulthood on such desistance patterns remains unclear. Clearly, more research is needed to examine whether the factors promoting desistance from sexual offending are age-graded. While these findings have not been validated, they do raise the issue of studying desistance in the current sociolegal context where sex offenders have been socially constructed has pariahs and monsters (Simon, 1998) which undoubtedly impacts at least some of the underlying processes responsible for desistance from sexual offending.

Summary

Several definitions of desistance from crime have been proposed and measured by researchers. These definitions somewhat overlap on certain aspects of desistance but also capture relatively distinctive ones. For example, recidivism studies capture probabilities of maintaining a non-offending state over time but does not inform about other aspects of offending (e.g., acceleration, deceleration). Offending trajectories inform about possible patterns of desistance but this perspective, while informative about long-term patterns, is somewhat limited when it comes to short-term predictions and interventions. Together, these viewpoints provide a more complete conceptualization of desistance from crime. As argued in this chapter, desistance is not a random process. It is relatively bounded to the precocity and the level of prior involvement in crime and delinquency. Of importance, offending trajectories characterized by a distinct pattern of desistance in terms of timing, deceleration and probabilities of reoffending have been identified. Clearly, therefore, the phenomenon of desistance from crime is diverse and complex and should be understood as being multifaceted involving multiple pathways. Desistance is best described as a process possibly involving a series of lapses and relapses. From this viewpoint, the presence of lapses and relapses highlight the limitation of a crude offending descriptor such as being a "recidivist." The developmental perspective suggests that this process involves deceleration and de-escalation of offending until termination. Deceleration is intrinsically related to the velocity of offending prior to the start of deceleration of offending. In other words, the more important and serious offending becomes, the longer the desistance phase will be. Considering the range of offending trajectories found for individuals involved in sexual offenses, this process is likely to be relatively short and abrupt for some and slow and gradual for others. Desistance implies the probability of maintaining a non-offending state over time. Recidivism studies have been insightful with respect to the presence of much heterogeneity as to the risk of recidivism at any given time across offenders. Young adult offenders who have maintained a non-offending state are among those most likely to move back to an offending state. Even in the presence of protective factors promoting the deceleration of offending in place, negative life events (e.g., alcohol/drug use, financial difficulties, significant interpersonal conflicts, and negative mood) may favor the movement away from a non-offending state back to an offending state. Given the heterogeneity in the probabilities of offending in adulthood and that these probabilities are not static, but dynamic and subject to several factors starting with the process of aging. In other words, with age, the probabilities of a relapse decrease. Finally, termination of offending or the maintenance of a non-offending state over time may be difficult to achieve for those whose prior offending involvement is more frequent, where the deceleration has not started, and the probabilities of reoffending remain relatively high. Taken together, this proposed unified concept of desistance encompasses the combination of population heterogeneity and state-dependent processes.

For the last three decades, policy development in the area of sexual violence and abuse has been limited to environment-focused interventions and measures to deter individuals from sexually reoffending (Lussier, Gress, Deslauriers-Varin, & Amirault, 2014). The sexual offender registry, public notification, denying/limiting parole, intensive supervision, and home residency restrictions are examples of risk-focused interventions that have little to do with desistance as it is currently understood from available research. In fact, Shover and Henderson (1995) have argued that crime control policies need not be only focused on deterrence and the threat of punishment, but also on increasing legitimate opportunities as increased opportunities extent the number of life options for these individuals. Important research and policy questions that arise are, among other things, whether (a) the current policy landscape regarding the prevention of sexual violence and abuse significantly limit offenders opportunities with respect to experiencing these hooks for change or turning points that are pivotal for desistance from crime, (b) the hooks for change and turning points that appear to play an important role on desistance from crime also operate more specifically for sexual offending. While there is little doubt that repressive policies focusing on neutralization and deterrence negatively impact social opportunities upon reentry, the mechanisms responsible for desistance from sexual offending remain unclear due mainly to the relative absence of research on this topic.

Explanations of desistance from crime and delinquency can be organized along three promising dimensions. The first dimension can be characterized by the role and importance of internal processes and individual factors, such as aging, maturity, and self-identity change. The second dimension refers to those models and hypotheses stressing the role and importance of the environmental factors, such as the opportunity structure, negative consequences of offending as well as the role and influence of peers. A third dimension refers to those models emphasizing person–environment interactions and the context in which these interactions take place, such as the developmental life course perspective and the role and importance of life transitions and turning points. This latter dimension is perhaps the most promising, theoretically as well as for policy development, especially for those individuals with more substantial involvement in crime and delinquency as well as high-risk offenders. The presence of hooks for change as suggested by Giordano et al. (2002) or turning points as formulated by Sampson and Laub (2003) that favor cognitive shifts and cognitive reappraisal as well as significant behavior and lifestyle changes are promising explanatory avenues that researchers have yet to fully describe, analyze, and understand. Furthermore, it is unclear whether such mechanisms also apply to sexual offending or individuals involved in sexual offenses, but emerging results are indicative of similar trends. After all, looking at the limited research, both Kruttschnitt et al. (2000) as well as Lussier and Gress (2014) both reported significant person–environment interactions effects associated with positive outcomes in different samples of individuals convicted for a sexual offense. The Kruttschnitt et al. (2000) study reiterated the importance of social factors (e.g., job) in combination with individual-focus interventions while the Lussier and Gress (2014) findings suggest that measures helping individuals cutting ties with negative peer influences, in line with Warr (1998) hypothesis, increased positive community reentry outcomes. Given the state of empirical research on desistance from crime, more generally, and desistance from sexual offending, more specifically, these conclusions should be seen as tentative.

References

Abel, G. G., Osborn, C. A., & Twigg, D. A. (1993). Sexual assault through the life span. In H. E. Barbaree, W. L. Marshall, & S. M. Hudson (Eds.), *The juvenile sex offender* (pp. 104–117). New York, NY: Guilford Press.

Akers, R. L., & Cochran, J. K. (1985). Adolescent marijuana use: A test of three theories of deviant behavior. *Deviant Behavior, 6*(4), 323–346.

Amirault, J., & Lussier, P. (2011). Population heterogeneity, state dependence and sexual offender recidivism: The aging process and the lost predictive impact of prior criminal charges over time. *Journal of Criminal Justice, 39*(4), 344–354.

Arnett, J. J. (2000). Emerging adulthood: A theory of development from the late teens through the twenties. *American Psychologist, 55*(5), 469.

Barbaree, H. E., Blanchard, R., & Langton, C. M. (2003). The development of sexual aggression through the life span. *Annals of the New York Academy of Sciences, 989*(1), 59–71.

Barbaree, H. E., Langton, C. M., & Blanchard, R. (2007). Predicting recidivism in sex offenders using the VRAG and SORAG: The contribution of age-at-release. *International Journal of Forensic Mental Health, 6*(1), 29–46.

Beech, A. R., & Ward, T. (2004). The integration of etiology and risk in sexual offenders: A theoretical framework. *Aggression and Violent Behavior, 10*(1), 31–63.

Becker, J. V. (1998). What we know about the characteristics and treatment of adolescents who have committed sexual offenses. *A theoretical framework. Aggression and Violent Behavior, 10*(1), 31-63.

Bergman, L. R., & Magnusson, D. (1997). A person-oriented approach in research on developmental psychopathology. *Development and Psychopathology, 9*(02), 291–319.

Bergman, L. R., & Trost, K. (2006). The person-oriented versus the variable-oriented approach: Are they complementary, opposites, or exploring different worlds? *Merrill-Palmer Quarterly, 52*(3), 601–632.

Blokland, A. A., & Nieuwbeerta, P. (2005). The effects of life circumstances on longitudinal trajectories of offending. *Criminology, 43*(4), 1203–1240.

Blokland, A. A. J., & van der Geest, V. (2015). Lifecourse transitions and desistance in sex offenders: An event history analysis. In A. Blokland & P. Lussier (Eds.), *Sex offenders: A criminal career approach*. Oxford: Wiley.

Blumstein, A., Cohen, J., Roth, J. A., & Visher, C. A. (1986). *Criminal careers and "career criminals"*. Washington, DC: National Academies, National Academy Press.

Blumstein, A., Cohen, J., & Farrington, D. P. (1988). Criminal career research: Its value for criminology. *Criminology, 26*(1), 1–35.

Bushway, S. D., Nieuwbeerta, P., & Blokland, A. (2011). The predictive value of criminal background checks: Do age and criminal history affect time to redemption? *Criminology, 49*(1), 27–60.

Bushway, S. D., Piquero, A. R., Broidy, L. M., Cauffman, E., & Mazerolle, P. (2001). An empirical framework for studying desistance as a process. *Criminology, 39*(2), 491–516.

Bushway, S. D., Thornberry, T. P., & Krohn, M. D. (2003). Desistance as a developmental process: A comparison of static and dynamic approaches. *Journal of Quantitative Criminology, 19*(2), 129–153.

Caldwell, M. F. (2010). Study characteristics and recidivism base rates in juvenile sex offender recidivism. *International Journal of Offender Therapy and Comparative Criminology, 54*(2), 197–212.

Cale J, Smallbone S, Rayment-McHugh S, Dowling C (2015) Offense trajectories, the unfolding of sexual and non-sexual criminal activity, and sex offense characteristics of adolescent sex offenders. *Sexual Abuse: A Journal of Research and Treatment*. doi:10.1177/1079063215580968.

Cernkovich, S. A., & Giordano, P. C. (2001). Stability and change in antisocial behavior: The transition from adolescence to early adulthood. *Criminology, 39*(2), 371–410.

Corrado, R. R. (Ed.). (2002). *Multi-problem violent youth: A foundation for comparative research on needs, interventions, and outcomes* (Vol. 324). Amsterdam: Ios Press.

Corrado, R. R., Cohen, I. M., Glackman, W., & Odgers, C. (2003). Serious and violent young offenders' decisions to recidivate: An assessment of five sentencing models. *Crime & Delinquency, 49*(2), 179–200.

Craig, L. A., Browne, K. D., Stringer, I., & Beech, A. (2005). Sexual recidivism: A review of static, dynamic and actuarial predictors. *Journal of Sexual Aggression, 11*(1), 65–84.

Craissati, J., & Beech, A. (2003). A review of dynamic variables and their relationship to risk prediction in sex offenders. *Journal of Sexual Aggression, 9*(1), 41–55.

Cusson, M. (2008). *La délinquance, une vie choisie: Entre plaisir et crime*. Montréal, QC: Les Éditions Hurtubise.

Cusson, M., & Pinsonneault, P. (1986). The decision to give up crime. In D. B. Cornish & R. V. Clarke (Eds.), *The reasoning criminal (rational choice perspectives on offending)*. New York, NY: Springer.

Dempster, R. J., & Hart, S. D. (2002). The relative utility of fixed and variable risk factors in discriminating sexual recidivists and nonrecidivists. *Sexual Abuse: A Journal of Research and Treatment, 14*(2), 121–138.

Doren, D. M. (2004). Toward a multidimensional model for sexual recidivism risk. *Journal of Interpersonal Violence, 19*(8), 835–856.

Doren, D. M. (2006). What do we know about the effect of aging on recidivism risk for sexual offenders? *Sexual Abuse: A Journal of Research and Treatment, 18*(2), 137–157.

Duncan, T. E., & Duncan, S. C. (2004). An introduction to latent growth curve modeling. *Behavior Therapy, 35*(2), 333–363.

Elder, G. H. (1998). The life course as developmental theory. *Child Development, 69*(1), 1–12.

Farmer, M., Beech, A. R., & Ward, T. (2012). Assessing desistance in child molesters: A qualitative analysis. *Journal of interpersonal Violence, 27*, 930–950.

Farrington, D. P. (1986). Age and crime. *Crime and Justice, 189–250*.

Farrington, D. P. (2003). Developmental and life-course criminology: Key theoretical and empirical issues—The 2002 Sutherland award address. *Criminology, 41*(2), 221–225.

Fazel, S., Sjöstedt, G., Långström, N., & Grann, M. (2006). Risk factors for criminal recidivism in older sexual offenders. *Sexual Abuse: A Journal of Research and Treatment, 18*(2), 159–167.

Feeley, M. M., & Simon, J. (1992). The new penology: Notes on the emerging strategy of corrections and its implications. *Criminology, 30*(4), 449–474.

Francis, B., Harris, D., Wallace, S., Soothill, K., & Knight, R. (2013). Sexual and general offending trajectories of men referred for civil commitment. *Sexual Abuse*. doi:10.1177/1079063213492341.

Francis B, Harris D, Wallace S, Soothill K, Knight R (2014) Sexual and general offending trajectories of men referred for civil commitment. *Sexual Abuse: A Journal of Research and Treatment*. doi:10.1177/1079063213492341.

Giordano, P. C., Cernkovich, S. A., & Rudolph, J. L. (2002). Gender, crime, and desistance: Toward a theory of cognitive transformation. *American Journal of Sociology, 107*(4), 990–1064.

Giordano, P. C., Cernkovich, S. A., & Holland, D. D. (2003). Changes in friendship relations over the life course: Implications for desistance from crime. *Criminology, 41*(2), 293–328.

Glueck, S., & Glueck, E. (1940). *Juvenile delinquents grown up*. Oxford, UK: Commonwealth Fund.

Glueck, S., & Glueck, E. T. (1974). *Of delinquency and crime: A panorama of years of search and research*. Springfield, IL: CC Thomas.

Gottfredson, M. R., & Hirschi, T. (1990). *A general theory of crime*. Palo Alto, CA: Stanford University Press.

Greenberg, D. F. (1985). Age, crime, and social explanation. *American of Journal Sociology, 1–21*.

Hanson, R. K. (2002). Recidivism and age: Follow-up data from 4,673 sexual offenders. *Journal of Interpersonal Violence, 17*(10), 1046–1062.

Hanson, R. K. (2006). Does Static-99 predict recidivism among older sexual offenders? *Sexual Abuse: A Journal of Research and Treatment, 18*(4), 343–355.

Hanson, R. K., & Bussière, M. T. (1998). Predicting relapse: A meta-analysis of sexual offender recidivism studies. *Journal of Consulting and Clinical Psychology, 66*(2), 348.

Hanson, R. K., & Harris, A. J. (2000). Where should we intervene? Dynamic predictors of sexual offense recidivism. *Criminal Justice and Behavior, 27*(1), 6–35.

Hanson, R. K., & Harris, A. J. (2001). A structured approach to evaluating change among sexual offenders. *Sexual Abuse: A Journal of Research and Treatment, 13*(2), 105–122.

Hanson, R., Morton, K. E., & Harris, A. J. R. (2003). Sexual offender recidivism risk. *Annals of the New York Academy of Sciences, 989*(1), 154–166.

Hanson, R. K., & Morton-Bourgon, K. E. (2005). The characteristics of persistent sexual offenders: A meta-analysis of recidivism studies. *Journal of Consulting and Clinical Psychology, 73*(6), 1154.

Hanson, R. K., & Thornton, D. (2000). Improving risk assessments for sex offenders: A comparison of three actuarial scales. *Law and Human Behavior, 24*(1), 119–136.

Harris, D. A. (2014). Desistance from sexual offending: Findings from 21 life history narratives. *Journal of Interpersonal Violence, 0886260513511532*.

Harris, G. T., & Rice, M. E. (2007). Adjusting actuarial violence risk assessments based on aging or the passage of time. *Criminal Justice and Behavior, 34*(3), 297–313.

Hirschi, T., & Gottfredson, M. (1983). Age and the explanation of crime. *American Journal of Sociology, 552–584*.

Kazemian, L. (2007). Desistance from crime theoretical, empirical, methodological, and policy considerations. *Journal of Contemporary Criminal Justice, 23*(1), 5–27.

Kazemian, L. (2014). Desistance from crime and antisocial behavior. In J. Morizot & L. Kazemian (Eds.), *The development of criminal and antisocial behavior: Theory, research and practical applications* (pp. 295–312). New York, NY: Springer.

Kazemian, L., & Maruna, S. (2009). Desistance from crime. In M. D. Krohn, A. J. Lizotte, & G. P. Hall (Eds.), *Handbook on crime and deviance* (pp. 277–295). New York, NY: Springer.

Knight, R. A., Ronis, S. T., & Zakireh, B. (2009). Bootstrapping persistence risk indicators for juveniles who sexually offend. *Behavioral Sciences & the Law, 27*(6), 878.

Kruttschnitt, C., Uggen, C., & Shelton, K. (2000). Predictors of desistance among sex offenders: The interaction of formal and informal social controls. *Justice Quarterly, 17*(1), 61–87.

Kurlychek, M. C., Brame, R., & Bushway, S. D. (2006). Scarlet letters and recidivism: Does an old criminal record predict future offending? *Criminology & Public Policy, 5*(3), 483–504.

Lalumière, M. L., Harris, G. T., Quinsey, V. L., & Rice, M. E. (2005). *The causes of rape: Understanding individual differences in male propensity for sexual aggression*. Washington, DC: American Psychological Association.

Langan, P. A., Schmitt, E. L., & Durose, M. R. (2003). *Recidivism of sex offenders released from prison in 1994*. Washington, DC: US Department of Justice, Bureau of Justice Statistics.

Laub, J. H., & Sampson, R. J. (2001). Understanding desistance from crime. *Crime and Justice, 28*, 1–69.

Laub, J. H., & Sampson, R. J. (2009). *Shared beginnings, divergent lives: Delinquent boys to age 70*. Cambridge, MA: Harvard University Press.

Laws, D. R., & Ward, T. (2011). *Desistance from sex offending: Alternatives to throwing away the keys*. New York, NY: Guilford Press.

Le Blanc, M., & Fréchette, M. (1989). *Male criminal activity, from childhood through youth: Multilevel and developmental perspectives*. New York, NY: Springer.

Letourneau, E. J., & Miner, M. H. (2005). Juvenile sex offenders: A case against the legal and clinical status quo. *Sexual Abuse: A Journal of Research and Treatment, 17*(3), 293–312.

Loeber, R., & Farrington, D. P. (Eds.). (1998). *Serious and violent juvenile offenders: Risk factors and successful interventions*. Thousand Oaks, CA: Sage.

Loeber, R., Farrington, D. P., Stouthamer-Loeber, M., & White, H. R. (Eds.). (2008). *Violence and serious theft: Development and prediction from childhood to adulthood*. London: Taylor & Francis.

Loeber, R., & Le Blanc, M. (1990). Toward a developmental criminology. *Crime and Justice, 12*, 375–473.

Lussier, P. (2005). The criminal activity of sexual offenders in adulthood: Revisiting the specialization debate. *Sexual Abuse, 17*(3), 269–292.

Lussier, P. (2015). Juvenile sex offending through a developmental life course criminology perspective: An agenda for policy and research. *Sexual Abuse: A Journal of Research and Treatment, pii*, 1079063215580966.

Lussier, P., & Blokland, A. (2014). The adolescence-adulthood transition and Robins's continuity paradox: Criminal career patterns of juvenile and adult sex offenders in a prospective longitudinal birth cohort study. *Journal of Criminal Justice, 42*(2), 153–163.

Lussier, P., Blokland, A., Mathesius, J., Pardini, D., & Loeber, R. (2015). The childhood risk factors of adolescent-onset and adult-onset of sex offending: Evidence from a prospective longitudinal study. In A. Blokland & P. Lussier (Eds.), *Sex offenders: A criminal career approach.* Oxford: Wiley.

Lussier, P., & Cale, J. (2013). Beyond sexual recidivism: A review of the sexual criminal career parameters of adult sex offenders. *Aggression and Violent Behavior, 18*(5), 445–457.

Lussier, P., Corrado, R. R., & McCuish, E. (2015). A criminal career study of the continuity and discontinuity of sex offending during the adolescence-adulthood transition: A prospective longitudinal study of incarcerated youth. *Justice Quarterly.* doi:10.1080/07418825.2015.1028966.

Lussier, P., & Davies, G. (2011). A person-oriented perspective on sexual offenders, offending trajectories, and risk of recidivism: A new challenge for policymakers, risk assessors, and actuarial prediction? *Psychology, Public Policy, and Law, 17*(4), 530.

Lussier, P., & Gress, C. L. (2014). Community re-entry and the path toward desistance: A quasi-experimental longitudinal study of dynamic factors and community risk management of adult sex offenders. *Journal of Criminal Justice, 42*(2), 111–122.

Lussier, P., Gress, C., Deslauriers-Varin, N., & Amirault, J. (2014). Community risk management of high-risk sex offenders in Canada: Findings from a quasi-experimental study. *Justice Quarterly, 31*(2), 287–314.

Lussier, P., & Healey, J. (2009). Rediscovering Quetelet, again: The "aging" offender and the prediction of reoffending in a sample of adult sex offenders. *Justice Quarterly, 26*(4), 827–856.

Lussier, P., Tzoumakis, S., Cale, J., & Amirault, J. (2010). Criminal trajectories of adult sex offenders and the age effect: Examining the dynamic aspect of offending in adulthood. *International Criminal Justice Review, 20*(2), 147–168.

Lussier, P., Van Den Berg, C., Bijleveld, C., & Hendriks, J. (2012). A developmental taxonomy of juvenile sex offenders for theory, research, and prevention: The adolescent-limited and the high-rate slow desister. *Criminal Justice and Behavior, 39*(12), 1559–1581.

Magnusson, D. (2003). The person approach: Concepts, measurement models, and research strategy. *New Directions for Child and Adolescent Development, 2003*(101), 3–23.

Maruna, S. (2001). *Making good: How ex-convicts reform and rebuild their Lives.* Washington, DC: American Psychological Association.

McCann, K., & Lussier, P. (2008). A meta-analysis of the predictors of sexual recidivism in juvenile offenders. *Youth Violence and Juvenile Justice, 6*, 363–385.

McCuish, E., Lussier, P., & Corrado, R. (2015). Criminal careers of juvenile sex and nonsex offenders: Evidence from a prospective longitudinal study. *Youth Violence and Juvenile Justice, 1541204014567541.*

Moffitt, T. E. (1993). Adolescence-limited and life-course-persistent antisocial behavior: A developmental taxonomy. *Psychological Review, 100*(4), 674–701.

Monahan, K. C., Steinberg, L., Cauffman, E., & Mulvey, E. P. (2009). Trajectories of antisocial behavior and psychosocial maturity from adolescence to young adulthood. *Developmental Psychology, 45*(6), 1654.

Morizot, J., & Le Blanc, M. (2005). Searching for a developmental typology of personality and its relations to antisocial behavior: A longitudinal study of a representative sample of men. *Journal of Personality, 73*(1), 139–182.

Mulvey, E. P., Steinberg, L., Fagan, J., Cauffman, E., Piquero, A. R., Chassin, L., …, Losoya, S. H. (2004). Theory and research on desistance from antisocial activity among serious adolescent offenders. *Youth Violence and Juvenile Justice, 2*(3), 213–236.

Murphy, L., Brodsky, D., Brakel, J., Petrunik, M., Fedoroff, J., & Grudzinskas, A. (2009). Community-based management of sex offenders: An examination of sex offender registries and community notification in the United States and Canada. In F. M. Saleh, A. J. Grudzinskas, J. M. Bradford, & D. J. Brodsky (Eds.), *Sex offenders: Identification, risk assessment, treatment, and legal issues* (pp. 412–441). Oxford: Oxford University Press.

Nagin, D. (2005). *Group-based modeling of development*. Cambridge, MA: Harvard University Press.

Nakamura, K., & Blumstein, A. (2015). Potential for redemption for sex offenders. In A. Blokland & P. Lussier (Eds.), *Sex offenders: A criminal career approach*. Oxford: Wiley.

Petrunik, M. G. (2002). Managing unacceptable risk: Sex offenders, community response, and social policy in the United States and Canada. *International Journal of Offender Therapy and Comparative Criminology, 46*(4), 483–511.

Petrunik, M. (2003). The hare and the tortoise: Dangerousness and sex offender policy in the United States and Canada. *Canadian Journal of Criminology and Criminal Justice, 45*(1), 43–72.

Piliavin, I., Gartner, R., Thornton, C., & Matsueda, R. L. (1986). Crime, deterrence, and rational choice. *American Sociological Review, 101–119.*

Piquero, A. R., Farrington, D. P., & Blumstein, A. (2003). The criminal career paradigm. *Crime and Justice, 359–506.*

Piquero, A. R., & Moffitt, T. E. (2005). Explaining the facts of crime: How the developmental taxonomy replies to Farrington's invitation. In D. P. Farrington (Ed.), *Integrated developmental & life-course theories of offending: Advances in criminological theory* (pp. 51–72). New Brunswick, NJ: Transaction.

Pogarsky, G., & Piquero, A. R. (2003). Can punishment encourage offending? Investigating the "resetting" effect. *Journal of Research in Crime and Delinquency, 40*(1), 95–120.

Prentky, R. A., & Lee, A. F. (2007). Effect of age-at-release on long term sexual re-offense rates in civilly committed sexual offenders. *Sexual Abuse: A Journal of Research and Treatment, 19*(1), 43–59.

Proulx, J., & Lussier, P. (2001). La prédiction de la récidive chez les agresseurs sexuels. *Criminologie, 34,* 9–29.

Quinsey, V. L., Harris, G. T., Rice, M. E., & Cormier, C. A. (1998). *Violent offenders: Appraising and managing risk*. Washington, DC: American Psychological Association.

Quinsey, V. L., Rice, M. E., & Harris, G. T. (1995). Actuarial prediction of sexual recidivism. *Journal of Interpersonal Violence, 10*(1), 85–105.

Robbé, M. D. V., Mann, R. E., Maruna, S., & Thornton, D. (2014). An exploration of protective factors supporting desistance from sexual offending. *Sexual Abuse: A Journal of Research and Treatment, 27*(1), 16–33.

Rosenfeld, R., White, H., & Esbensen, F. (2012). *Special categories of serious and violent offenders: Drug dealers, gang members, homicide offenders, and sex offenders. From juvenile delinquency to adult crime: Criminal careers, justice policy, and prevention* (pp. 118–149). New York, NY: Oxford University Press.

Sample, L. L., & Bray, T. M. (2003). Are sex offenders dangerous? *Criminology & Public Policy, 3*(1), 59–82.

Sampson, R. J., & Laub, J. H. (1995). *Crime in the making: Pathways and turning points through life*. Cambridge, MA: Harvard University Press.

Sampson, R. J., & Laub, J. H. (2003). Life-course desisters? Trajectories of crime among delinquent boys followed to age 70. *Criminology, 41*(3), 555–592.

Sampson, R. J., & Laub, J. H. (2005). A life-course view of the development of crime. *The Annals of the American Academy of Political and Social Science, 602*(1), 12–45.

Shover, N., & Henderson, B. (1995). Repressive crime control and male persistent thieves. In H. Barlow (Ed.), *Crime and public policy*. Oxford: Westview Press.

Shover, N., & Thompson, C. Y. (1992). Age, differential expectations, and crime desistance. *Criminology, 30*(1), 89–104.

Simon, J. (1998). Managing the monstrous: Sex offenders and the new penology. *Psychology, Public Policy, and Law, 4*(1–2), 452.

Soothill, K., Fitzpatrick, C., & Francis, B. (2013). *Understanding criminal careers*. London: Routledge.

Steinberg, L. (2010). A behavioral scientist looks at science of adolescent brain development. *Brain and Cognition, 72,* 160–164.

Stouthamer-Loeber, M., Wei, E., Loeber, R., & Masten, A. S. (2004). Desistance from persistent serious delinquency in the transition to adulthood. *Development and Psychopathology, 16*(4), 897–918.

Sutherland, E. H. (1947). *Principles of criminology* (4th ed.). Philadelphia, PA: J. B. Lippincott.

Tewksbury, R., & Jennings, W. G. (2010). Assessing the impact of sex offender registration and community notification on sex-offending trajectories. *Criminal Justice and Behavior, 37*(5), 570–582.

Thornberry, T. P., Lizotte, A. J., Krohn, M. D., Farnworth, M., & Jang, S. J. (1994). Delinquent peers, beliefs, and delinquent behavior: A longitudinal test of interactional theory. *Criminology, 32*(1), 47–83.

Thornton, D. (2006). Age and sexual recidivism: A variable connection. *Sexual Abuse: A Journal of Research and Treatment, 18*(2), 123–135.

Tolan, P. H., & Gorman-Smith, D. (1998). Development of serious and violent offending careers. In R. Loeber & D. P. Farrington (Eds.), *Serious and violent juvenile offenders: Risk factors and successful interventions* (pp. 68–85). Thousand Oaks, CA: Sage.

Tremblay, P. (1999). Attrition, récidive et adaptation. *Revue Internationale de Criminologie et de Police Technique, 52*, 163–178.

Tzoumakis, S., Lussier, P., Le Blanc, M., & Davies, G. (2012). Onset, offending trajectories, and crime specialization in violence. *Youth Violence and Juvenile Justice, 1541204012458440.*

Uggen, C. (2000). Work as a turning point in the life course of criminals: A duration model of age, employment, and recidivism. *American Sociological Review, 65*, 529–546.

von Eye, A., & Bogat, G. A. (2006). Person-oriented and variable-oriented research: Concepts, results, and development. *Merrill-Palmer Quarterly, 52*(3), 390–420.

Warr, M. (1993). Parents/peers, and delinquency. *Social Forces, 72*(1), 247–264.

Warr, M. (1998). Life-course transitions and desistance from crime. *Criminology, 36*(2), 183–216.

Wolfgang, M. E., Figlio, R. M., & Sellin, T. (1972). *Delinquency in a birth cohort.* Chicago, IL: University of Chicago Press.

Wollert, R. (2006). Low base rates limit expert certainty when current actuarials are used to identify sexually violent predators: An application of Bayes's theorem. *Psychology, Public Policy, and Law, 12*(1), 56.

Wollert, R., Cramer, E., Waggoner, J., Skelton, A., & Vess, J. (2010). Recent research (N = 9,305) underscores the importance of using age-stratified actuarial tables in sex offender risk assessments. *Sexual Abuse: A Journal of Research and Treatment, 22*(4), 471–490.

Worling, J. R., & Langton, C. M. (2014). A prospective investigation of factors that predict desistance from recidivism for adolescents who have sexually offended. *Sexual Abuse: A Journal of Research and Treatment, 27*(1), 127–142.

Zamble, E., & Quinsey, V. L. (1997). *The criminal recidivism process.* New York, NY: Cambridge University Press.

Zimring, F. E., Piquero, A. R., & Jennings, W. G. (2007). Sexual delinquency in Racine: Does early sex offending predict later sex offending in youth and young adulthood? *Criminology & Public Policy, 6*(3), 507–534.

Chapter 14
Changing Course: From a Victim/Offender Duality to a Public Health Perspective

Joan Tabachnick, Kieran McCartan, and Ryan Panaro

Sexual Violence: Definitions and Understandings

In the last few decades, there has been a growing recognition of the depth and extent of sexual violence globally (UNICEF, 2014). This recognition is related to the increased investment in sexual violence education, an increase in the reporting of historical cases, the growing recognition that anyone can be a victim or perpetrator (including, but not limited to, celebrities, politicians, and, most recently, our sons and daughters on college campuses and even younger children and adolescents), and an increased media profile for sexual violence cases nationally in the USA as well as internationally (especially from countries like India and Egypt which have been historically silent on this matter). Internationally, studies of sexual violence found that lifetime prevalence of sexual violence by an intimate partner ranged from 6 to 59 %; by a non-partner in those older than 15 ranged from 1 to 12 %; and in those younger than 15 ranged from 1 to 21 % (World Health Organization, 2014). Research also suggests that sexual violence varies widely between and within countries (Jewkes, 2012; UNICEF, 2014), especially in respect to the size, culture, and economic status of the country. In the USA, certain populations within their defined

J. Tabachnick (✉)
DSM Consultants, 16 Munroe Street, Northampton, MA 01060, USA
e-mail: info@joantabachnick.com

K. McCartan
Health and Applied Social Science, University of the West of England,
Frenchay Campus, Coldharbour Lane, Bristol BS16 1QY, UK
e-mail: Kieran.mccartan@uwe.ac.uk

R. Panaro
LCSW, 5 Eastern Ave, Boston, MA 02026, USA
e-mail: panarory@gmail.com

© Springer International Publishing Switzerland 2016   323
D.R. Laws, W. O'Donohue (eds.), *Treatment of Sex Offenders*,
DOI 10.1007/978-3-319-25868-3_14

community (e.g., college women) are at greater risk for rape and other forms of sexual violence than women in the general population of the same age and income (Fenton et al., 2014; Fisher, Cullen, & Turner, 2000). Although male victimization is difficult to determine due to poor reporting and recording rates (UNICEF, 2014), studies indicate that there are higher levels of male victimization in countries with greater gender equality and higher income/industrialized countries (Archer, 2006).

Research has also documented the lifelong damaging impact of sexual abuse on the physical, mental, reproductive, and sexual health of so many men, women, boys, and girls (Felitti & Anda, 2009). The short-term and long-term consequences of sexual violence include physical injuries, depression, post-traumatic stress disorder, chronic pain, suicide attempts, substance abuse, unwanted pregnancy, gynecological disorders, sexually transmitted infections, increased risk for HIV/AIDS, and others (Felitti & Anda, 2009; Harvey, Garcia-Morena, & Butchart, 2007; DeGue et al., 2012a, 2012b).

Years of research have brought us closer to defining the problem of sexual violence (Wilson & Prescott, 2014). The US Centers for Disease Control and Prevention recently released a revised definition of sexual violence (Basile, Smith, Breiding, Black, & Mahendra, 2014). This new document defines sexual violence as:

> A sexual act that is committed or attempted by another person without freely given consent of the victim or against someone who is unable to consent or refuse. It includes: forced or alcohol/drug facilitated penetration of a victim; forced or alcohol/drug facilitated incidents in which the victim was made to penetrate a perpetrator or someone else; nonphysically pressured unwanted penetration; intentional sexual touching; or non-contact acts of a sexual nature. Sexual violence can also occur when a perpetrator forces or coerces a victim to engage in sexual acts with a third party.

Many of the challenges of defining the scope of sexual violence are linked to the fundamental question about how to consistently define sexual violence (Harrison, Manning, & McCartan, 2010). Estimates of sexual violence will vary widely depending upon how broadly or narrowly the term is defined (Zeuthen & Hagelskjaer, 2013), especially as there is a broad range of legal and clinical categories of sexual violence, both nationally and internationally. One group of researchers explained that, "rape and other forms of sexual violence are probably the most difficult experiences to measure. They are rarely observed and occur in private places" (Cook, Gidycz, Koss, & Murphy, 2011, p. 203). In general, a public health approach defines sexual violence more broadly and includes touching and non-touching offenses as well as attempts as well as completed rapes. Even within the criminal justice system, statutory definitions of sex offenses vary from jurisdiction to jurisdiction, and what is considered a sex crime in one place may not be prosecuted in another (Wiseman, 2014). Another example of conflagration of definitions is between child sexual abuse and pedophilia. The two terms are often used interchangeably in society (McCartan, 2010), when in fact we are talking about two distinct populations (Harrison et al., 2010), one that is primarily based on breaking social norms as well as laws (child sexual abuse) and the other primarily viewed as being a clinical issue (pedophilia). Someone who commits a child sexual offense can be pedophilic or hebephilic but does not have to be, and a pedophile does have to commit a contact offense to be labeled as such. The confusion surrounding definitions of sexual violence in society may distort the issue for the general population and make it difficult to respond to as well as prevent (McCartan, Kemshall, & Tabachnick, 2015; Harris & Socia, 2015), with the label of being a sex offender having a negative impact on all offenders, especially adolescents and children (Pittman, 2013).

Even with these varying definitions, some clear information has emerged from the research. Both criminal justice reports and surveys of victims consistently identify males as the primary perpetrators of sexual violence (Ministry of Justice, Home Office & the Office for National Statistics 2013; Wilson & Prescott, 2014), although women also commit sexual abuse (Eliott & Bailey, 2014; Gannon & Cortoni, 2010). The majority of these crimes are perpetrated by someone the victim knows. In cases of child sexual abuse, one-third of the cases are perpetrated by a family member and two-thirds by someone the victim knows (Snyder, 2000). In addition, it is clear that, although the majority of sex offenses are committed by adults, a significant proportion (20–50 %) is committed by adolescents (Barbaree & Marshall, 2006; Finkelhor, Ormrod, & Chaffin, 2009; Knight & Prentky, 1993). Because research is beginning to clearly demonstrate considerable differences between adults and adolescents who sexually abuse (Przybylski & Lobanov-Rostovsky, 2015), decidedly different intervention and prevention strategies are needed for these distinct populations.

The Baseline Issue and the Impact on Responding to Sexual Violence

Because the majority (80–90 %) of sexual violence remains unreported to authorities (Hanson, Resnick, Saunders, Kilpatrick, & Best, 1999; Tjaden & Thoennes, 2006), defining the scope of sexual violence remains a significant challenge (Saied-Tessier, 2014). This means that there is no reliable baseline to start from in measuring the reality of sexual violence either nationally or internationally. Therefore, the available data and related analysis is always contextual (e.g., to the time and location of recording) and relational (e.g., to the previous year's recorded data). Shame, fear, and threats of physical violence are among the many reasons why victims do not report these crimes (London, Bruck, Ceci, & Shuman, 2005; UNICEF, 2014). In addition, only a small percentage of reported sex crimes ever go to trial and are successfully prosecuted (Abel et al., 1987; Ministry of Justice, 2013; Stroud, Martens, & Barker, 2000) (see Fig. 14.1). Consequently, many researchers use retrospective surveys of adult men and women to better understand and measure the prevalence of sexual violence over the life span.

We do know something about reported cases of sexual violence: based upon the National Crime Victimization Survey, an estimated 243,800 rapes were perpetrated in 2011 (Truman, Langton, & Planty, 2013), and the Federal Bureau of Investigation records over 100,000 local and state arrests for sex crimes each year (FBI, 2010). Given the number of cases that are unreported to authorities, the scope of sexual violence is almost certainly much larger than these numbers indicate (Ministry of

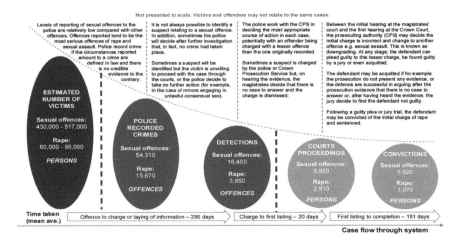

Fig. 14.1 Flow of sexual offense cases from victimization to conviction (*figures displayed are 3-year averages*)

Justice, 2013), especially in countries with poor recording practices and/or a lack of trust in the criminal justice system (UNICEF, 2014).

Retrospective studies have explored what is known about the victims of sexual abuse, and the study questions typically only asked about victimization experiences. Looking at victimization through the incidence of sexual violence across the life span, nearly one in five (18.3 %) women and one in 71 men (1.4 %) reported experiencing rape at some time in their lives. For those under 18, 26.6 % of girls and 5.1 % of boys experienced sexual abuse and/or sexual assault. Sexual abuse and sexual assault experienced exclusively by adults across the life span was 11.2 % for females and 1.9 % for males (Finkelhor, Shattuck, Turner, & Hamby, 2013). Key research findings from the National Survey of Children's Exposure to Violence found that 9.8 % of children had been a victim of sexual violence in their lifetime and 6.1 % had been sexually victimized in the past year. These numbers are echoed internationally. UNICEF (2014) recently produced a report from across 190 countries focusing on child sexual abuse showing that:

- Sexual abuse against children is not just limited to girls.
- Most victims were harmed between the ages of 15–19.
- In most cases the perpetrator was an intimate partner.
- The abuse occurred in everyday locations.

In addition, victims of childhood sexual abuse delayed any disclosure of their victimization, if they disclosed at all, with the main reason being is fear of reprisals, guilt, shame, lack of confidence, and/or lack of awareness of support services. The report indicated that in some countries girls (15–19) are less likely to seek help and support than adult women, with boys and men consistently seeking less help than girls or women.

Measuring Rates of Sexual Violence Perpetration

Historically, most prevention programs have focused on the victims of sexual violence rather than the perpetrators. As described above, the extent of sexual victimization has been well documented and essential for responding to sexual violence after someone is harmed. In contrast, little has been learned about the rates of sexual assault perpetration (Abbey, 2005), and there are no large national studies of sexual violence perpetration. In fact, understanding the scope of perpetration in the USA and internationally could dramatically change the way intervention and prevention programs are created and evaluated (Fenton et al., 2014; Mann, 2014; Saied-Tessier, 2014).

In general, questions about the perpetration of sexual violence are not typically asked for many valid reasons. How a question is asked (e.g., which behaviors are included in the definition of sexual abuse) and what method is used (e.g., telephone survey versus paper survey or computer-assisted survey) clearly affects how it is answered. Furthermore, there appears to be significant hesitation in asking questions about perpetration of sexual violence because it is too complicated (e.g., the respondent needs to understand the concept and be able to remember whether consent was actively obtained), there may be too much shame to recall the events, it might be hard to remember sexual events in previous years or decades, and/or the respondent does not view his (or her) actions as sexually abusive behaviors.

Given the difficulties in asking the questions, there is currently a wide range of responses. The results of studies conducted in the USA asking about attempted rape and completed rape range from 4 to 9 % of adolescents (Ybarra & Mitchell, 2013), and for adults, the rates of completed rapes were as high as 15 % and attempted rape/sexual assault as high as 61 % (Abbey, 2005; Widman, Olson, & Bolen, 2013). International studies do not appear to make the same distinctions between the legal definitions of rape and more general definitions of forced/coerced sex, typically using what the USA would consider the legal definition of rape. Internationally, the rates of perpetration in adult men ranged from 2.5 % in Botswana (Tsai et al., 2011) and up to 37 % of men in South Africa (Jewkes et al., 2013) giving South Africa the name of "rape capital of the world" (Interpol, 2012). When looking at the perpetration of sexual violence across the life span, 16 years old was the most common age of an offender's first sexual perpetration (Ybarra & Mitchell, 2013). Rape of a woman in marriage was more prevalent than non-partner rape (Jewkes et al., 2013), and 73 % of victims were a romantic partner in this adolescent survey (Ybarra & Mitchell, 2013). The young age for first-time perpetration (age 16) suggests that school-based education programs relating to healthy sexual functioning, relationships, prevention, and bystander intervention would be optimally placed at this age-group or slightly younger (Fenton, McCartan, Rumney, & Jones, 2013; Ybarra & Mitchell, 2013).

With this growing focus on preventing the perpetration of sexual violence, the information about the prevalence of perpetration becomes more urgent to help define the program parameters, identify the ideal age for intervention, and ultimately measure the effectiveness of prevention programs.

The Need for a Paradigm Shift

With growing public attention to sexual violence over the past few decades, legislators have responded with numerous laws directed at those who have sexually abused; these have generally been reactive to a single, horrific case and the response has been focused on primarily punitive solutions (e.g., Adam Walsh Act, Megan's Law, etc.). Because most of these laws have been built on the concept of "stranger danger," they either increase the length of incarceration or increase the level of monitoring, tracking, or restrictions once the offender returns to their community (Levenson & D'Amora, 2007; Tabachnick & Klein, 2010). Although these laws have helped to increase the visibility of this issue and hopefully increase victim access services and justice, research also seems to indicate some unintentional consequences. These consequences include family members' struggles with the shame and stigma of public notification, families being less likely to seek help fearing the possible consequences they may face, and families possibly being less likely to see sexual abuse when most offenders are portrayed as monsters by the media (McCartan et al., 2015; McLean & Maxwell, 2015; Tabachnick & Klein, 2010; Pittman, 2013; Tewksbury & Levenson, 2009).

There appears to be growing consensus in the research literature that to truly end sexual violence, it is unlikely that approaches which focus exclusively on a justice solution or even on changing individual behaviors will have a significant impact on this problem (DeGue et al., 2012a, 2012b; Dodge, 2009). Research suggests that only a more comprehensive approach to sexual violence that includes prevention will be successful to ending this global problem (Lee, Guy, Perry, Keoni-Sniffen, & Mixson, 2007; Nation et al., 2003). A more comprehensive approach will help to integrate existing efforts to incarcerate offenders and provide services to victims into broader strategies to educate communities and change the very circumstances that allow sexual abuse to be perpetrated.

One of the largest shifts in focus over the last 10 years has been the growing attention on how to implement strategies before anyone is harmed (Banyard, Eckstein, & Moynihan, 2010). Increasingly the CDC and other public health agencies have focused their research and programming priorities to stopping the perpetration of sexual violence before anyone is harmed, which is also a message and strategy used internationally by Stop it Now! in the UK (Now!, 2014) as well as Project Dunkelfeld in Germany (Project Dunkelfeld, 2015). In fact, there is a growing trend toward preventing first-time perpetration of sexual abuse—focusing on those at risk to abuse and those who have abused to prevent further assaults (Zeuthen & Hagelskjaer, 2013; DeGue et al., 2012a, 2012b). This focus maximizes the opportunities to achieve population level reductions in the prevalence of sexual violence (DeGue et al., 2012a, 2012b). An expanded view to focus on perpetration has the additional benefit of taking the burden of prevention off of victims and off of those individuals at risk to be victimized and places it squarely on those who are at risk to cause the harm. But to prevent sexual violence before anyone is harmed, strategies must include a focus on those who might be at risk to perpetrate sexual violence, a strategy which has been applied to other at risk and vulnerable populations (Hoggett et al., 2014).

According to the World Health Organization (Harvey et al., 2007), when people become truly aware of the full extent of sexual violence, especially with a focus on those who abuse, the instinct is to demand justice and care for the victim while increasing the harsh punishment for the perpetrators. In fact, most of the responses have been to enact legislation to increase the penalties for these crimes (e.g., civil commitment, offender registration, chemical castration, residency restrictions, etc.), which can create more problems than solutions or are at best ineffective (Zgoba et al., 2015). In many countries, the approach to prevention has been to develop education programs to increase awareness of the problem or change attitudes (DeGue et al., 2012a, 2012b; Gidycz, Rich, & Marioni, 2002; Lonsway, 1996). The media has also responded with stories that increase fear and anger and portray the abusers as a monster and encourage simple solutions that punish the individual. However, there have been some alternative news stories over the past 12–18 months that have started to create a more nuanced view in the media including the UK (Humphries, 2014), the USA (Malone, 2014), and India (Philip, 2014). It is difficult to look beyond the urgency of so many children and other vulnerable adults and the safety of their families and communities to take the larger public health view—but this larger nuanced view of the issue allows society to alter the very factors that can prevent people at harm from acting on it. Hence, a shift from a simplistic victim/perpetrator duality to a broader public health paradigm opens a view of the trends, social norms, circumstances, and structures that inadvertently encourage and allow sexual violence to continue, therefore allowing us to attempt to combat them (McCartan et al., 2015).

Public Health Approach to Preventing Sexual Violence

Public health offers a unique insight into ending sexual violence by focusing on the safety and benefits for the largest group of people possible (Laws, 2000; Smallbone, Marshall, & Wortley, 2008; Wortley & Smallbone, 2006; CDC, 2004; McCartan et al., 2015). While it is essential that society respond to the urgency and crisis of sexual violence, a public health focus on prevention expands that response to address the health of an entire population (Laws, 2000; Centers for Disease Control and Prevention, 2004). A public health multi-disciplinary scientific approach to large health problems involves the perspectives offered by medicine, epidemiology, sociology, psychology, criminology, education, and economics among others. It is this access to a broad knowledge base that allows the public health approach to effectively respond to a large number of health issues around the world (Laws, 2000; Wortley & Smallbone, 2006). Although many have written about the importance of using a public health approach to complement existing criminal justice strategies (Laws, 2000; Longo, 1997; McMahon, 2000; Mercy, Rosenberg, Powell, Broome, & Roper, 1993; Smallbone et al., 2008), as each year passes, our understanding of how to apply public health to sexual violence becomes more evidence based and ultimately more effective.

The CDC describes a public health approach to prevention through three prevention categories based upon when the intervention occurs (Centers for Disease Control and Prevention, 2004). These levels include:

- Primary prevention: Approaches that take place before sexual violence has occurred in order to prevent initial perpetration or victimization
- Secondary prevention: An immediate response after sexual violence has occurred to deal with the short-term consequences of violence
- Tertiary prevention: A long-term response that follows sexual violence, designed to deal with the lasting consequences of violence and provide treatment to perpetrators

The aim of these levels is to effectively position the appropriate interventions to prevent harmful behavior and the subsequent negative consequences. In regard to sexual violence prevention, the core aim of these three levels is to stop offending and reduce the impact of sexual violence (Laws, 2000; McCartan et al., 2015; Smallbone et al., 2008).

The social-ecological model (Krug, Dahlberg, Mercy, Zwi, & Lozano, 2002) is orientated around four levels of intervention: individuals, relationships, communities, and society. Prevention programs that address all four levels are more likely to successfully change the targeted behavior(s). This social-ecological model expands prevention efforts beyond typical education and individual self-help or treatment models to describe a broader range of activities. Those who use this model argue that to address complex public health problems, no single solution will work. Rather, multiple interventions need to be targeted at each of these levels. In fact, the authors suggest that prevention programs that address all four levels are more likely to change the targeted behavior(s).

Combining these two public health frameworks (see Table 14.1) would mean that prevention strategies would need to: (1) target behaviors before they are perpetrated as well as interventions targeting sexually abusive behavior after it is perpetrated combined with (2) interventions that target all the four levels of the social-ecological model to be successful in reducing sexually abusive behaviors. Taken together, these strategies encompass a large spectrum of sexual violence interventions stretching from healthy sexuality educational curricula for adoles-

Table 14.1 Suggested framework for preventing the perpetration of sexual violence

	Individual/relationship	Community/society
Before	Healthy sexuality education (e.g., bystander interventions such as Green Dot and Bringing in the Bystanders) and programs targeting at risk individuals (e.g., Project Dunkelfeld)	Programs targeting at risk populations (e.g., Safe Dates program, Shifting Boundaries, growing number of consent laws, child safety policies within youth serving organizations)
After	Programs for those who have harmed or been harmed (e.g., treatment) as well as the criminal justice system to prosecute those who have abused	Policies and programs responding to sexual violence and targeting sex offenders in the community (e.g., sex offender management laws, Circles of Support and Accountability)

cents as a means of promoting primary prevention, secondary prevention immediately reaching the victims and abuser after sexual abuse has occurred to ensure treatment and heal, to tertiary prevention public policies that allow for the registration requirements, community supervision strategies, and community-based programming for convicted adult sex offenders (McCartan et al., 2015).

However, most perpetration prevention initiatives are aimed at the tertiary levels of prevention, preventing further sexually abusive behavior—interventions that are least likely to be effective in promoting healthy communities (Laws, 2008). With this in mind, this discussion will focus attention primarily on what is known about preventing first-time perpetration at all levels of the social-ecological model.

Risk and Protective Factors: A Foundation for Prevention

One of the most significant areas of recent research regarding the adults, adolescents, and children who sexually abuse is the growing understanding of the factors that put someone at risk to abuse again and the protective factors that may decrease the likelihood of sexually abusive behaviors (Wilson & Prescott, 2014). Understanding both the risk and the protective factors for sexually abusive behaviors and especially for first-time perpetration is an essential building block for developing evidence-based prevention programs that can reduce the prevalence of sexual violence over time (Graffunder, Lang, & Mercy, 2010; Whitaker et al., 2008).

Risk factors are defined as any variable that increases the likelihood that a person will commit a sexual offense (Jewkes, 2012). Complementing the presence of risk factors is the presence of protective factors. Although the research about protective factors is very limited (Tharp et al., 2012), they are commonly recognized to be "the factors in personal, social, and external support systems, which modify, ameliorate, compensate, or alter a person's response to risk factors for any maladaptive life event and thus reduce the probability of those outcomes" (Klein, Rettenberger, Yoon, Kohler, & Briken, 2014, p. 2). Furthermore, Tharp et al. (2012) suggest that individual protective factors may develop or "activate" according to certain periods of psychosocial development. This relationship could have important implications for developing comprehensive, effective prevention programming targeting specifically to age and developmental level. This early intervention may have lifelong impact because the majority of sexually abusive behavior begins in adolescence and the balance of risk and protective factors can be changed at various levels of the social-ecological model.

Given the higher and lower rates of sexual violence in various communities (Ministry of Justice, 2013; UNICEF, 2014), some of the most promising new research explores the risk factors at the community level. These community level factors would allow programs and initiatives to utilize a larger population-based approach. The emerging factors include the following: gender dynamics (e.g., the level of education for females and male attitudes toward gender roles), poverty, societal tolerance for violence, lack of accountability for perpetrators, and patriarchal and rape-supportive social norms (Casey & Lindhorst, 2009; World Health Organization & London School of Hygiene and Tropical Medicine, 2010).

Practical Applications of Perpetration Prevention Strategies

Other public health problems such as smoking, drinking and driving, and HIV transmission have been successful because they moved beyond a simple educational component targeting individuals to develop a multilevel comprehensive approach to prevention (Banyard, Plante, & Moynihan, 2004; CDC, 2004; Davis, Parks, & Cohen, 2006). Experts in the field are calling for a paradigm shift in sexual violence prevention that: "moves us away from low-dose educational programs in adulthood and towards investment in the development and rigorous evaluation of more comprehensive multi-level strategies that target younger populations and seek to modify community and/or contextual supports for violence" (DeGue et al., 2014). In fact, growing consensus indicates that in order to sustain long-term changes within individual's, families', and communities' attitudes to violence, these changes must first take place at a societal level (Lee et al., 2007); therefore, it is about comprehensive, sustained societal change rather than piecemeal individual change.

In recent years there has been a growing movement toward a more comprehensive public health understanding and response to sexual violence, focusing on the importance of prevention efforts (Casey & Lindhorst, 2009; DeGue et al., 2014; Lee et al., 2007; Nation et al., 2003; Tabachnick and Klein 2011). As awareness of and interest in prevention efforts increase, the public has become more engaged and asking for more accurate information about those who abuse, supporting the need for programs that prevent the perpetration of sexual abuse. In fact, according to a survey conducted by the Center for Sex Offender Management (2010), "The vast majority of [the public] (83 %) expressed a desire for more information than they currently have regarding how to prevent sex offending in their communities." These survey results suggest that the timing may be right to support a shift toward primary prevention programs focusing on preventing the perpetration of sexual violence.

The section below outlines a number of evidence-based programs that have undergone a rigorous evaluation; each will be briefly described below. Also below are promising practices, initiatives that are still being evaluated and/or that have been evaluated with a less rigorous research design (e.g., did not measure impact on sexually violent behavior), may not yet show significant changes in behavior, or may not have completed their evaluations over time. These promising programs include: bystander programs, structural interventions, early childhood and family-based interventions, school-based programs, youth serving organization interventions, as well as social norm and social marketing campaigns (CDC, 2004; Lee et al., 2007; DeGue et al., 2014). All of these programs show promise in the field, despite not having extensive and/or outcome data, contributing at a ground level to prevention. It is important to state that given the early stage that we are at in developing and evaluating public health approaches to sexual violence, 15 years since the concept was initially introduced (Laws, 2000; McMahon, 2000) with most programs only having run for less than 10 years (see below), there is no robust evidence for impact and success of any given initiative. As it is not possible to be inclusive of all prevention programs, brief descriptions of select programs with more rigorous research are included.

Safe Dates is a 10 session prevention curriculum about dating violence for middle and high school students. After four years, students participating in the program were significantly less likely to have been victimized or to perpetrate sexual violence involving a dating partner (Foshee et al.,2004).

Shifting Boundaries is a building-level intervention using temporary building-level restraining orders, poster campaign, and "hotspot" mapping to identify unsafe areas of the school for increased monitoring. Results showed that the initiative reduced both exposure to and perpetration of sexually harassing behaviors and peer violence as well as sexual violence victimization. This intervention did not have a significant impact on the perpetration of sexual violence by a dating partner.

US Violence Against Women Act of 1994 (VAWA) targets the increase in prosecution and penalties for sexual violence as well as funding research and education programs in this area. Quasi-experimental evaluation indicates an annual reduction of 0.66% in rapes reported (DeGue et al., 2014). Many of the programs outlined in this section are funded through VAWA.

Fig. 14.2 Three evidence-based interventions to prevent the perpetration of sexually violent behaviors (DeGue et al., 2014)

Evidence-Based Primary Prevention Programs

Based upon the first systematic review of 140 initiatives to prevent the perpetration of sexual violence, DeGue et al. (2014) identified three primary prevention strategies that used a rigorous outcome evaluation to demonstrate a decrease in sexually violent behavior: *Safe Dates* (Foshee et al., 2004), *Shifting Boundaries* (Taylor, Stein, Woods, & Mumford, 2011), and funding associated with the *1984 US Violence Against Women Act* (Boba & Lilley, 2009) (see Fig. 14.2).

Two of these programs are aimed at younger audiences and speak to the need to be appropriately timed which is consistent with other violence intervention strategies and research that suggest early adolescences as a critical window for intervention (DeGue et al., 2014; Lee et al., 2007). Given the research which indicates that the average age for initial perpetration is 16, interventions targeting ages prior to the age of 16 offer a unique opportunity to influence future developmental trajectories (Ybarra & Mitchell, 2013).

Promising Practices

Bystander Intervention Programs

Bystander programs have begun to demonstrate a significant impact on reducing victimization and sexually aggressive behaviors (Foubert, 2005) and on participant's willingness to intervene (Banyard, Moynihan, & Plante, 2007). Consistently across the various models, communities with higher levels of engagement (e.g., trust that the system will work) had more young adults who reported bystander action and interventions (Coker et al., 2014). Most effective when there is community ownership, repeated exposure through multiple channels and multiple components delivered in a variety of community settings (World Health Organization, 2007). Three programs which have been closely evaluated are as follows: (1) *Bringing in the Bystanders* (Banyard et al., 2007) is a multi-session program (4.5 h) focusing on skills to help participants act when they see behaviors that put others at risk for victimization or perpetration. Research on this program showed that it was effective in increasing knowledge, decreasing rape-supportive attitudes, and increasing bystander behavior over time (Banyard et al., 2007). Although there were no direct questions which would measure the decrease in sexually abusive behaviors, it is an ideal place to begin to monitor the impact on those at risk to abuse. (2) *Coaching Boys into Men* (Miller et al., 2012) provides 11 brief 10–15-min sessions on dating violence and respectful relationships delivered by athletic coaches to young men. Initial results showed a positive effect on reducing dating violence generally and increasing high school young men's intention to intervene in situations that they see might be abusive. The link to sexually abusive behaviors is clear. Unfortunately, the research did not ask direct questions about sexual violence perpetration. (3) The US Office of Violence against Women has required all grantees to include evidence-informed bystander prevention programming in their work and develop both targeted and universal prevention strategies. The *Green Dot* program involves both a motivational speech by key leadership and a 4–6-h curriculum delivered by peer opinion leaders. Initial evaluation results indicate that both victimization and perpetration rates were lower among college students attending the campuses that received the *Green Dot* intervention (Coker et al., 2014).

Social Marketing Programs

Social marketing is a relatively new campaign approach that involves the "application of commercial marketing principles … to influence the voluntary behavior of target audiences in order to improve their personal welfare and that of their society" (Andreasen, 1995). There have been promising results shown when applied to both domestic and sexual violence initiatives. One of the first applications of social marketing to a domestic violence initiative was the Western Australia *Freedom from Fear Campaign*. This innovative campaign was designed to motivate those at risk to abuse and those who have abused to call a helpline and voluntarily attend counseling program. In the first 7 months, they found a significant shift in attitude by the men exposed to the campaign (e.g., 52 % agreed that "occasional slapping of their partner" is never justified, compared with 38 % before the campaign), and during this time, 1385 men from the target audience called the helpline (Donovan & Vlais, 2005). This same social marketing concept was used by *Stop It Now!* in the USA, the UK, and parts of Europe as well as by the *Prevention Project Dunkelfeld* in Germany (Beier et al., 2009; Tabachnick & Newton-Ward, 2010). The *Prevention*

Project of Dunkelfeld, based in Berlin, Germany, developed a program that offered treatment and pharmaceutical options to anyone who stepped forward to seek help with sexually abusive behaviors. With funding from a private foundation, bus ads and other campaign materials were developed targeting those who are sexually attracted to children with the primary slogan that asks, "Do you like children in ways you shouldn't?" Even with a limited public outreach campaign, between 2005 and 2008, over 800 individuals contacted the program. Approximately 40 of these individuals traveled to the program's outpatient clinic for a full assessment, and 200 were invited to participate in a one-year treatment program (Beier et al., 2009). The same approach was developed by *Stop It Now!* in an attempt to reach a broader range of adults and adolescents who might be at risk to sexually abuse a child. These programs were developed with different approaches and campaigns and tested in a variety of countries and jurisdictions. Because some of these locations had mandated reporting requirements, the structure also had to be slightly different. However, promising results were found in each of these pilot programs. For example, in a pilot test in Vermont, USA, a campaign was carried out from 1995 to 1997. At the end of this period, Vermont sex offender treatment providers reported that 50 persons self-reported sexual abuse before entering the legal system. Of these, 11 were adults who self-reported, and 39 were adolescents who entered treatment as a result of a parent or guardian soliciting help (Chasan-Taber & Tabachnick, 1999). Each of the social marketing campaigns has demonstrated that there are adults and adolescents who are willing to seek help in order to control and ideally prevent sexually abusive behaviors. Not only are they affecting those at risk to sexually abuse, but they have the potential for a greater impact by affecting the families and communities that surround these individuals.

The Cost and Savings of a Public Health Approach

The prevention of sexual violence, especially child sexual abuse, is important given the social stigma attached to victims and perpetrators, the impact on victims, and its cost to the state in terms of legal, health, and social care responses to victims and offenders. Generally, the sexual violence public health discourse is prevention based upon education, engagement, and awareness raising (Kemshall, McCartan, & Hudson, 2012); however, this message does not always get effectively conveyed by the state and/or professionals to the public, especially in terms of what happens at secondary and tertiary levels, and when it does the public do not always receive it well. When it comes to public health, there are a multitude of campaigns throughout society which have effectively changed people's attitudes to certain harmful behaviors, the most obvious ones being alcohol, smoking, and obesity (Health Development Agency, 2004). A public health approach would then seem to work, so it seems logical that it would work with child sexual abuse/pedophilia as well because as a topic area it shares similar triggers like mental health outcomes, health outcomes, interpersonal outcomes, and socioeconomic outcomes.

Unfortunately, the funding for prevention initiatives has been lacking in the field of sexual violence especially in relation to other areas of public health (DeGue et al., 2012a, 2012b). Even less funding is available for evaluation of these limited number of innovative prevention strategies (Letourneau, Eaton, Bass, Berlin, & Moore, 2014). For example, the Centers for Disease Control and Prevention has funded more than 27 research projects with $19 million over 10 years (DeGue et al., 2012a, 2012b). While this represents a significant investment, the amount pales in comparison to the billions of dollars representing the real cost of sexual violence as well as the funding available for the arrest and prosecution of sexual abusers and the billions of dollars spent on containing the offender or monitoring their activities including options such as prison, GPS bracelet, civil commitment, and other sex offender management strategies. It also pales in terms of the impact of not fully responding to this problem—and the impacts have been seismic across the USA and around the world. Although it is hard to estimate the cost of ignoring the problem, the US National Institutes of Justice has estimated that the cost of victimization from sexual violence may total as much as $126 billion annually in the USA alone (Miller, Cohen, Wiersema, & Justice, 1996). Estimates of child sexual abuse internationally echo these numbers with figures calculated at $124 billion in the USA (Fang, Brown, Florence, & Mercy, 2012), $3.9 billion in Australia (Taylor et al., 2008), and £3.2 billon in the UK (Saied-Tessier, 2014), therefore suggesting that effective prevention has the capacity to not only reduce sexual violence but also to reduce the attached cost. Given the volume of money spent, nationally and internationally, on sexual violence perpetrators as well as victims, the benefits of investing in prevention, purely from a monetary point of perspective, seem apparent.

Conclusion

Until fairly recently, the primary challenge facing advocates for sexual abuse prevention was getting the public and public officials to recognize the enormity of the problem. Through the efforts of these advocates, the courage of survivors speaking out about their experiences, the investment of many organizations in prevention, a closer examination of which initiatives are having an impact, and the growing media attention to this issue, there have been an incredible number of positive changes over time. Some of the key shifts in our understanding and our investment in primary prevention over the last few decades include:

- Expanding the focus from teaching children to protect themselves to also involve the caring adults in the lives of each child and putting the responsibility of prevention on those adults
- Expanding the focus from individual choices and decisions to also examine the role and influence of peers, communities, and policies on preventing sexual violence
- Shifting away from a restrictive, reactive victim/offender paradigm for understanding sexual violence to a more proactive, inclusive, and engaged public health paradigm, which involves the family and the larger community in prevention

- Shifting away from the concept of a single information session (single dosage) to a more comprehensive approach that involves multiple education sessions tied to other structural strategies and policies
- Including a stronger focus on preventing the perpetration of sexual violence to address sexual abuse before any child, teen, or vulnerable adult is harmed

Certainly, the field continues to face an incredible number of challenges—most evident is the immense complexity of this issue. Other challenges include the lack of information about risk factors for first-time perpetration and the protective factors that might limit that risk (DeGue et al., 2012a; 2012b), the separation of research, academic journals, government centers, and even conferences for those working with victims and those working with perpetrators of sexual abuse (Letourneau et al., 2014), the lack of theoretical guidance to identify promising programs and policies at the community level (DeGue et al., 2012a, 2012b), the continued media framing of sexual violence as a sex crime story that promotes angry and fearful responses or introduces skepticism that allows the public to ignore the problem (Letourneau et al., 2014; McCartan et al., 2015), and the continued lack of funding streams for primary prevention programs (Cohen, David, & Graffunder, 2006). However, even with these seemingly insurmountable challenges, government agencies are exerting new leadership and focusing resources on primary prevention through stopping initial perpetration of sexual violence, new initiatives are beginning to open small and important funding streams for child sexual abuse prevention, and a growing number of programs are able to demonstrate successful outcomes building a base of promising practices for sexual violence prevention.

The challenge of sexual violence is also the future strength of this work. The complexity of sexual violence is widely recognized, and the answer therefore demands a thoughtful and comprehensive response—this cannot be a single-agency issue. Literally hundreds of organizations and agencies and individuals are working together to prevent sexual violence around the world. This points to the need for a strong, coherent, coordinated, and engaged public policy and well-funded evidence-based strategies to prevent sexual violence. These efforts are supported by core human values that it is ultimately more humane to prevent sexual violence than to wait and respond after a child, adolescent, or adult has been exposed to and harmed by the trauma of sexual abuse.

References

Abbey, A. (2005). Lessons learned and unanswered questions about sexual assault perpetration. *Journal of Interpersonal Violence, 20*(1), 39–42. doi:10.1177/0886260504268117.

Abel, G. G., Becker, J. V., Cunningham-Rathner, J., Mittleman, M. S., Murphy, M. S., & Rouleou, J. L. (1987). Self-reported crimes of non-incarcerated paraphiliacs. *Journal of Interpersonal Violence, 2*, 3–25.

Andreasen, A. (1995). *Marketing social change*. San Francisco, CA: Josey-Bass Publishers.

Archer, J. (2006). Cross-cultural differences in physical aggression between partners: A social-role analysis. *Personality and Social Psychology Review, 10*, 133–153.

Banyard, V. L., Eckstein, R. P., & Moynihan, M. M. (2010). Sexual violence prevention: The role of stages of change. *Journal of Interpersonal Violence, 25*, 111–135.

Banyard, V. L., Moynihan, M. M., & Plante, E. G. (2007). Sexual violence prevention through bystander education: An experimental evaluation. *Journal of Community Psychology, 35*, 463–481. doi:10.1002/jcop.20159.

Banyard, V. L., Plante, E. G., & Moynihan, M. M. (2004). Bystander education: Bringing a broader community perspective to sexual violence prevention. *Journal of Community Psychology, 32*, 61–79.

Barbaree, H. E., & Marshall, W. L. (2006). An introduction to the juvenile sexual offender: Terms, concepts, and definitions. In H. E. Barbaree & W. L. Marshall (Eds.), *The juvenile sex offender* (pp. 1–18). New York, NY: Guilford Press.

Basile, K. C., Smith, S. G., Breiding, M. J., Black, M. C., & Mahendra, R. R. (2014). *Sexual violence surveillance: Uniform definitions and recommended data elements, Version 2.0*. Atlanta, GA: National Center for Injury Prevention and Control, Centers for Disease Control and Prevention.

Beier, M., Neutze, J., Mundt, I. A., Ahlers, C. J., Goecker, D., Konrad, A., & Schaefer, G. E. (2009). Encouraging self-identified pedophiles and hebephiles to seek professional help: First results of the Prevention Project Dunkelfeld (PPD). *Child Abuse and Neglect, 33*, 545–549.

Boba, R., & Lilley, D. (2009). Violence against women act (VAWA) funding: A nationwide assessment of effects on rape and assault. *Violence Against Women, 15*, 168–185.

Bumby, K., Carter, M., Gilligan, L., & Talbot, T. (2010). *Exploring public awareness and attitudes about sex offender management: Findings from a national public opinion poll*. Silver Spring, MD: Center for Sex Offender Management, Center for Effective Public Policy.

Casey, E. A., & Lindhorst, T. P. (2009). Toward a multi-level, ecological approach to the primary prevention of sexual assault: Prevention in peer and community contexts. *Trauma Violence Abuse, 10*(2), 91–114. doi:10.1177/1524838009334129.

Centers for Disease Control and Prevention. (2004). *Sexual violence prevention: Beginning the dialogue*. Atlanta: Author.

Chasan-Taber, L., & Tabachnick, J. (1999). Evaluation of a child sexual abuse prevention program. *Sexual Abuse: A Journal of Research and Treatment, 4*, 279–292.

Cohen, L., David, R., & Graffunder, C. (2006). Before it occurs: Primary prevention of intimate partner violence and abuser. In P. Salber & E. Taliaferro (Eds.), *The physician's guide to intimate partner violence and abuser* (pp. 89–100). Volcano, CA: Volcano Press.

Coker, A. L., Fisher, B. S., Bush, H. M., Swan, S. C., Williams, C. M., Clear, E. R., & DeGue, S. (2014). Evaluation of the Green Dot bystander intervention to reduce interpersonal violence among college students across three campuses. *Violence Against Women*. doi:10.177/1077801214545284.

Cook, S. L., Gidycz, C. A., Koss, M. P., & Murphy, M. (2011). Emerging issues in the measurement of rape victimization. *Violence Against Women, 17*, 201–218.

Davis, R., Parks, L. F., & Cohen, L. (2006). *Sexual violence and the spectrum of prevention: Towards a community solution*. Retrieved from http://www.preventioninstitute.org.

DeGue, S., Holt, M. K., Massetti, G. M., Matjasko, J. L., Tharp, A. T., & Valle, L. A. (2012). Looking ahead toward community-level strategies to prevent sexual violence. *Journal of Women's Health, 22*(1), 1–3. doi:10.1089/jwh.2011.3263.

DeGue, S., Simon, T. R., Basile, K. C., Yee, S. L., Lang, K., & Spivak, H. (2012). Moving forward by looking back: Reflecting on a decade of CDC's work in sexual violence prevention, 2000–2010. *Journal of Women's Health, 21*(12), 1211–1218. doi:10.1089/jwh.2012.3973.

DeGue, S., Valle, L. A., Holt, M. K., Massetti, B. M., Matjasko, J. L., & Tharp, A. T. (2014). A systematic review of primary prevention strategies for sexual violence perpetration. *Aggression and Violence Behavior, 19*, 346–362.

Dodge, K. A. (2009). Community intervention and public policy in the prevention of antisocial behavior. *Journal of Child Psychology and Psychiatry, 50*, 194–200.

Donovan, R. J., & Vlais, R. (2005). *VicHealth review of communication components of social marketing/public education campaigns focusing on violence against women*. Melbourne, VIC: Victorian Health Promotion Foundation.

Eliott, I., & Bailey, A. (2014). Female sex offenders: Gender, risk and risk perception. In K. McCartan (Ed.), *Responding to sexual offending: Perceptions, risk management and public protection* (pp. 206–226). Hampshire: Palgrave Macmillan.

Fang, X., Brown, D. S., Florence, C. S., & Mercy, J. A. (2012). The economic burden of child maltreatment in the United States and implications for prevention. *Child Abuse & Neglect, 36,* 156–165.

Federal Bureau of Investigation. (2010). *Uniform crime reports.* Washington, DC: US Department of Justice.

Felitti, V., & Anda, R. (2009). The relationship of adverse childhood experiences to adult medical disease, psychiatric disorders, and sexual behavior: Implications for healthcare. In R. Lanius & E. Vermetten (Eds.), *The hidden epidemic: The impact of early life trauma on health and disease.* Cambridge: Cambridge University Press.

Fenton, R., McCartan, K., Rumney, P., & Jones, J. (2013). Myths, reality, and sexual violence: Changing attitudes, changing practice. *ATSA Forum, 25,* 3–4.

Fenton, R., Mott, H., McCartan, K. & Rumney, P. (2014) The Intervention Initiative. UWE and Public Health England, Bristol. Available from http://eprints.uwe.ac.uk/25530.

Finkelhor, D., Ormrod, R, & Chaffin, M. (2009). Juveniles who commit sex offenses against minors. *Juvenile Justice Bulletin.* Retrieved from http://www.ncjrs.gov/pdffiles1/ojjdp/227763. pdf

Finkelhor, D., Shattuck, A., Turner, H. A., & Hamby, S. L. (2013). The lifetime prevalence of child sexual abuse and sexual assault assessed in late adolescence. *Journal of Adolescent Health, 55*(3), 329–333.

Fisher, B., Cullen, F., & Turner, M. (2000). *The sexual victimization of college women.* Washington, DC: National Institute of Justice and the Bureau of Justice Statistics.

Foshee, V. A., Baiam, L. E., Emmett, S. T., Linder, G. F., Benefield, T., & Suchindran, C. (2004). Assessing the long-term effects of the safe dates program and a booster in preventing and reducing adolescent dating violence victimization and perpetration. *American Journal of Public Health, 94,* 619–624.

Foubert, J. D. (2005). *The men's program: A peer education guide to rape prevention.* New York, NY: Routledge.

Gannon, T., & Cortoni, F. (2010). *Female sexual offenders: Theory, assessment and treatment.* New York, NY: John Wiley & Sons.

Gidycz, C. A., Rich, C. L., & Marioni, M. L. (2002). Interventions to prevent rape and sexual assault. In J. Petrak & B. Hedge (Eds.), *The trauma of sexual assault: Treatment, prevention and policy* (pp. 235–260). New York, NY: Wiley.

Graffunder, C. M., Lang, K. S., & Mercy, J. A. (2010). Advancing a federal sexual violence prevention agenda: Research and program. In K. Kaufman (Ed.), *The prevention of sexual violence: A practitioner's sourcebook* (pp. 207–220). Holyoke, MA: NEARI Press.

Hanson, R. F., Resnick, H. S., Saunders, B. E., Kilpatrick, D. G., & Best, C. (1999). Factors related to the reporting of childhood rape. *Child Abuse and Neglect, 23,* 559–569.

Harris, A. J., & Socia, K. (2015). What's in a name? Evaluating the effects of the "sex offender" label on public opinions and beliefs. *Sexual Abuse: A Journal of Research and Treatment.* Retrieved from http://sax.sagepub.com/content/early/2014/12/24/1079063214564391.abstract.

Harrison, K., Manning, R., & McCartan, K. (2010). Multi-disciplinary definitions and understandings of 'paedophilia'. *Social and Legal Studies, 19,* 481–496.

Harvey, A., Garcia-Morena, C., & Butchart, A. (2007). *Primary prevention of intimate-partner violence and sexual violence.* Geneva: World Health Organization. Background paper for WHO expert meeting, May 2–3, 2007.

Health Development Agency. (2004). *The effectiveness of public health campaigns.* HDA Briefing No. 7, Consumers and Markets.

Hoggett, J., Ahmad, Y., Frost, E., Kimberlee, R., McCartan, K., Solle, J., & Bristol City Council. (2014). *The troubled families programme: A process, impact and social return on investment analysis.* Project Report. University of the West of England, UWE repository.

Humphries, S. (2014, November 25). *The pedophile next door* [Documentary]. Retrieved from http://www.channel4.com/programmes/the-paedophile-next-door.

Interpol. (2012, April 19). South Africa, world's rape capital. *SABC*. Retrieved from http://www.sabc.co.za/news/a/a424c0804af19b5e9583fd7db529e2d0/SouthAfrica,-worlds-rape-capital:-Interpol-20121904.

Jewkes, R. (2012). *Rape perpetration: A review*. Pretoria: Sexual Violence Research Initiative.

Jewkes, R., Fulu, E., Roselli, T., & Garcia-Moreno, C. (2013). Prevalence of and factors associated with non-partner rape perpetration: Findings from the UN Multi-country Cross-sectional Study on Men and Violence in Asia and the Pacific. thelancet.com. Vol 1, 208–218.

Kemshall, H., McCartan, K., & Hudson, K. (2012). International approaches to understanding and responding to sexual abuse. *ATSA Forum, 25*, 2.

Klein, V., Rettenberger, M., Yoon, D., Kohler, N., & Briken, P. (2014). Protective factors and recidivism in accused juveniles who sexually offended. *Sexual Abuse: A Journal of Research and Treatment*. doi:10.1177/1079063214554958.

Knight, R. A., & Prentky, R. A. (1993). Exploring characteristics for classifying juvenile sex offenders. In H. E. Barbaree, W. L. Marshall, & S. M. Hudson (Eds.), *The juvenile sex offender* (pp. 45–83). New York, NY: Guilford Press.

Krug, E., Dahlberg, L., Mercy, J., Zwi, A. & Lozano, R. (Eds.). (2002). Violence — A global public health problem. In *World report on violence and health* (pp. 3–21). Geneva: World Health Organization.

Laws, D. R. (2000). Sexual offending as a public health problem: A North American perspective. *Journal of Sexual Aggression, 5*, 30–44.

Laws, R. (2008). Sexual offending as a public health problem: A North American perspective. *Journal of Sexual Aggression, 5*(1), 173–191.

Lee, D. S., Guy, L., Perry, B., Keoni-Sniffen, C., & Mixson, S. A. (2007). Sexual violence prevention. *The Prevention Researcher, 14*, 15–20.

Letourneau, E. J., Eaton, W. W., Bass, J., Berlin, F., & Moore, S. G. (2014). The need for a comprehensive public health approach to preventing child sexual abuse. *Public Health Reports, 129*(3), 222–228.

Levenson, J. S., & D'Amora, D. (2007). Social policies designed to prevent sexual violence: The emperor's new clothes? *Criminal Justice Policy Review, 18*, 168–199.

London, K., Bruck, M., Ceci, S. J., & Shuman, D. W. (2005). Disclosure of child sexual abuse: What does the research tell us about the ways that children tell? *Psychology, Public Policy, and Law, 11*, 194–226.

Longo, R. (1997). Reducing sexual abuse in America: Legislating tougher laws or public education and prevention. *New England Journal on Criminal and Civil Confinement, 23*, 303.

Lonsway, K. (1996). Preventing acquaintance rape through education: What do we know? *Psychology of Women Quarterly, 20*, 229–265.

McLean, S., & Maxwell, J. (2015). Sex offender re-integration into the community: realities and challenges. *Journal of Sexual Aggression, 21*(1), 16–27.

Malone, L. (2014). *Help wanted. On This American Life* [Audio]. Retrieved from http://www.thisamericanlife.org/radio-archives/episode/522/tarred-and-feathered?act=2.

Mann, R. (2014). Defining and developing good evidence for policy and practice. Keynote presentation at *The importance of effective evidence based policy and practice in sex offender work*. Conference conducted at University of the West of England, Bristol.

McCartan, K. (2010). Media constructions and reactions to, paedophilia in modern society. In K. Harrison (Ed.), *Managing high-risk sex offenders in the community: Risk management, treatment and social responsibilities*. Cullompton: Willan Publishing.

McCartan, K., Kemshall, H., & Tabachnick, J. (2015). The construction of community understandings of sexual violence: Rethinking public, practitioner and policy discourses. *Journal of Sexual Aggression, 21*(1), 100–116. doi:10.1080/13552600.2014.945976.

McMahon, P. (2000). A public health approach to the prevention of sexual violence. *Sexual Abuse: A Journal of Research and Treatment, 12*, 27–36.

Mercy, J. A., Rosenberg, M. L., Powell, K. E., Broome, C. V., & Roper, W. L. (1993). Public health policy for preventing violence. *Health Affairs, 12*(4), 7–29. doi:10.1377/hlthaff.12.4.7.

Miller, T. R., Cohen, M. A., Wiersema, B., & Justice, N. I. (1996). *Victim costs and consequences: A new look* (Vol. 3). Washington, DC: US Department of Justice, Office of Justice Programs, National Institute of Justice.

Miller, E., Tancredi, D. J., McCauley, H. L., Decker, M. R., Virata, M. C. D., Andersona, H. A., …, Silverman, J. G. (2012). Coaching boys into men: A cluster-randomized controlled trial of a dating violence prevention program. *Journal of Adolescent Health, 51*, 431–438.

Ministry of Justice, Home Office & the Office for National Statistics (2013). *An Overview of Sexual Offending in England and Wales*. Ministry of Justice, Home Office and Office for National Statistics. Accessed on 14th February 2014 via https://www.gov.uk/government/uploads/system/uploads/attachment_data/file/214970/sexual-offending-overview-jan-2013.pdf.

Nation, M., Crusto, C., Wandersman, A., Kumpfer, K. L., Seybolt, D., Morrrissey-Kane, E., & Davino, K. (2003). What works in prevention: Principles of effective prevention programs. *American Psychologist, 58*, 449.

Stop it Now! (2014). *Stop it Now!* Retrieved from http://www.stopitnow.org.uk/.

Philip, C. M. (2014) 93 women are being raped in India every day, NCRB data show. The Times of India. Accessed on 17th November 2014 via http://timesofindia.indiatimes.com/india/93-women-are-being-raped-in-India-every-day-NCRB-data-show/articleshow/37566815.cms.

Pittman, N. (2013). *Raised on the registry: The irreparable harm of placing children on sex offender registries in the U.S.* Human Rights Watch. Retrieved from http://www.opensocietyfoundations.org/reports/raised-registry-irreparable-harm-placing-children-sex-offender-registries-us.

Project Dunklefeld. (2015). *Project Dunklefeld*. Retrieved from https://www.dont-offend.org/.

Przybylski, R., & Lobanov-Rostovsky, C. (2015). *Unique considerations regarding juveniles who commit sexual offenses*. Sex offender management assessment and planning initiative, SMART Office, DOJ. Retrieved from http://www.smart.gov/SOMAPI/sec2/ch1_overview.html.

Saied-Tessier, A. (2014). *Estimating the cost of child sexual abuse in the UK*. London: NSPCC. Retrieved from http://www.nspcc.org.uk/globalassets/documents/research-reports/estimating-costschild-sexual-abuse-uk.pdf.

Smallbone, S., Marshall, W. L., & Wortley, R. (2008). *Preventing child sexual abuse: Evidence, policy and practice*. Cullompton: Willan Publishing.

Snyder, H. N. (2000, July). *Sexual assault of young children as reported to law enforcement: Victim, incident, and offender characteristics*. Retrieved from Bureau of Justice Statistics website http://bjs.ojp.usdoj.gov/content/pub/pdf/saycrle.pdf.

Stroud, D., Martens, S. L., & Barker, J. (2000). Criminal investigation of child sexual abuse: A comparison of cases referred to the prosecutor to those not referred. *Child Abuse & Neglect, 24*, 689–700.

Tabachnick, J., & Klein, A. (2010). *A reasoned approach: Reshaping sex offender policy to prevent child sexual abuse*. Beaverton, OR: Association for the Treatment of Sexual Abusers.

Tabachnick, J., & Klein, A. (2011). *A reasoned approach: Reshaping sex offender policy to prevent child sexual abuse*. Beaverton, OR: Association for the Treatment of Sexual Abusers.

Tabachnick, J., & Newton-Ward, I. (2010). Using social marketing for effective sexual violence prevention. In K. Kaufman (Ed.), *Sexual violence prevention* (pp. 135–146). Holyoke, MA: NEARI Press.

Taylor, P., Moore, P., Pezzullo, L., Tucci, J., Goddard, C., & De Bortoli, L. (2008). *The cost of child abuse in Australia*. Melbourne, VIC: Australian Childhood Foundation and Child Abuse Prevention Research.

Taylor, B., Stein, N., Woods, D., & Mumford, E. (2011). *Shifting boundaries: Final report on an experimental evaluation of a youth dating violence prevention program in New York City middle schools*. Washington, DC: US Department of Justice.

Tewksbury, R., & Levenson, J. (2009). Street experiences of family members of registered sex offenders. *Behavioral Sciences and the Law, 27*, 1–16.

Tharp, A. T., Degue, S., Valle, L. A., Brookmeyer, K. A., Massetti, G. M., & Matjaso, J. L. (2012). A systematic qualitative review of risk and protective factors for sexual violence perpetration. *Trauma, Violence and Abuse, 14*, 133–167.

Tjaden, P., & Thoennes, N. (2006). *Extent, nature, and consequences of rape victimization: Findings from the national violence against women survey. NIJ special report*. Washington, DC: National Institute of Justice.

Truman, J., Langton, L., & Planty, M. (2013). *Criminal victimization*. Washington, DC: Bureau of Justice Statistics Bulletin, Bureau of Justice Statistics. Retrieved from http://www.bjs.gov/content/pub/pdf/cv12.pdf.

Tsai, A. C., Leiter, K., Heisler, M., JIacopino, V., Wolfe, W., Shannon, K., …, Weiser, S. D. (2011). Prevalence and correlates of forced sex perpetration and victimization in Botswna and Swaziland. *American Journal of Public Health, 101*, 1068–1074.

UNICEF. (2014). *Hidden in plain sight*. Retrieved from http://files.unicef.org/publications/files/Hidden_in_plain_sight_statistical_analysis_EN_3_Sept_2014.pdf.

Whitaker, D. J., Le, B., Hanson, K., Baker, C. K., McMahon, P., Ryan, G., …, Rice, D. D. (2008). Risk factors for the perpetration of child sexual abuse: A review and meta-analysis. *Child Abuse & Neglect, 32*, 529–548.

Widman, L., Olson, M. A., & Bolen, R. M. (2013). Self-reported sexual assault in convicted sex offenders and community men. *Journal of Interpersonal Violence, 28*, 1519–1536.

Wilson, R., & Prescott, D. (2014). Community-based management of sexual offender risk: Options and opportunities. In K. McCartan (Ed.), *Responding to sexual offending: Perceptions, risk management and public protection* (pp. 206–226). Hampshire: Palgrave Macmillan.

Wiseman, J. (2014). *Incidence and prevalence of sexual offending*. Sex offender management assessment and planning initiative, SMART Office, DOJ. Retrieved from http://www.smart.gov/SOMAPI/sec1/ch1_incidence.html.

World Health Organization. (2014). *Global status report on violence prevention 2014*. Retrieved from http://www.who.int/violence_injury_prevention/violence/status_report/2014/report/report/en/.

World Health Organization & London School of Hygiene and Tropical Medicine. (2010). *Preventing intimate partner and sexual violence against women: taking action and generating evidence*. Geneva: World Health Organization.

Wortley, R., & Smallbone, S. (Eds.). (2006). *Situational prevention of child sexual abuse*. Monsey, NY: Criminal Justice Press.

Ybarra, M. L., & Mitchell, K. J. (2013). Prevalence rates of male and female sexual violence perpetrators in a national sample of adolescents. *JAMA Pediatrics, 167*(12), 1125–1134.

Zeuthen, K., & Hagelskjaer, M. (2013). Prevention of child sexual abuse: Analysis and discussion of the field. *Journal of Child Sexual Abuse, 22*, 742–760. doi:10.1080/10538712.2013.811136.

Zgoba, K. M., Miner, M., Levenson, J., Knight, R., Letourneau, E., & Thornton, D. (2015). The Adam Walsh Act: An examination of sex offender risk classification systems. *Sexual Abuse: A Journal of Research and Treatment*. doi:10.1177/1079063215569543.

Index

© Springer International Publishing Switzerland 2016
D.R. Laws, W. O'Donohue (eds.), *Treatment of Sex Offenders*,
DOI 10.1007/978-3-319-25868-3

Lightning Source UK Ltd.
Milton Keynes UK
UKHW02n0040240418

321527UK00007B/42/P